Neurosurgical Anesthesia

Guest Editors

ANSGAR M. BRAMBRINK, MD, PhD
JEFFREY R. KIRSCH, MD

ANESTHESIOLOGY CLINICS

www.anesthesiology.theclinics.com

Consulting Editor
LEE A. FLEISHER, MD, FACC

June 2012 • Volume 30 • Number 2

SAUNDERS an imprint of ELSEVIER, Inc.

W.B. SAUNDERS COMPANY
A Division of Elsevier Inc.

1600 John F. Kennedy Boulevard, Suite 1800 • Philadelphia, PA 19103-2899

http://www.theclinics.com

ANESTHESIOLOGY CLINICS Volume 30, Number 2
June 2012 ISSN 1932-2275, ISBN-13: 978-1-4557-4837-2

Editor: Pamela Hetherington

Anesthesiology Clinics (ISSN 1932-2275) is published quarterly by Elsevier Inc., 360 Park Avenue South, New York, NY 10010-1710. Months of issue are March, June, September, and December. Periodicals postage paid at New York, NY and at additional mailing offices. Subscription prices are $154.00 per year (US student/resident), $313.00 per year (US individuals), $383.00 per year (Canadian individuals), $496.00 per year (US institutions), $615.00 per year (Canadian institutions), $216.00 per year (Canadian and foreign student/resident), $434.00 per year (foreign individuals), and $615.00 per year (foreign institutions). To receive student and resident rate, orders must be accompanied by name of affiliated institution, date of term, and the *signature* of program/residency coordinator on institutions letterhead. Orders will be billed at individual rate until proof of status is received. Foreign air speed delivery is included in all *Clinics'* subscription prices. All prices are subject to change without notice. POSTMASTER: Send address changes to *Anesthesiology Clinics,* Elsevier Health Sciences Division, Subscription Customer Service, 3251 Riverport Lane, Maryland Heights, MO 63043. Customer Service (orders, claims, online, change of address): Elsevier Health Sciences Division, Subscription Customer Service, 3251 Riverport Lane, Maryland Heights, MO 63043. Tel: 1-800-654-2452 (U.S. and Canada); 314-447-8871 (outside U.S. and Canada). Fax: 314-447-8029. E-mail: journalscustomerservice-usa@elsevier.com (for print support); journalsonlinesupport-usa@elsevier.com (for online support).

Reprints. For copies of 100 or more of articles in this publication, please contact the Commercial Reprints Department, Elsevier Inc., 360 Park Avenue South, New York, NY 10010-1710. Tel.: 212-633-3812; Fax: 212-462-1935; E-mail: reprints@elsevier.com.

Anesthesiology Clinics, is also published in Spanish by McGraw-Hill Inter-americana Editores S. A., P.O. Box 5-237, 06500 Mexico D. F., Mexico.

Anesthesiology Clinics, is covered in *MEDLINE/PubMed (Index Medicus), Current Contents/Clinical Medicine, Excerpta Medica, ISI/BIOMED,* and *Chemical Abstracts.*

Printed and bound by CPI Group (UK) Ltd, Croydon, CR0 4YY

Transferred to Digital Print 2012

Contributors

CONSULTING EDITOR

LEE A. FLEISHER, MD, FACC
Robert D. Dripps Professor and Chair of Anesthesiology and Critical Care, University of Pennsylvania, Perelman School of Medicine, Philadelphia, Pennsylvania

GUEST EDITORS

ANSGAR M. BRAMBRINK, MD, PhD
Professor, Director, Neurosciences Intensive Care Unit, Department of Anesthesiology and Perioperative Medicine, Oregon Health and Science University, Portland, Oregon

JEFFREY R. KIRSCH, MD
Professor and Chair, Department of Anesthesiology and Perioperative Medicine, Oregon Health and Science University; Associate Dean, Clinical and Veteran's Affairs, Portland, Oregon

AUTHORS

MICHAEL AZIZ, MD
Assistant Professor, Department of Anesthesiology and Perioperative Medicine, Oregon Health and Science University, Portland, Oregon

AUDRÉE A. BENDO, MD
Professor and Executive Vice Chair, Department of Anesthesiology, State University of New York, Downstate Medical Center, Brooklyn, New York

ANSGAR M. BRAMBRINK, MD, PhD
Professor, Director, Neurosciences Intensive Care Unit, Department of Anesthesiology and Perioperative Medicine, Oregon Health and Science University, Portland, Oregon

J. RICARDO CARHUAPOMA, MD
Associate Professor of Neurology, Neurosurgery, and Anesthesiology and Critical Care Medicine, Division of Neurosciences Critical Care Medicine, Department of Anesthesiology and Critical Care Medicine, The Johns Hopkins Hospital, The Johns Hopkins University, Baltimore, Maryland

TIFFANY R. CHANG, MD
Fellow, Division of Neurosciences Critical Care Medicine, Department of Anesthesiology and Critical Care Medicine, The Johns Hopkins Hospital, The Johns Hopkins University, Baltimore, Maryland

DANIEL J. COLE, MD
Professor of Anesthesiology, Department of Anesthesiology, Mayo Clinic College of Medicine, Rochester, Minnesota; Chair, Department of Anesthesiology, Mayo Clinic Hospital, Mayo Clinic Arizona, Phoenix, Arizona

DENISE CRUTE, MD
Fellow in Neurosurgery and Neurocritical Care, Department of Neurosurgery, Mount Sinai School of Medicine, New York, New York

ANNE L. DONOVAN, MD
Resident, Department of Anesthesia and Perioperative Care, University of California, San Francisco, San Francisco, California

BRIAN EGAN, MD
Fellow, Division of Pediatric Anesthesiology, Department of Anesthesiology and Perioperative Medicine, Oregon Health and Science University, Portland, Oregon

KIRSTIN M. ERICKSON, MD
Consultant, Assistant Professor of Anesthesiology, Department of Anesthesiology, Mayo Clinic College of Medicine, Rochester, Minnesota

ALANA M. FLEXMAN, MD, FRCPC
Clinical Assistant Professor, Department of Anesthesiology, Pharmacology and Therapeutics, Vancouver General Hospital, University of British Columbia, Vancouver, British Columbia, Canada

ADRIAN W. GELB, MBChB, FRCPC
Professor, Department of Anesthesia and Perioperative Care, University of California, San Francisco, San Francisco, California

LESLIE C. JAMESON, MD
Department of Anesthesiology, University of Colorado, Anschutz Medical Campus, Aurora, Colorado

MATTHEW A. KIRKMAN, MBBS, BSc
Honorary Fellow in Neurocritical Care, The National Hospital for Neurology and Neurosurgery, University College London Hospitals; National Institute for Health Research, Academic Clinical Fellow in Neurosurgery, Imperial College London, London, United Kingdom

JEFFREY R. KIRSCH, MD
Professor and Chair, Department of Anesthesiology and Perioperative Medicine, Oregon Health and Science University; Associate Dean, Clinical and Veteran's Affairs, Portland, Oregon

W. ANDREW KOFKE, MD, MBA, FCCM
Department of Neurosurgery; Department of Anesthesiology and Critical Care, University of Pennsylvania, Philadelphia, Pennsylvania

JEFFREY L. KOH, MD, MBA
Professor of Anesthesiology and Pediatrics, Department of Anesthesiology and Perioperative Medicine, Doernbecher Children's Hospital/Oregon Health and Science University, Portland, Oregon

LAWRENCE T. LAI, MD
Clinical Assistant Professor, Department of Anesthesiology, State University of New York, Downstate Medical Center, Brooklyn, New York

SHIH-SHAN LANG, MD
Department of Neurosurgery, University of Pennsylvania, Philadelphia, Pennsylvania

CHANHUNG Z. LEE, MD, PhD
Associate Professor of Anesthesiology, Department of Anesthesia and Perioperative Care, University of California, San Francisco, San Francisco, California

GEORGE A. MASHOUR, MD, PhD
Assistant Professor of Anesthesiology and Neurosurgery, Departments of Anesthesiology, and Neurosurgery, University of Michigan Medical School; Faculty, Neuroscience Graduate Program Center for Sleep Science, University of Michigan, Ann Arbor, Michigan

TERRENCE MCGRAW, MD
Associate Professor of Anesthesiology and Pediatrics, Department of Anesthesiology and Perioperative Medicine, Doernbecher Children's Hospital/Oregon Health and Science University, Portland, Oregon

NEERAJ S. NAVAL, MD
Assistant Professor of Neurology, Neurosurgery, and Anesthesiology and Critical Care Medicine, Division of Neurosciences Critical Care Medicine, Department of Anesthesiology and Critical Care Medicine, The Johns Hopkins Hospital, The Johns Hopkins University, Baltimore, Maryland

ANDREA ORFANAKIS, MD
Assistant Professor, Department of Anesthesiology and Perioperative Medicine, Oregon Health and Science University, Portland, Oregon

JOSE R. ORTIZ-CARDONA, MD
Clinical Assistant Instructor, Department of Anesthesiology, University of Puerto Rico, San Juan, Puerto Rico

IRENE P. OSBORN, MD
Associate Professor of Anesthesiology, Department of Anesthesiology, Mount Sinai School of Medicine, New York, New York

DINESH PAL, PhD
Research Investigator, Department of Anesthesiology, University of Michigan Medical School, Ann Arbor, Michigan

JOSEPH SEBEO, MD, PhD
Resident in Anesthesiology, Department of Neurosurgery, Mount Sinai School of Medicine, New York, New York

DEEPAK SHARMA, MD, DM
Departments of Anesthesiology and Pain Medicine, and Neurological Surgery, University of Washington, Seattle, Washington

TOD B. SLOAN, MD, MBA, PhD
Department of Anesthesiology, University of Colorado, Anschutz Medical Campus, Aurora, Colorado

MARTIN SMITH, MBBS, FRCA, FFICM
Consultant and Honorary Professor in Neurocritical Care, The National Hospital for Neurology and Neurosurgery, University College London Hospitals, London, United Kingdom

MICHAEL F. STIEFEL, MD, PhD
Department of Neurosurgery, Westchester Medical Center, New York Medical College, Valhalla, New York

MICHAEL M. TODD, MD
Professor and Head, Department of Anesthesia, University of Iowa Carver College of Medicine, Iowa City, Iowa

MONICA S. VAVILALA, MD
Departments of Anesthesiology and Pain Medicine, Neurological Surgery, Pediatrics, and Radiology, University of Washington; Professor, Department of Anesthesiology, Harborview Medical Center, Seattle, Washington

WILLIAM L. YOUNG, MD
Professor and Vice Chair, Department of Anesthesia and Perioperative Care, University of California, San Francisco, San Francisco, California

Contents

with acute intracranial bleeding, including packed red blood cell transfusion, platelet transfusion, and reversal of coagulopathy; (2) indications for seizure prophylaxis and choice of antiepileptic agent; and (3) the role of specialized neurocritical care units and specialists in the care of critically ill neurology and neurosurgery patients.

George A. Mashour and Dinesh Pal

In the past decades there has been an increasing focus on the relationship of sleep and anesthesia. This relationship bears on the fundamental scientific questions in anesthesiology, such as the mechanism of anesthetic-induced unconsciousness. However, given the increasing prevalence of sleep disorders in surgical patients, the interfaces of sleep and anesthesia are now a pressing clinical concern. This article discusses sleep and anesthesia from the perspective of phenotype, mechanism and function, with some concluding thoughts on the relevance to neuroanesthesiology.

Michael M. Todd

Although there is a huge body of literature concerning the cerebrovascular and cerebrometabolic effects of anesthetics, it is unclear how much of this high-quality physiology and pharmacology actually applies to the clinical care of neurosurgical patients, in particular those with intracranial mass lesions or those at risk for intraoperative cerebral ischemia. This article attempts to review the clinical aspects of the care of such patients and to define when our physiologic understanding is important and when it is largely irrelevant.

ANESTHESIOLOGY CLINICS

DOWNLOAD
Free App!

Review Articles
THE CLINICS

NOW AVAILABLE FOR YOUR iPhone and iPad

Foreword

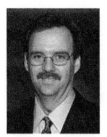

Lee A. Fleisher, MD
Consulting Editor

It has been almost over 20 years since President George Bush designated the 1990s as the decade of the brain to enhance public awareness of the benefits to be derived from brain research. These past two decades have seen exciting developments related to both new discoveries and new interventions. This has led to a great expansion in the number of neurosurgical procedures within the operating room and importantly in the catheterization laboratory. Therefore, we have created an issue of *Anesthesiology Clinics of North America* that includes timely articles including anesthesia for endovascular neurosurgery and the awake craniotomy. The authors also discuss basic science issues including anesthetic toxicity and have incorporated issues of controversy in critical care and the important expanding area of knowledge related to sleep in anesthesia. Finally, they asked questions regarding outcome after neuroanesthesia and neurosurgery. These articles will help prepare the anesthesia community to take care of increasingly complex patients in the operating room, the catheterization lab, and the intensive care unit.

We are fortunate to have two outstanding editors for this issue. Ansgar Brambrink, MD, PhD is currently Professor of Anesthesiology and Perioperative Medicine, with joint appointments in neurology and neurologic surgery at Oregon Health and Science University. He is currently director of the neuroscience intensive care unit. He is an established clinician scientist whose primary interest is dedicated to translational research regarding anesthesia-induced developmental neurotoxicity. His area of research has resulted in his being awarded the Frontiers in Anesthesia and Research Award from the International Anesthesia Research Society in 2012. Jeffrey Kirsch, MD is currently Professor and Chair of Anesthesiology and Perioperative Medicine and Associate Dean for Clinical and Veterans Affairs at the Oregon Health and Science University. He has been an active researcher in the area of neurotrauma and neuroprotection and has published extensively in this area. He has also been President of the Society of Neurosurgical Anesthesia and Critical Care in 1999 and has held numerous

Anesthesiology Clin 30 (2012) xiii–xiv
http://dx.doi.org/10.1016/j.anclin.2012.06.004
1932-2275/12/$ – see front matter © 2012 Elsevier Inc. All rights reserved.

leadership positions in the specialty. Together they have assembled an outstanding group of authors to advance our knowledge in the care of the neurosurgical patient.

Lee A. Fleisher, MD
University of Pennsylvania Perelman School of Medicine
3400 Spruce Street, Dulles 680
Philadelphia, PA 19104, USA

E-mail address:
lee.fleisher@uphs.upenn.edu

Preface

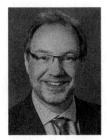 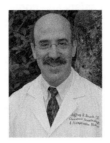

Ansgar M. Brambrink, MD, PhD   Jeffrey R. Kirsch, MD
Guest Editors

The practice of perioperative neuroanesthesiology is constantly evolving because therapeutic and diagnostic options are changing. Patients who have to undergo neurosurgical and neurointerventional procedures in many centers are treated by neuroanesthesiologists during the perioperative period, which frequently includes close involvement in the critical care phase of their recovery. In other institutions the same patients are treated by anesthesiologists who are not specialized and provide neuroanesthesiology as part of their diverse general practice as anesthesiologists and perioperative physicians. We hope that the information found in this issue will improve the fund of knowledge for both of these groups of anesthesia providers.

In addition, anesthesiologists in any subspecialty of our profession tailor perioperative patient management to the well-being of the nervous system. And many patients who present in nonneurosurgical practice will frequently present with specific concerns that require a "brain-focused" intervention. These situations include, but are not limited to, patient after head trauma who now require general or orthopedic surgery, patients with arteriosclerosis who have an increased perioperative stroke risk, and pregnant patients or the very young who may require multiple anesthetic exposures.

We believe that all anesthesia providers should have a clear understanding of (1) the physiology and pathophysiology of the central nervous system (CNS) as well as specific diagnostics and treatment options; (2) the means necessary to provide safe and comfortable anesthesia and perioperative care for patients who undergo either interventions targeting the CNS or who are at risk for developing CNS injury during other types of surgery. In addition, we also believe that a constant critical appraisal of currently practiced and newly proposed anesthetic techniques and concepts will help the anesthesia provider understand which therapies are likely to be most beneficial for their patients.

Our goal as guest editors was to provide an update of the key topics in neurosurgical anesthesiology and perioperative care. The 2012 issue on Neurosurgical Anesthesia and Critical Care compiles outstanding new review articles that cover the most interesting and controversial topics in the field. We are convinced that clinicians

Anesthesiology Clin 30 (2012) xv–xvii
http://dx.doi.org/10.1016/j.anclin.2012.06.005
1932-2275/12/$ – see front matter © 2012 Elsevier Inc. All rights reserved.

anesthesiology.theclinics.com

in private practice and academic medicine will enjoy reading with the likely result of improved patient care at the bedside. Our primary aim was to provide information that will help to further improve the safety and comfort of patients who unfortunately suffer from injury or disease of the CNS and require surgical or interventional procedure in order to improve their outcome.

Ansgar M. Brambrink, MD, PhD
Department of Anesthesiology and Perioperative Medicine
Oregon Health and Science University
3181 SW Sam Jackson Park Road, UHS-2
Portland, OR 97239-3098, USA

Jeffrey R. Kirsch, MD
Department of Anesthesiology and Perioperative Medicine
Oregon Health and Science University
3181 SW Sam Jackson Park Road, KPV 5A
Portland, OR 97239-3098, USA

E-mail addresses:
brambrin@ohsu.edu (A.M. Brambrink)
kirschje@ohsu.edu (J.R. Kirsch)

DEDICATION

The Editors would like to thank their mentors for instilling in them the ability to explore their questions deeply and receive their answers with an appropriate amount of skepticism. We would specifically like to recognize the mentorship by Drs Nelly Tsouyopoulos (deceased), Wolfgang F. Dick and John W. Olney for Ansgar Brambrink and Drs Louis G. D'Alecy and Richard J. Traystman for Jeffrey Kirsch.

Anesthesia for Endovascular Neurosurgery and Interventional Neuroradiology

Chanhung Z. Lee, MD, PhD*, William L. Young, MD

KEYWORDS

- Brain injury • Brain vascular malformation • Intracranial hemorrhage • Thrombolysis

KEY POINTS

- Choice of anesthetics is based on the individual patient and the specific procedure. Patient immobility during the procedure facilitates imaging. Careful management of coagulation is required.
- Complications during endovascular instrumentation can be rapid and life threatening and require a multi-disciplinary approach.
- Although it is generally agreed that ruptured lesions need treatment, the aggregate risks for treating all unruptured cases may exceed the potential benefit from protecting against future hemorrhage.
- Active angiogenesis and vascular remodeling in intracranial vascular malformations may open new clinical paradigms in which pharmacologic interventions are proposed to stabilize these abnormal blood vessels and prevent further growth or hemorrhage.

This article discusses the roles of the anesthesiologist in the management of patients undergoing invasive endovascular procedures to treat vascular diseases, primarily of the central nervous system (**Table 1**). This practice is usually termed interventional neuroradiology (INR) or endovascular neurosurgery. The article emphasizes perioperative and anesthetic management strategies to prevent complications and minimize their effects, if they occur. There are several fundamental management principles of affording protection from injury (**Box 1**). Planning the anesthetic and perioperative management is predicated on understanding the goals of the therapeutic intervention and anticipating potential problems.

INR is firmly established in the management of cerebrovascular disease, most notably in the management of intracranial aneurysm[1] because there is level 1 evidence for aneurysm coiling offering advantages compared with surgical clipping. Because

Department of Anesthesia and Perioperative Care, University of California, San Francisco, San Francisco, CA, USA
* Corresponding author. Department of Anesthesia, University of California, San Francisco, 1001 Potrero Avenue, Building 10, Room 1206, Box 1363, San Francisco, CA 94110.
E-mail address: ccr@anesthesia.ucsf.edu

Anesthesiology Clin 30 (2012) 127–147
http://dx.doi.org/10.1016/j.anclin.2012.05.009   anesthesiology.theclinics.com

---

Box 1
Management of intracranial catastrophes[a]

Initial resuscitation

Communicate with endovascular therapy team

Assess need for assistance; call for assistance

Secure the airway ventilate with 100% O_2

Determine whether problem is hemorrhagic or occlusive

Hemorrhagic: immediate heparin reversal (1 mg protamine for each 100 units of heparin given) and low normal mean arterial pressure

Occlusive: deliberate hypertension, titrated to neurologic examination, angiography, or physiologic imaging studies; or to clinical context

Further resuscitation

Head up 15° in neutral position, if possible

Arterial carbon dioxide tension ($Paco_2$) manipulation consistent with clinical setting, otherwise normocapnia

Mannitol 0.5 g/kg, rapid intravenous (IV) infusion

Titrate IV agent to electroencephalography burst suppression

Passive cooling to 33°C to 34°C

Consider ventriculostomy for treatment or monitoring of increased intracranial pressure

Consider anticonvulsants (eg, phenytoin or phenobarbital)

[a] These are only general recommendations and drug doses that must be adapted to specific clinical situations and in accordance with a patient's preexisting medical condition. In some cases of asymptomatic or minor vessel puncture or occlusion, less aggressive management may be appropriate.

---

the practice of INR has evolved, the physician delivering the treatment may be a specially trained radiologist, neurologist, or neurosurgeon.

There are several anesthetic concerns that are particularly important for INR procedures, including (1) maintaining immobility during the procedure to facilitate imaging; (2) rapid recovery from anesthesia at the end of the case to facilitate neurologic examination and monitoring, or provide for intermittent evaluation of neurologic function during the procedure; (3) managing anticoagulation; (4) treating and managing sudden unexpected procedure-specific complications during the intervention (eg, hemorrhage or vascular occlusion), which may involve manipulating systemic or regional blood pressures; (5) guiding the medical management of critical care patients during transport to and from the radiology suites (or hybrid operating room); (6) self-protection issues related to radiation safety.[2,3]

PREOPERATIVE PLANNING AND PATIENT PREPARATION

Baseline blood pressure and cardiovascular reserve should be assessed carefully. This statement is almost axiomatic and is particularly important for several reasons. Blood pressure manipulation is commonly required and treatment-related perturbations should be anticipated. Therefore, a clear sense of the patient's normal range of blood pressure variation needs to be established. Autoregulation, as presented in textbooks, is a description of a population and, as such, may not predict blood

Table 1
Interventional neuroradiologic procedures and primary anesthetic considerations

Procedure	Possible Anesthetic Considerations
Therapeutic embolization of vascular malformation	
Intracranial AVMs	Deliberate hypotension, postprocedure NPPB
Dural AVM	Existence of venous hypertension; deliberate hypercapnia
Extracranial AVMs	Deliberate hypercapnia
Carotid cavernous fistula (CCF)	Deliberate hypercapnia, postprocedure NPPB
Cerebral aneurysms	Aneurysmal rupture, blood pressure control[a]
Ethanol sclerotherapy for arteriovenous or venous malformations	Brain swelling, airway swelling, hypoxemia, hypoglycemia, intoxication from ethanol, cardiorespiratory arrest
Balloon angioplasty and stenting of occlusive cerebrovascular disease	Cerebral ischemia, deliberate hypertension, concomitant coronary artery disease, bradycardia, hypotension
Balloon angioplasty of cerebral vasospasm secondary to aneurysmal SAH	Cerebral ischemia, blood pressure control[a]
Therapeutic carotid occlusion for giant aneurysms and skull base tumors	Cerebral ischemia, blood pressure control[a]
Thrombolysis of acute thromboembolic stroke	Postprocedure ICH (NPPB), concomitant coronary artery disease, blood pressure control[a]
Intra-arterial chemotherapy for head and neck tumors	Airway swelling, intracranial hypertension
Embolization for epistaxis	Airway control

Abbreviations: AVM, arteriovenous malformation; ICH, intracranial hemorrhage; NPPB, normal perfusion pressure breakthrough; SAH, subarachnoid hemorrhage.
[a] Blood pressure control refers to deliberate hypotension and/or hypertension.

pressure needs for individuals to stay in their own autoregulatory range.[4,5] Stated another way, each point on the usual autoregulation curve has a 95% confidence interval associated with it in both x and y directions. It was recently suggested that the lower limit of the conceptual autoregulation curve of the mean arterial pressure (MAP) should be increased from 50 mm Hg to 70 mm Hg.[6] This change may have important implications in the delivery of deliberate hypotension, because it would be essential to ensure adequate cerebral perfusion during the manipulations of blood pressure. For procedures involving the intracranial, intraspinal, or circle of Willis vasculature, beat-to-beat blood pressure monitoring (ie, placement of an arterial catheter specifically for the purpose of continuous blood pressure monitoring) is useful, considering the rapid time constants in this setting for changes in systemic or cerebral hemodynamics. In those cases where intra-arterial catheters are used, the concordance between blood pressure cuff and intra-arterial readings needs to be considered because the safe preoperative blood pressure range is likely only to be known through blood pressure cuff values.

Preoperative calcium channel blockers may have been administered either orally or intravenously in an attempt to prevent cerebral ischemia and can affect hemodynamic management during the interventional procedure. In addition, these agents, or transdermal nitroglycerin applied to patients' upper chests after securing femoral access, are sometimes used to lessen the incidence of catheter-induced cerebral vasospasm during the procedure, adding to the need for close (beat-to-beat) monitoring of blood pressure.

For cases managed with an unsecured airway, routine evaluation of the potential ease of laryngoscopy in an emergent situation should take into account that direct access to the airway may be limited by table or room logistics. In addition, recent pterional craniotomy can sometimes result in impaired temporomandibular joint mobility, limited mouth opening, and an unexpectedly difficult emergent tracheal intubation.

For sedation cases, careful padding of pressure points and working with the patient to obtain final comfortable positioning may assist in the patient's ability to tolerate a long period of lying supine and motionless, and may decrease the requirement for sedation, anxiolysis, and analgesia. Likewise, placement of a bladder catheter not only assists in fluid management, it facilitates patient comfort, because these procedures often require that the patient receive a significant volume of heparinized flush solution and radiographic contrast agent. The possibility of pregnancy in female patients and a history of adverse reactions to radiographic contrast agents should be explored, and this information should be used in planning anesthetic management.

Secure intravenous (IV) access must be available in all patients for INR, with adequate extension tubing to allow drug and fluid administration at maximal distance from the image intensifier during fluoroscopy. Because access to intravenous or arterial catheters can be difficult when the patient is draped and the arms are restrained at the sides, connections between infusion tubing and the catheter should be secure. Infusions of anticoagulant, primary anesthetics, or vasoactive agents should be through proximal ports with minimal dead space. The anesthesiologist must always be ready to quickly administer resuscitation drugs through an intravenous catheter to treat acute deterioration of the patient during the procedure.

In addition to standard monitors, capnography sampling via the sampling port of a nasal cannula is useful for IV sedation cases. Loss or reduced detection of expired carbon dioxide is often the first sign of complete or impending airway obstruction (from oversedation or a complication related to the INR). A pulse oximeter probe can be placed on the great toe of the leg that will receive the femoral introducer sheath to provide an early warning of femoral artery obstruction or distal thromboembolism.

For intracranial procedures and postoperative care, beat-to-beat arterial pressure monitoring and blood sampling can be facilitated by placement of an intra-arterial catheter. A side port of the femoral artery introducer sheath can be used for beat-to-beat monitoring of blood pressure during the procedure, but the sheath is usually removed immediately after the procedure. Therefore, it is appropriate to place a radial arterial catheter in patients who require continuous blood pressure monitoring or frequent blood sampling following completion of the procedure.

Placement of a coaxial or triaxial catheter system by the interventionalist allows measurement of arterial pressure at the carotid artery, vertebral artery, and the distal cerebral circulation. Pressures in these distal catheters usually underestimate systolic and overestimate diastolic pressure; however, mean pressures are reliable.

A fundamental knowledge of radiation safety is essential for all staff members working in an INR suite. Radiation safety is a critical part of preoperative planning. It is reasonable to assume that the x-ray machine is always on. There are 3 sources of radiation in the INR suite: direct radiation from the x-ray tube, leakage (through the collimators' protective shielding), and scattered radiation (reflected from the patients and the area surrounding the body part to be imaged). The amount of exposure decreases proportionally to the inverse of the square of the distance from the source of radiation (inverse square law). Digital subtraction angiography (DSA), which is commonly used in INR, delivers more radiation than fluoroscopy. During DSA, interventionalists often move away from patients and position themselves behind a glass shield. It is therefore advised that anesthesiologists also take maximum precautions for themselves during DSA, by increasing their distance from the x-ray source or moving behind a portable glass shield.

Optimal protection includes the use of lead aprons, thyroid shields, and radiation exposure badges. Members of the anesthesiology team should do their best to wear aprons that cover both the front and back of their bodies, because it is easy to forget that the radiation source is still providing a dangerous environment when their backs are turned to the patients to chart or draw up drugs. The lead aprons should be periodically evaluated for any cracks in the lead lining that may allow accidental radiation exposure. Movable lead glass screens may provide additional protection for the anesthesia team. Recent data have also indicated the danger of accumulation of radiation to the eyes of anesthesiologists working for a significant time in the INR suite, suggesting the importance of appropriate eye protection.[7] Clear communication between the INR and anesthesia teams is also crucial for limiting radiation exposure (eg, receiving adequate warning before starting DSA). With proper precautions, the anesthesia team should be exposed to less than the annual recommended limit for health care workers (see URL http://pdg.lbl.gov/).

ANESTHETIC TECHNIQUE
Choice of Anesthetic Technique

Most centers routinely involved use general endotracheal anesthesia for complex procedures or procedures that are of prolonged duration. Choice of anesthetic technique varies among centers, with no clearly superior method, and generally follows the dictates of the well-described considerations for operative neuroanesthesia. This article summarizes benefits and disadvantages for different anesthetic choices first, and then explores the analyses of evidence and procedural and technical aspects for individual INR therapies.

General Anesthesia

The primary reasons for using general anesthesia (GA) are to minimize motion artifacts to improve the quality of image, and to facilitate navigation of endovascular catheters with the continuously evolving therapeutic devices and interventions. The inability to continuously assess neurologic status is a major drawback for procedure performed under GA. The other claimed disadvantages, including delaying start of the interventional procedures and fluctuations of hemodynamics, are manageable, depending on the institutional organization of procedure planning and predefined hemodynamic goals, respectively. In a survey of neurointerventionalists,[8] the top reasons that made GA appealing were eliminating movement and saving intraoperative time (65.3% of respondents), increased procedural safety (59.2%), and increased procedure efficacy (42.9%). The most common perceived complications of GA were time delay (71.4% of respondents) and hypotension (44.9%). Relative normocapnia or modest hypocapnia consistent with the safe conduct of positive pressure ventilation should be maintained unless intracranial pressure is a concern. The specific choice of anesthesia may be guided primarily by other cardiovascular and cerebrovascular considerations. There is no clear superiority of one modern anesthetic rather than another in terms of pharmacologic protection against neuronal injury. Total intravenous anesthetic techniques, or combinations of inhalational and intravenous methods, may optimize postprocedure rapid emergence. An argument could be made for avoiding N_2O because of the possibility of introducing air emboli into the cerebral circulation and reports that it worsens outcome after experimental brain injury.

It is important to distinguish between 2 general settings in which hyperventilation is used in anesthetic practice. First, it is used to treat intracranial hypertension. Hyperventilation is an important mainstay of the acute management of an intracranial catastrophe to acutely reduce cerebral blood volume. The second, and more common, application is to provide brain relaxation after the skull is open, with the intent of providing better surgical access and presumably a lesser degree of brain retraction for a given surgical approach. The former indication may be critical in crisis management; the latter is not relevant to endovascular procedures. Therefore, $Paco_2$ management should try to achieve normocapnia or mild hypocapnia to a degree consistent with the safe conduct of positive pressure ventilation. If a patient has increased intracranial pressure, prophylactic mild hypocapnia may be indicated during induction and maintenance of GA.

There are some special circumstances in which induced hypercapnia may be indicated, such as embolization of extracranial vascular malformations that drain into the intracranial venous system. In these cases, induction of hypercapnia can promote high venous outflow from the cerebral venous system and help minimize the risk of inadvertent movement of embolic material into the intracranial compartment (discussed later).

Intravenous Sedation

A major benefit of intravenous sedation is to allow continuous assessment of neurologic functions during the procedure. Goals of anesthetic choice for intravenous sedation are to alleviate pain, anxiety, and discomfort, provide patient immobility, and allow rapid recovery. There may be discomfort associated with injection of contrast into the cerebral arteries (burning) and with distention or traction on them (headache). A long period of lying motionless in the supine position can cause significant discomfort for the patient.

A variety of sedation regimens are available, and specific choices are based on the experience of the practitioner and the goals of anesthetic management. Common to all intravenous sedation techniques is the desire to avoid upper airway obstruction. Although placement of a nasopharyngeal airway is common in anesthetic practice to treat upper airway obstruction, placement of a nasopharyngeal airway in patients having INR may cause troublesome bleeding because of their anticoagulated state and is generally avoided. Dexmedetomidine is a new agent that may be applicable in the setting of INR. It is a potent, selective α_2-agonist with sedative, anxiolytic, and analgesic properties, with recent regulatory approval for sedation. Dexmedetomidine is especially noteworthy for its ability to produce a state of patient tranquility without depressing respiration. However, there are 2 caveats to consider. First, there are still unclear effects on cerebral perfusion.[9] More importantly, there is a tendency for patients managed with dexmedetomidine to have low blood pressure in the postanesthesia recovery period.[10] Because patients with aneurysmal subarachnoid hemorrhage (SAH) may be critically dependent on adequate collateral perfusion pressure, use of regimens that may result in blood pressure decreases should be used with caution.

There is a phenomenon that is inadequately characterized and lacks a good terminology. It is well known that patients, even with full recovery of a prior fixed neurologic deficit, may emerge from anesthesia with a reemergence of a prior fixed deficit.[11] These observations are consistent with functional neuroimaging studies that suggest that rewiring (an inadequately mechanistic metaphor) occurs to compensate for neurologic injury.[12] Why anesthetics cause a temporary reversal of the repair or compensatory process is unknown. For example, Thal and colleagues[11] showed that small doses of either midazolam or fentanyl induced transient focal motor deterioration in patients with prior motor deficits. Lazar and colleagues[13] used more sophisticated methodology to show that not only motor but also language and spatial functions can be affected by this process. They extended their observations to include patients who had suffered recent transient cerebral ischemic episodes and were neurologically intact with negative diffusion-weighted imaging. Midazolam caused reemergence of prior focal deficits that had been transient and fully resolved.[14]

There are therefore potentially important effects of IV sedative agents that may complicate neurologic monitoring, especially if functional testing of endovascular manipulations is desirable.

ANTICOAGULATION
Heparin

Careful management of coagulation is required to prevent thromboembolic complications during and after the INR procedure. After a baseline activated clotting time (ACT) is obtained, intravenous heparin (70 units/kg) is generally given to a target prolongation of approximately 2 to 3 times the baseline value. Then heparin can be given continuously or as an intermittent bolus with hourly monitoring of ACT. A patient may occasionally be refractory to attempts to obtain adequate anticoagulation. When this occurs, the anesthesiologist should consider switching from bovine to porcine heparin or vice versa. If antithrombin III deficiency is suspected, administration of fresh frozen plasma may be necessary to allow heparin to have its desired anticoagulant effect.

Direct Thrombin Inhibitors

Heparin-induced thrombocytopenia (HIT) is a rare but important adverse event for heparin anticoagulation. Development of heparin-dependent antibodies after initial exposure leads to a prothrombotic syndrome. In high-risk patients, direct thrombin inhibitors can be applied, although there are inherent adverse events associated with their use, such as anaphylaxis. Direct thrombin inhibitors inhibit free and clot-bound thrombin, and their effect can be monitored by either aPTT or ACT. Lepirudin and bivalirudin, a synthetic derivative, have half-lives of 40 to 120 minutes and about 25 minutes, respectively. Because these drugs undergo renal elimination, dose adjustments may be needed in patients with renal dysfunction. Argatroban is an alternative agent that undergoes primarily hepatic metabolism. A recent report described bivalirudin as a potential alternative to heparin for intravenous anticoagulation and intra-arterial thrombolysis during INR procedures.[15]

Antiplatelet Agents

Although still controversial in the acute setting,[16] antiplatelet agents (aspirin, the glycoprotein IIb/IIIa receptor antagonists, and the thienopyridine derivatives) are increasingly being used for cerebrovascular disease management.[17,18] For example, abciximab (Rheopro) has been used to treat thromboembolic complications. Activation of the platelet membrane glycoprotein (GP) IIb/IIIa leads to fibrinogen binding and is a final common pathway for platelet aggregation. Abciximab, eptifibatide, and tirofiban are glycoprotein IIb/IIIa receptor antagonists. The long duration and potent effect of abciximab also increase the likelihood of major bleeding. The smaller molecular agents, eptifibatide and tirofiban, are competitive blockers and have a shorter half-life of approximately 2 hours. Thienopyridine derivatives (ticlopidine and clopidogrel) bind to the platelet's adenosine diphosphate receptors and permanently alter the receptor; therefore, the duration of action is the life span of the platelet. The addition of clopidogrel to the antiplatelet regimen is commonly used for procedures that require placement of devices, such as stents, coiling, or stent-assisted coiling, primarily in patients who have not had an acute event such as unruptured aneurysms.

Reversal of Anticoagulation

At the end of the procedure or at the occurrence of a hemorrhagic complication, heparin may be reversed with protamine. Because there is no specific antidote for the direct thrombin inhibitors or the antiplatelet agents, the biologic half-life is one of the major considerations in drug choice, and platelet transfusion is required as a nonspecific therapy should reversal be indicated. There is currently no readily available accurate test to measure platelet function in patients taking the newer antiplatelet drugs. Intravenous desmopressin (DDAVP) has been reported to shorten the prolonged bleeding time of individuals taking antiplatelet agents such as aspirin and ticlopidine. There are also recent reports on using specific clotting factors, including recombinant factor VIIa and factor IX complex, to rescue severe life-threatening bleeding, including intracranial hemorrhage, uncontrolled by standard transfusion therapy. The safety and efficacy of these coagulation factors remain to be investigated.

DELIBERATE HYPERTENSION

During acute arterial occlusion or vasospasm, the only practical way to increase collateral blood flow may be an augmentation of the collateral perfusion pressure by increasing the systemic blood pressure. The circle of Willis is a primary collateral pathway in the cerebral circulation. However, in as many as 21% of otherwise normal subjects, the circle may not be complete. There are also secondary collateral channels that bridge adjacent major vascular territories, most importantly for the long circumferential arteries that supply the hemispheric convexities. These pathways are known as the pial-to-pial collateral or leptomeningeal pathways.

The extent to which the blood pressure has to be increased depends on the condition of the patient and the nature of the disease. During deliberate hypertension, the systemic blood pressure is increased by 30% to 40% more than the baseline in the absence of some direct outcome measure, such as resolution of ischemic symptoms or imaging evidence of improved perfusion. Intravenous phenylephrine is usually the first-line agent to produce deliberate hypertension and is titrated to achieve the desired level of blood pressure. The electrocardiogram and ST segment monitor should be carefully inspected for signs of myocardial ischemia during deliberate hypertension because the increase in afterload produced by the intervention could cause an imbalance of myocardial oxygen supply and demand.

During deliberate hypertension, the risk of causing hemorrhage into an ischemic area must be weighed against the benefits of improving perfusion, but augmentation of blood pressure in the face of acute cerebral ischemia is probably protective in most settings. There is also a risk of rupturing an aneurysm or arteriovenous malformation (AVM) with induction of hypertension. There are no data that speak to this concern directly, other than older case series that report rupture during anesthetic induction in the range of about 1% and are presumably caused by acute hypertension. For AVMs, cautious extrapolation of observations for head-frame application suggests the rarity of AVM rupture from acute blood pressure increases. Szabo and colleagues[19] measured blood pressure changes noninvasively in 56 conscious, unpremedicated patients undergoing local anesthetic injection and pin insertion; the maximum MAP was 118 ± 7 mm Hg, representing an increase of 37% from baseline. They concluded that, because none of the 56 patients, nor any of the more than 1000 patients treated in a similar fashion, suffered a hemorrhage, moderate arterial hypertension does not cause spontaneous AVM hemorrhage.

DELIBERATE HYPOTENSION

The 2 primary indications for induced hypotension are (1) to test cerebrovascular reserve in patients undergoing carotid occlusion, and (2) to slow flow in a feeding artery of brain arteriovenous malformations (BAVMs) before glue injection (sometimes termed flow arrest). The most important factor in choosing a hypotensive agent is the ability to safely and expeditiously achieve the desired reduction in blood pressure while maintaining the patient physiologically stable, and, if awake, not interfere with neurologic assessment.

The choice of agent should be determined by the experience of the practitioner, the patient's medical condition, and the goals of the blood pressure reduction in a particular clinical setting. Intravenous adenosine has been used to induce transient cardiac pause and may be a viable method of partial flow arrest.[20]

MANAGEMENT OF NEUROLOGIC AND PROCEDURAL CRISES

A well-thought-out plan, coupled with rapid and effective communication between the anesthesia and interventional teams, is critical for good outcomes. The primary responsibility of the anesthesia team is to preserve pulmonary gas exchange and, if indicated, secure the airway. Simultaneous with airway management, the first branch in the decision-making algorithm is for the anesthesiologist to communicate with the INR team and determine whether the problem is hemorrhagic or occlusive.

In the setting of vascular occlusion, the goal is to increase distal perfusion by blood pressure augmentation with or without direct thrombolysis. If the problem is hemorrhagic, immediate cessation of heparin and reversal with intravenous protamine is indicated. As an emergency reversal dose, 1 mg protamine can be given for each 100 units of initial heparin dosage that resulted in therapeutic anticoagulation. The ACT can then be used to fine-tune the final protamine dose. Complications of protamine administration include hypotension, true anaphylaxis, and pulmonary hypertension. With the advent of new, long-acting, direct thrombin inhibitors such as bivalirudin, new strategies for emergent reversal of anticoagulation will need to be developed.

Bleeding catastrophes are usually heralded by headache, nausea, vomiting, and vascular pain related to the area of perforation. Sudden loss of consciousness is not always caused by intracranial hemorrhage. Seizures, as a result of contrast reaction or transient ischemia, and the resulting postictal state, can also result in an obtunded patient. In the anesthetized or comatose patient, the sudden onset of bradycardia and hypertension (Cushing response) or the endovascular therapist's diagnosis of extravasation of contrast may be the only clues to a developing hemorrhage. Most cases of vascular rupture can be managed in the angiography suite. The INR team can attempt to seal the rupture site endovascularly and abort the procedure. A ventriculostomy catheter may be placed emergently in the angiography suite to drain cerebrospinal fluid to treat intracranial hypertension. Patients with suspected rupture require emergent computed tomography (CT) scan, but emergent craniotomy is usually not indicated.

SPECIFIC PROCEDURES
Intracranial Aneurysm Ablation

The 2 basic approaches for INR therapy for cerebral aneurysms are occlusion of proximal parent arteries and obliteration of the aneurysmal sac. With the publication of the

International Subarachnoid Aneurysm Trial (ISAT) trial,[21] coil embolization of intracranial aneurysms has become a routine first-choice therapy for many lesions. Patients who are unruptured or for whom stent placement is contemplated may be placed on antiplatelet agents before surgery.

There is great interest in the development of stent-assisted coiling methods. The stent can provide protection of the parent vessel. Stent placement requires a greater degree of instrumentation and manipulation, probably increasing the ever-present intraprocedural risk of parent vessel occlusion, thromboembolism, or vascular rupture.

Anesthetic management should proceed with the usual considerations in the care of a patient with an intracranial aneurysm.[22–24] The anesthesiologist should be prepared for aneurysmal rupture and acute SAH at all times, from spontaneous rupture of a leaky sac, direct injury of the aneurysm wall by the vascular manipulation, perianeurysmal thrombus formation, or arterial branch occlusion.

Most of the reported endovascular treatments of intracranial aneurysm have been performed under GA, especially in the care of patients with aneurysmal SAH. These patients often have either increased intracranial pressure or decreased intracranial compliance, secondary to the mass of SAH, or secondary parenchymal injury from ischemia or from hydrocephalus. GA may facilitate control of intracranial pressure and necessary blood pressure manipulations. Some recently published and ongoing studies advocate that sedation for endovascular embolization might be safe and feasible in unruptured aneurysms and low-grade ruptured aneurysms. However, in a series of 496 attempted coiling procedures for unruptured aneurysms under sedation and local anesthesia, 25.4% of the procedures were reported as either aborted or associated with medical or technical events.[23] Therefore, GA is always the backup for patients who cannot tolerate sedation or are technically challenging cases, and is safer and more efficient for managing intraprocedural complications.

Angioplasty of Cerebral Vasospasm from Aneurysmal SAH

Roughly 1 out of 4 patients with SAH develop symptomatic vasospasm. Angioplasty, either mechanical (balloon) or pharmacologic (intra-arterial vasodilators), may be used as a treatment.[25] Angioplasty is ideally done in patients who have already had the symptomatic lesion surgically clipped, and for patients in the early course of symptomatic ischemia to prevent hemorrhagic transformation of an ischemia region.

A balloon catheter is guided under fluoroscopy into the spastic segment and inflated to mechanically distend the constricted area. It is also possible to perform a pharmacologic angioplasty by direct intra-arterial infusion of a vasodilator. There is the greatest experience with papaverine as the intra-arterial vasodilator, but there are potential central nervous system toxic effects of this approach.[26] Other agents such as calcium channel blockers (nicardipine and verapamil) are also being used.[27] It is important to consider that intra-arterial vasodilators may have systemic effects (bradycardia and hypotension) which require rapid treatment to prevent systemic hypoperfusion complications.

Patients who come for angioplasty are often critically ill with a variety of challenging comorbidities including neurocardiac injury, volume overload from triple-H therapy, hydrocephalus, brain injury from recent craniotomy, and residual effects of the presenting hemorrhage. Procedural complications include arterial rupture, reperfusion hemorrhage, thromboembolism, and arterial dissection.

Given the combination of technical demands of the intervention and concerns for patients' neurologic and hemodynamic status before and after intervention, endovascular treatment of cerebral vasospasm is considered a high-risk procedure. GA is often performed to facilitate these procedures.

In patients who are symptomatic from vasospasm, it is common to increase MAP to a value 30% to 50% more than the baseline, with the goal of improving perfusion to ischemic brain regions. If the aneurysm is unsecured, this target may be tempered. Although phenylephrine is commonly administered for this purpose, if myocardial dysfunction is present from neurogenic injury, addition of an inotrope may be appropriate. Unless specifically trying to treat increased intracranial pressure, hyperventilation should be avoided.

Carotid Test Occlusion and Therapeutic Carotid Occlusion

Large or otherwise unclippable aneurysms may be partly or completely treated by proximal vessel occlusion. In order to assess the consequences of carotid occlusion in anticipation of surgery, the patient may be scheduled for a test occlusion in which cerebrovascular reserve is evaluated in several ways. A multimodal combination of angiographic, clinical, and physiologic tests can be used to arrive at the safest course of action for a given patient's clinical circumstances. The judicious use of deliberate hypotension can increase the sensitivity of the test.[28] The most important factor in choosing a hypotensive agent is the ability to safely and expeditiously achieve the desired reduction in blood pressure while maintaining the patient physiologically stable. The choice of agent should be determined by the experience of the practitioner, the patient's medical condition, and the goals of the blood pressure reduction in a particular clinical setting.

BAVMs

Also called cerebral or pial AVMs, BAVMs are typically large, complex lesions made up of a tangle of abnormal vessels (called the nidus), frequently containing several discrete fistulae served by multiple feeding arteries and draining veins. The goal of the therapeutic embolization is to obliterate as many of the fistulae and their respective feeding arteries as possible. BAVM embolization is usually an adjunct, and completed before surgery or radiotherapy.

Passage of glue into a draining vein can result in acute cerebral hemorrhage. In addition, in smaller patients, pulmonary embolism of glue can be symptomatic. For these reasons, deliberate hypotension may increase the safety of glue delivery. There is no compelling reason to choose any particular method to achieve the hypotension. The flow through the fistula is a pressure-dependent phenomenon.[29] For AVM evaluation, some centers use superselective Wada testing before therapeutic embolization to test the eloquence of regions adjacent to the lesion. In this test, the interventionalist administers an intravenous anesthetic through an arterial catheter placed in close proximity to the area of brain being anesthetized. Therefore, it is important to consider using a sedation regimen for such cases that will minimally affect cognitive or motor examinations (see earlier comments regarding reemergence phenomena). The purpose of such testing is to establish treatment risk (ie, removing perfusion to particular brain region) in individual patients. Such Wada testing, functional imaging studies, and intrasurgical cortical mapping have shown redistribution of language and memory to unpredictable regions.[30,31] Further, developmental cognitive history in these patients indicates that most have at least some background of learning problems during the school-age years with varying degrees of severity,[32] reflecting a time when brain reorganization may be occurring.

In the embolization of AVMs, the navigation of catheters, in combination with potential attempts of deliberate hypotension and/or temporary cardiovascular arrest to facilitate safe delivery of glue materials, which may affect the consciousness, would be better facilitated under GA.

Dural AVMs

Dural AVM is considered an acquired lesion resulting from venous dural sinus stenosis or occlusion, opening of potential atrioventricular (AV) shunts, and subsequent recanalization. Intracranial dural AV fistulae account for about 10% to 15% of all intracranial vascular malformations. Symptoms are variable according to which sinus is involved. Venous hypertension of pial veins is a risk factor for intracranial hemorrhage. Dural AVMs may be fed by multiple meningeal vessels, and, therefore, multistaged embolization is often necessary. Dural AV fistulae can induce markedly increased venous pressure and decreased net cerebral perfusion pressure. Therefore, presence of venous hypertension should be factored into management of systemic arterial and cerebral perfusion pressure. This aspect of dural AV fistulae perioperative management is critical. It is often assumed that the venous hypertension induces the angiogenic phenotype by acting through its causing cerebral ischemia, but newer evidence suggests that venous hypertension may be a direct stimulus for angiogenesis.[33] Dural AV fistulae are unique in that there are promising animal models of their pathogenesis,[34,35] unlike most other hemorrhagic brain diseases.

Vein of Galen malformations are a special case of dural AV fistulae that are beyond the scope of this article.[36] These are uncommon but complicated lesions that are present in infants and require a multidisciplinary approach. The patients may have intractable congestive heart failure, intractable seizures, hydrocephalus, and mental retardation. Several approaches for ablation have been attempted, including transarterial and transvenous. In infants with high-output failure, preexisting right-to-left shunts and pulmonary hypertension, a small pulmonary glue embolism resulting from an attempt to place glue in the dural AV fistula can be fatal.

Venous Malformations

Craniofacial venous malformations are congenital disorders and, in addition to causing significant cosmetic deformities, may impinge on the upper airway and interfere with swallowing. Many of these lesions are resistant to conventional surgery, cryosurgery, or laser surgery. In this procedure, United States Pharmacopeia–grade 95% ethanol opacified with contrast is injected percutaneously into the lesion under fluoroscopic guidance, resulting in a chemical burn to the lesion and eventually shrinking it. Sclerotherapy alone may be adequate treatment or may be combined with surgery.[37]

This therapy has several inter-reactions with anesthetic management.[2] Because marked swelling occurs immediately after ethanol injection, the ability of the patient to maintain a patent airway after surgery must be carefully considered.[37] Desaturation on the pulse oximeter is frequently noted after injection. Cardiopulmonary arrest has been reported.[38] The predictable intoxication and other side effects of ethanol may be evident after emergence from anesthesia, particularly postemergence agitation in children.

Venous malformations of the face or dural fistulas have the potential to drain into intracerebral veins or sinuses. By increasing the $Paco_2$ to 50 to 60 mm Hg, cerebral venous outflow will greatly exceed extracranial venous outflow, and the pressure gradient will favor movement of a sclerosing agent, chemotherapeutic agent, or glue away from vital intracranial drainage pathways. Although pressure gradients have never been studied, increased intracranial outflow is readily demonstrable in clinical practice with angiography. Addition of CO_2 gas to the inspired gas mixture is the easiest and safest way to achieve hypercapnia. Airway collapse and atelectasis are prevented by maintaining adequate tidal volume. However, hypoventilation may be used if CO_2 gas is not available. If hypoventilation is the method used to create hypercapnia, addition of positive end-expiratory pressure may be useful to maintain oxygenation.

Angioplasty and Stenting for Atherosclerotic Lesions

Angioplasty and stenting as a treatment of atherosclerotic disease involving the cervical and intracranial arteries continues to supplant open surgical management.[39,40] Risk of distal thromboembolism is a major issue in this procedure. Catheter systems using some kind of trapping system distal to the angioplasty balloon are being developed. There are multiple ongoing trials to compare the usefulness of stenting with carotid endarterectomy for extracranial carotid disease.[41,42]

Preparation for anesthetic management may include placement of transcutaneous cardiac pacing leads, in case of severe bradycardia or asystole from carotid body stimulation during angioplasty. Intravenous atropine or glycopyrrolate may be also used to mitigate against bradycardia, which almost always occurs to some degree with inflation of the balloon. This powerful negative chronotropic response may be difficult or impossible to prevent or control by conventional means. Adverse effects of increasing myocardial oxygen demand need to be considered in antibradycardia interventions. According to the 2010 American Heart Association Guidelines for Advanced Cardiovascular Life Support, atropine is not recommended for routine use in the management of PEA/asystole. For the treatment of the adult with symptomatic and unstable bradycardia, chronotropic drug infusions are recommended as an alternative to external transcutaneous pacing when atropine is ineffective.

Potential complications of cerebral angioplasty include vessel occlusion, perforation, dissection, spasm, thromboemboli, occlusion of adjacent vessels, transient ischemic episodes, and stroke. Similar to carotid endarterectomy, there is about a 5% risk of symptomatic cerebral hemorrhage and/or brain swelling after carotid angioplasty.[43] Although the cause of this syndrome is unknown, it has been associated with cerebral hyperperfusion, and it may be related to poor postoperative blood pressure control.[44]

Angioplasty and stent placement for cerebral artery stenosis have been successfully performed under GA or sedation with local anesthesia.[44] However, in certain specific lesions, such as basilar artery stenosis, GA is preferred to provide airway control when vascular occlusion from balloon inflation can cause loss of consciousness and apnea. In published studies of intracranial angioplasty and stenting in awake patients, alterations of intervention techniques secondary to intolerance of procedures have been described, although the analyses did not reveal the percentage of intraprocedure complications that occurred in lesions of basilar arteries.[45,46]

Thrombolysis of Acute Thromboembolic Stroke

In acute occlusive stroke, it is possible to recanalize the occluded vessel by superselective intra-arterial thrombolytic therapy. Thrombolytic agents can be delivered in high concentration by a microcatheter navigated close to the clot. Neurologic deficits may be reversed without additional risk of secondary hemorrhage if treatment is completed within several hours from the onset of carotid territory ischemia, and longer in vertebrobasilar territory. Intra-arterial thrombolysis is currently an off-label use. Despite an increased frequency of early symptomatic hemorrhagic complications, treatment with intra-arterial prourokinase within 6 hours of the onset of acute ischemic stroke with middle cerebral artery occlusion significantly improved clinical outcome at 90 days.[47]

A newer and promising approach is use of mechanical retrieval devices to physically remove the offending thromboembolic material from the intracranial vessel, as reviewed by Smith and colleagues.[48,49] This device seems to be efficacious in recanalizing occluded vessels. Whether outcome is also affected is less clear.

Both t-PA and mechanical retrieval have an inherent risk of promoting hemorrhagic transformation, just as in the case of IV thrombolysis. This area for investigation is important because hemorrhagic transformation, or its threat, has a great impact on clinical practice. t-PA promotes expression and activity of matrix metalloproteinase (MMP)-9, a key protease for tissue remodeling that is involved in various kinds of vascular injury that can damage the neurovascular unit and promote hemorrhage.[50] t-PA can increase MMP-9 expression in brain endothelium, acting through the low-density lipoprotein receptor–related protein (LRP), and promotes upregulation after focal cerebral ischemia.[51] Patient MMP-9 plasma levels are also increased after treatment.[52]

Details of anesthetic management are reviewed elsewhere.[53] There are Several challenges in the hyperacute care of a patient population that is generally elderly with frequent medical comorbidity, especially if little knowledge of patient history is available before treatment (because many of these patients will be brought to a regional referral center without family members). The choice of IV sedation versus GA must be carefully considered depending on local practices, and the potential for patient agitation versus the ability to monitor neurologic status. Intravascular volume management may be challenging for several reasons. Because many of these patients have preexisting systemic hypertension and associated intravascular volume depletion, they may become severely volume depleted because of an acute ictus. This depletion complicates management to address a request to maintain MAP at supranormal levels to increase collateral perfusion secondary to the acute arterial obstruction. The risk of vessel rupture or clot propagation is omnipresent.

Recent publications on the association of anesthesia for endovascular treatment in acute ischemic stroke and patient outcome have elicited extensive debates on choice of anesthetic techniques in INR procedures.[54,55] Although both studies were limited in part by the retrospective data, they did raise many important questions. The study by Abou-Chebl and colleagues,[54] a multicenter cohort of 980 patients, suggested that the use of GA was associated with poorer neurologic outcome at 90 days and higher mortality. However, this conclusion did not take account of various periprocedure variables, including the patients' baseline comorbidities and severity of the stroke, or any anesthesia and hemodynamic parameters. The more recently published retrospective review of the charts of 129 patients by Davis and colleagues[55] made the significant step of including patients' baseline characteristics, as well as the time to treatment, periprocedure blood pressure, and glucose measurements into their analyses. Their findings suggest that hypotension might be contributing to the worse neurologic outcome associated with GA. A crucial caveat was that hypotension was defined as the lowest systolic blood pressure less than 140 mm Hg at any point in the periprocedure period. It has been the general opinion in anesthesia practice that individual patients' baseline blood pressures set the base for guiding variation limits for perioperative care. Further, duration of hemodynamic changes would have no less weight on patient outcome than some transient deviations. In contrast, in the trials of patients undergoing endovascular treatment using mechanical devices, the study showed that the ability to remove the clot was negatively influenced by systolic blood pressure ($\geq$150 mm Hg) on presentation.[56] A similar phenomenon was observed in a few other studies.[57,58] The hypothesized underlying mechanisms include that (1) high systolic pressure, a marker for poor collateral flow, can cause a high-pressure gradient across the clot, resulting in more clot impaction and therefore more difficult mechanical retrieval; (2) greater clot impaction leads to vascular spasm that further hamper clot removal; and (3) in thrombolysis attempts, the higher impaction of the clots may prevent penetration of plasminogen activator into the thrombus, and decrease the influx of new plasminogen into the clot matrix. These controversial observations again highlight the need for future investigations on hemodynamic parameters in acute stroke patients.

POSTOPERATIVE MANAGEMENT

Patients who have had endovascular surgery pass the immediate postoperative period in a monitored setting to watch for signs of hemodynamic instability or neurologic deterioration. Control of blood pressure may be necessary during transport and postoperative recovery (eg, induced hypertension, if indicated). In particular, patients undergoing treatment of extracranial carotid disease are prone to postprocedural hemodynamic instability, similar to patients after carotid endartectomy.[59]

Abrupt restoration of normal systemic pressure to a chronically hypotensive (ischemic) vascular bed may overwhelm autoregulatory capacity and result in hemorrhage or swelling (normal perfusion pressure breakthrough).[43,60] The pathophysiologic mechanism is unclear, but it is probably not simply a hemodynamic effect, and the loss of neurovascular unit integrity is probably related to the pathways involved in postreperfusion hemorrhage in the setting of acute stroke (described earlier).

Nonetheless, cerebral hyperemia is probably exacerbated by uncontrolled increases in systemic arterial blood pressure. In the absence of collateral perfusion pressure inadequacy, fastidious attention to preventing hypertension is warranted. Complicated cases may go first to CT or some other kind of tomographic imaging; critical care management may need to be extended during transport and imaging. Symptomatic hyperemic complications are more uncommon than silent hyperemic states, and, with use of more sensitive MR imaging, ischemic events are probably more common than previously suspected.[61]

FUTURE DIRECTIONS

For the overall management approach to the patient with cerebrovascular disease, there is increasing interest and discussion of the appropriate management of asymptomatic or unruptured lesions. Anesthesiologists are not traditionally directly involved with these management dilemmas. However, optimal provision of perioperative care and effective resource allocation would benefit from active involvement of all practitioners involved in the management of these patients, because the questions concern the effects of anesthesia on patient outcome after acute ischemic stroke.

The indications for invasive therapy for unruptured AVMs[62] and aneurysms[63,64] are currently undergoing critical discussion. Although it is generally agreed that ruptured lesions need treatment, the aggregate risks for treating all unruptured cases may exceed the potential benefit from protecting against future hemorrhage. For example, A Randomized Trial of Unruptured Brain Arteriovenous Malformations is an international multicenter randomized controlled trial that will test whether functional outcome and the risk of spontaneous AVM rupture at 5 years for best medical therapy is superior to procedural intervention, including embolization, microsurgical resection, or radiosurgery (http://clinicaltrials.gov/ct/show/NCT00389181). Similarly, the International Study of Unruptured Intracranial Aneurysms (ISUIA) is a long-standing effort to document the natural history and treatment outcomes for unruptured lesions.[63,65]

Future research directions for vascular disease of the brain present opportunities for neuroanesthesia, perioperative management, and neurocritical care. Basic or translational questions include the interaction of angiogenesis and vascular remodeling on pathogenesis and clinical course. There is growing evidence suggesting that some of these lesions undergo active angiogenesis and vascular remodeling in the adult life. This new concept of active angiogenesis and vascular remodeling in intracranial vascular malformations may open new clinical paradigms in which pharmacologic interventions are proposed to stabilize these abnormal blood vessels and prevent further growth or hemorrhage. Recent research on intracranial vascular malformations has focused on identifying the roles of angiogenic and antiangiogenic factors in their pathophysiology.[66]

Abnormal vascular remodeling mediated by inflammatory cells has been identified as a key pathologic component of various vascular diseases, including abdominal aortic aneurysms, BAVMs, and atherosclerosis.[67–70] This concept may provide a new treatment strategy to use agents to inhibit inflammation or cytokines produced by inflammatory cells such as MMPs. Based on findings from observational studies that analyzed human intracranial aneurysms, and experimental studies that used animal models, an emerging concept suggests that a key component of the pathophysiology of intracranial aneurysms is sustained abnormal vascular remodeling coupled with inflammation.[71–73]

Consistent with a background contribution of a ubiquitous process such as inflammation, aneurismal disease may be better conceived of as a process, rather than an event. For example, the long-term durability of aneurysm treatment is often assumed. There is growing appreciation that the traditional notion of disease treatment should not necessarily be construed as a cure, although it may be in many cases. Although treatment decreases new rupture rates, there is a measurable rebleed rate after treatment (surgery or coiling).[1] The risk of further hemorrhage continues for up to 30 years after SAH.[74] The Dutch Aneurysm Screening After Surgical Treatment for Ruptured Aneurysms (ASTRA) group reported follow-up CT angiography on 610 patients 1 to 15 years after surgical clipping of a ruptured aneurysm, and found an incidence of 16% of new aneurysms.[75] In 24 patients, aneurysms were present at the site of the previous clipping and, in 3 of these, the postoperative angiogram had shown complete aneurysm occlusion. Taken together with observations that a significant fraction of aneurysms enlarge over time,[74–76] aneurismal disease may be a process characterized by generalized vascular dysfunction rather than a sporadic focal event.

Proinflammatory influence on disease susceptibility[77,78] and clinical course[79,80] seems to apply to AVMs as well. Tissue IL-6 expression is associated with the IL-6-174G>C genotype and linked to downstream targets involved in angiogenesis and vascular instability.[81] Further, IL-6 induced MMP-3 and MMP-9 expression and activity in the mouse brain and increased proliferation and migration of cerebral endothelial cells. Taken together, such observations are consistent with the hypothesis that inflammatory processes influence angiogenic and proteolytic activity, thus contributing to the pathogenesis of intracranial hemorrhage.

In the future, genetic variation has the potential to be developed to help predict new intracranial hemorrhage in the natural course after presentation[79,80] or used to stratify risk for postoperative complications.[82] Genetic variation or plasma cytokine assays[83,84] have the potential for development to affect multiple aspects of perioperative management.

In the discussion of anesthetic management and its effects on outcome from interventional procedures, various preoperative and perioperative factors have been proposed to have potential influences, including medical comorbidities, choice of anesthesia techniques, length of time before the start of therapeutic interventions, and hemodynamic control. Future well-designed prospective clinical studies are needed to investigate the influence of such factors on patient outcome and provide critical evidence to guide clinical practice.

ACKNOWLEDGMENTS

The author would like to thank the members of the UCSF Brain AVM Study Project and the Center for Cerebrovascular Research (www.avm.ucsf.edu) for the opportunities to learn more about cerebrovascular disease and anesthetic management.

REFERENCES

1. Molyneux AJ, Kerr RS, Yu LM, et al. International Subarachnoid Aneurysm Trial (ISAT) of neurosurgical clipping versus endovascular coiling in 2143 patients with ruptured intracranial aneurysms: a randomised comparison of effects on survival, dependency, seizures, rebleeding, subgroups, and aneurysm occlusion. Lancet 2005;366(9488):809–17.
2. Young WL, Pile-Spellman J. Anesthetic considerations for interventional neuroradiology. Anesthesiology 1994;80(2):427–56.
3. Young WL, Pile-Spellman J, Hacein-Bey L, et al. Invasive neuroradiologic procedures for cerebrovascular abnormalities: anesthetic considerations. Anesthesiol Clin North Am 1997;15(3):631–53.
4. Strandgaard S, Olesen J, Skinhoj E, et al. Autoregulation of brain circulation in severe arterial hypertension. BMJ 1973;1(5852):507–10.
5. Drummond JC. The lower limit of autoregulation: time to revise our thinking? Anesthesiology 1997;86(6):1431–3.
6. Patel PM, Drummond JC. Cerebral physiology and the effects of anesthetic drugs. In: Miller RD, et al, editors. Miller's anesthesia. New York: Churchill Livingstone; 2010. p. 305–39. Chapter 13.
7. Anastasian ZH, Strozyk D, Meyers PM, et al. Radiation exposure of the anesthesiologist in the neurointerventional suite. Anesthesiology 2011;114(3):512–20.
8. McDonagh DL, Olson DM, Kalia JS, et al. Anesthesia and sedation practices among neurointerventionalists during acute ischemic stroke endovascular therapy. Front Neurol 2010;1:118.
9. Prielipp RC, Wall MH, Tobin JR, et al. Dexmedetomidine-induced sedation in volunteers decreases regional and global cerebral blood flow. Anesth Analg 2002;95(4):1052–9.
10. Arain SR, Ebert TJ. The efficacy, side effects, and recovery characteristics of dexmedetomidine versus propofol when used for intraoperative sedation. Anesth Analg 2002;95(2):461–6.
11. Thal GD, Szabo MD, Lopez-Bresnahan M, et al. Exacerbation or unmasking of focal neurologic deficits by sedatives. Anesthesiology 1996;85(1):21–5 [discussion: 29A–30A].
12. Chollet F, DiPiero V, Wise RJ, et al. The functional anatomy of motor recovery after stroke in humans: a study with positron emission tomography. Ann Neurol 1991;29(1):63–71.
13. Lazar RM, et al. Reemergence of stroke deficits with midazolam challenge. Stroke 2002;33(1):283–5.
14. Lazar RM, Fitzsimmons BF, Marshall RS, et al. Midazolam challenge reinduces neurological deficits after transient ischemic attack. Stroke 2003;34(3):794–6.
15. Harrigan MR, Levy EI, Bendok BR, et al. Bivalirudin for endovascular intervention in acute ischemic stroke: case report. Neurosurgery 2004;54(1):218–22 [discussion: 222–3].
16. Ciccone A, Abraha I, Santilli I. Glycoprotein IIb-IIIa inhibitors for acute ischaemic stroke. Cochrane Database Syst Rev 2006;4:CD005208.
17. Hashimoto T, Gupta DK, Young WL. Interventional neuroradiology–anesthetic considerations. Anesthesiol Clin North Am 2002;20(2):347–59.
18. Fiorella D, Albuquerque FC, Han P, et al. Strategies for the management of intraprocedural thromboembolic complications with abciximab (ReoPro). Neurosurgery 2004;54(5):1089–97 [discussion: 1097–8].

19. Szabo MD, Crosby G, Sundaram P, et al. Hypertension does not cause spontaneous hemorrhage of intracranial arteriovenous malformations. Anesthesiology 1989;70(5):761–3.

20. Hashimoto T, Young WL, Aagaard BD, et al. Adenosine-induced ventricular asystole to induce transient profound systemic hypotension in patients undergoing endovascular therapy. Dose-response characteristics. Anesthesiology 2000; 93(4):998–1001.

21. Molyneux A, Kerr R, Stratton I, et al. International Subarachnoid Aneurysm Trial (ISAT) of neurosurgical clipping versus endovascular coiling in 2143 patients with ruptured intracranial aneurysms: a randomised trial. Lancet 2002; 360(9342):1267–74.

22. Drummond JC, Patel PM. Neurosurgical anesthesia. In: Miller RD, et al, editors. Miller's anesthesia. New York: Churchill Livingstone; 2010. p. 2045–87. Chapter 63.

23. Ogilvy CS, Yang X, Jamil OA, et al. Neurointerventional procedures for unruptured intracranial aneurysms under procedural sedation and local anesthesia: a large-volume, single-center experience. J Neurosurg Anesthesiol 2011; 114(1):120–8.

24. Kimball MM, Velat GJ, Hoh BL. Critical care guidelines on the endovascular management of cerebral vasospasm. Neurocrit Care 2011;15(2):336–41.

25. Newell DW, Eskridge JM, Mayberg MR, et al. Angioplasty for the treatment of symptomatic vasospasm following subarachnoid hemorrhage. J Neurosurg 1989;71(5 Pt 1):654–60.

26. Smith WS, Dowd CF, Johnston SC, et al. Neurotoxicity of intra-arterial papaverine preserved with chlorobutanol used for the treatment of cerebral vasospasm after aneurysmal subarachnoid hemorrhage. Stroke 2004;35(11):2518–22.

27. Feng L, Fitzsimmons BF, Young WL, et al. Intraarterially administered verapamil as adjunct therapy for cerebral vasospasm: safety and 2-year experience. AJNR Am J Neuroradiol 2002;23(8):1284–90.

28. Marshall RS, Lazar RM, Pile-Spellman J, et al. Recovery of brain function during induced cerebral hypoperfusion. Brain 2001;124(Pt 6):1208–17.

29. Gao E, Young WL, Pile-Spellman J, et al. Deliberate systemic hypotension to facilitate endovascular therapy of cerebral arteriovenous malformations: a computer modeling study. Neurosurg Focus 1997;2(6):e3.

30. Lazar RM, Marshall RS, Pile-Spellman J, et al. Interhemispheric transfer of language in patients with left frontal cerebral arteriovenous malformation. Neuropsychologia 2000;38(10):1325–32.

31. Lazar RM, Marshall RS, Pile-Spellman J, et al. Anterior translocation of language in patients with left cerebral arteriovenous malformations. Neurology 1997;49(3): 802–8.

32. Lazar RM, Connaire K, Marshall RS, et al. Developmental deficits in adult patients with arteriovenous malformations. Arch Neurol 1999;56(1):103–6.

33. Zhu Y, Lawton MT, Du R, et al. Expression of hypoxia-inducible factor-1 and vascular endothelial growth factor in response to venous hypertension. Neurosurgery 2006;59(3):687–96 [discussion: 687–96].

34. Lawton MT, Jacobowitz R, Spetzler RF. Redefined role of angiogenesis in the pathogenesis of dural arteriovenous malformations. J Neurosurg 1997;87(2):267–74.

35. Terada T, Higashida RT, Halbach VV, et al. Development of acquired arteriovenous fistulas in rats due to venous hypertension. J Neurosurg 1994;80(5):884–9.

36. Fullerton HJ, Aminoff AR, Ferriero DM, et al. Neurodevelopmental outcome after endovascular treatment of vein of Galen malformations. Neurology 2003;61(10): 1386–90.

37. Lasjaunias P, Berenstein A. Endovascular treatment of the craniofacial lesions. In: Surgical neuroangiography, vol 2. Heidelberg (Germany): Springer-Verlag; 1987. p. 389–97.
38. Yakes WF, Rossi P, Odink H. How I do it. Arteriovenous malformation management. Cardiovasc Intervent Radiol 1996;19(2):65–71.
39. Higashida RT, et al. Intracranial angioplasty & stenting for cerebral atherosclerosis: a position statement of the American Society of Interventional and Therapeutic Neuroradiology, Society of Interventional Radiology, and the American Society of Neuroradiology. AJNR Am J Neuroradiol 2005;26(9):2323–7.
40. Goodney PP, Schermerhorn ML, Powell RJ. Current status of carotid artery stenting. J Vasc Surg 2006;43(2):406–11.
41. Yadav JS, Wholey MH, Kuntz RE, et al. Protected carotid-artery stenting versus endarterectomy in high-risk patients. N Engl J Med 2004;351(15):1493–501.
42. Mas JL, Chatellier G, Beyssen B, et al. Endarterectomy versus stenting in patients with symptomatic severe carotid stenosis. N Engl J Med 2006; 355(16):1660–71.
43. Meyers PM, Higashida RT, Phatouros CC, et al. Cerebral hyperperfusion syndrome after percutaneous transluminal stenting of the craniocervical arteries. Neurosurgery 2000;47(2):335–43 [discussion: 343–5].
44. Schumacher HC, Meyers PM, Higashida RT, et al. Reporting standards for angioplasty and stent-assisted angioplasty for intracranial atherosclerosis. Stroke 2009;40(5):e348–65.
45. Abou-Chebl A, Krieger DW, Bajzer CT, et al. Intracranial angioplasty and stenting in the awake patient. J Neuroimaging 2006;16(3):216–23.
46. Chamczuk AJ, Ogilvy CS, Snyder KV, et al. Elective stenting for intracranial stenosis under conscious sedation. Neurosurgery 2010;67(5):1189–93 [discussion: 1194].
47. Furlan A, Higashida R, Wechsler L, et al. Intra-arterial prourokinase for acute ischemic stroke. The PROACT II study: a randomized controlled trial. Prolyse in Acute Cerebral Thromboembolism. JAMA 1999;282(21):2003–11.
48. Smith WS. Safety of mechanical thrombectomy and intravenous tissue plasminogen activator in acute ischemic stroke. Results of the multi Mechanical Embolus Removal in Cerebral Ischemia (MERCI) trial, part I. AJNR Am J Neuroradiol 2006; 27(6):1177–82.
49. Smith WS, Sung G, Starkman S, et al. Safety and efficacy of mechanical embolectomy in acute ischemic stroke: results of the MERCI trial. Stroke 2005;36(7): 1432–8.
50. Wang X, Lee SR, Arai K, et al. Lipoprotein receptor-mediated induction of matrix metalloproteinase by tissue plasminogen activator. Nat Med 2003;9(10):1313–7.
51. Tsuji K, Aoki T, Tejima E, et al. Tissue plasminogen activator promotes matrix metalloproteinase-9 upregulation after focal cerebral ischemia. Stroke 2005; 36(9):1954–9.
52. Horstmann S, Kalb P, Koziol J, et al. Profiles of matrix metalloproteinases, their inhibitors, and laminin in stroke patients: influence of different therapies. Stroke 2003;34(9):2165–70.
53. Lee CZ, Litt L, Hashimoto T, et al. Physiologic monitoring and anesthesia considerations in acute ischemic stroke. J Vasc Interv Radiol 2004;15(1 Pt 2):S13–9.
54. Abou-Chebl A, Lin R, Hussain MS, et al. Conscious sedation versus general anesthesia during endovascular therapy for acute anterior circulation stroke: preliminary results from a retrospective, multicenter study. Stroke 2010;41(6): 1175–9.

55. Davis MJ, Menon BK, Baghirzada LB, et al. Anesthetic management and outcome in patients during endovascular therapy for acute stroke. Anesthesiology 2012;116(2):396–405.
56. Nogueira RG, Liebeskind DS, Sung G, et al. Predictors of good clinical outcomes, mortality, and successful revascularization in patients with acute ischemic stroke undergoing thrombectomy: pooled analysis of the Mechanical Embolus Removal in Cerebral Ischemia (MERCI) and Multi MERCI Trials. Stroke 2009;40(12): 3777–83.
57. Mattle HP, Kappeler L, Arnold M, et al. Blood pressure and vessel recanalization in the first hours after ischemic stroke. Stroke 2005;36(2):264–8.
58. Tsivgoulis G, Saqqur M, Sharma VK, et al. Association of pretreatment blood pressure with tissue plasminogen activator-induced arterial recanalization in acute ischemic stroke. Stroke 2007;38(3):961–6.
59. Qureshi AI, Luft AR, Sharma M, et al. Frequency and determinants of postprocedural hemodynamic instability after carotid angioplasty and stenting. Stroke 1999;30(10):2086–93.
60. Young WL, Kader A, Ornstein E, et al. Cerebral hyperemia after arteriovenous malformation resection is related to "breakthrough" complications but not to feeding artery pressure. Columbia University AVM Study Project. Neurosurgery 1996;38(6):1085–93 [discussion: 1093–5].
61. Cronqvist M, Wirestam R, Ramgren B, et al. Endovascular treatment of intracerebral arteriovenous malformations: procedural safety, complications, and results evaluated by MR imaging, including diffusion and perfusion imaging. AJNR Am J Neuroradiol 2006;27(1):162–76.
62. Stapf C, Mohr JP, Choi JH, et al. Invasive treatment of unruptured brain arteriovenous malformations is experimental therapy. Curr Opin Neurol 2006;19(1): 63–8.
63. Wiebers DO, Whisnant JP, Huston J 3rd, et al. Unruptured intracranial aneurysms: natural history, clinical outcome, and risks of surgical and endovascular treatment. Lancet 2003;362(9378):103–10.
64. Wiebers DO. Patients with small, asymptomatic, unruptured intracranial aneurysms and no history of subarachnoid hemorrhage should generally be treated conservatively. Stroke 2005;36(2):408–9.
65. International Study of Unruptured Intracranial Aneurysms Investigators. Unruptured intracranial aneurysms–risk of rupture and risks of surgical intervention. International Study of Unruptured Intracranial Aneurysms Investigators. N Engl J Med 1998;339(24):1725–33.
66. Hashimoto T, Young WL. Roles of angiogenesis and vascular remodeling in brain vascular malformations. Semin Cerebrovasc Dis Stroke 2004;4(4):217–25.
67. Hashimoto T, Wen G, Lawton MT, et al. Abnormal expression of matrix metalloproteinases and tissue inhibitors of metalloproteinases in brain arteriovenous malformations. Stroke 2003;34(4):925–31.
68. Knox JB, Sukhova GK, Whittemore AD, et al. Evidence for altered balance between matrix metalloproteinases and their inhibitors in human aortic diseases. Circulation 1997;95(1):205–12.
69. Goodall S, Crowther M, Hemingway DM, et al. Ubiquitous elevation of matrix metalloproteinase-2 expression in the vasculature of patients with abdominal aneurysms. Circulation 2001;104(3):304–9.
70. Loftus IM, Naylor AR, Goodall S, et al. Increased matrix metalloproteinase-9 activity in unstable carotid plaques. A potential role in acute plaque disruption. Stroke 2000;31(1):40–7.

71. Chyatte D, Bruno G, Desai S, et al. Inflammation and intracranial aneurysms. Neurosurgery 1999;45(5):1137–46 [discussion: 1146–7].
72. Frosen J, Piippo A, Paetau A, et al. Remodeling of saccular cerebral artery aneurysm wall is associated with rupture: histological analysis of 24 unruptured and 42 ruptured cases. Stroke 2004;35(10):2287–93.
73. Hashimoto T, Meng H, Young WL. Intracranial aneurysms: links between inflammation, hemodynamics and vascular remodeling. Neurol Res 2006;28(4): 372–80.
74. Juvela S, Porras M, Poussa K. Natural history of unruptured intracranial aneurysms: probability of and risk factors for aneurysm rupture. J Neurosurg 2000; 93(3):379–87.
75. Wermer MJ, van der Schaaf IC, Velthuis BK, et al. Follow-up screening after subarachnoid haemorrhage: frequency and determinants of new aneurysms and enlargement of existing aneurysms. Brain 2005;128(Pt 10):2421–9.
76. Mangrum WI, Huston J 3rd, Link MJ, et al. Enlarging vertebrobasilar nonsaccular intracranial aneurysms: frequency, predictors, and clinical outcome of growth. J Neurosurg 2005;102(1):72–9.
77. Simon M, Franke D, Ludwig M, et al. Association of a polymorphism of the ACVRL1 gene with sporadic arteriovenous malformations of the central nervous system. J Neurosurg 2006;104(6):945–9.
78. Pawlikowska L, Tran MN, Achrol AS, et al. Polymorphisms in transforming growth factor-B-related genes ALK1 and ENG are associated with sporadic brain arteriovenous malformations. Stroke 2005;36(10):2278–80.
79. Achrol AS, Pawlikowska L, McCulloch CE, et al. Tumor necrosis factor-alpha-238G>A promoter polymorphism is associated with increased risk of new hemorrhage in the natural course of patients with brain arteriovenous malformations. Stroke 2006;37(1):231–4.
80. Pawlikowska L, Poon KY, Achrol AS, et al. Apoliprotein E epsilon2 is associated with new hemorrhage risk in brain arteriovenous malformation. Neurosurgery 2006;58(5):838–43 [discussion: 838–43].
81. Chen Y, Pawlikowska L, Yao JS, et al. Interleukin-6 involvement in brain arteriovenous malformations. Ann Neurol 2006;59(1):72–80.
82. Achrol AS, Kim H, Pawlikowska L, et al. TNF-alpha polymorphism is associated with intracranial hemorrhage (ICH) after arteriovenous malformation (AVM) treatment [abstract]. Stroke 2007;38(2):597–8.
83. Castellanos M, Leira R, Serena J, et al. Plasma metalloproteinase-9 concentration predicts hemorrhagic transformation in acute ischemic stroke. Stroke 2003;34(1): 40–6.
84. Tung PP, Olmsted EA, Kopelnik A, et al. Plasma B-type natriuretic peptide levels are associated with early cardiac dysfunction after subarachnoid hemorrhage. Stroke 2005;36(7):1567–9.

Neuroimaging for the Anesthesiologist

Denise Crute, MD[a], Joseph Sebeo, MD, PhD[a],
Irene P. Osborn, MD[b,*]

KEYWORDS

- Computed tomography • Magnetic resonance imaging • Anesthesiology

KEY POINTS

- Fluoroscopy and plain radiography provide good 2-dimensional visualization of bone and hardware, and are the mainstays of intraoperative localization in spinal surgery.
- Computed tomography (CT) provides excellent visualization of bone and good visualization of neural elements.
- Magnetic resonance imaging (MRI) provides excellent imaging of neural elements.
- Positron emission tomography, single-photon emission CT, and functional MRI provide direct information about localized cerebral perfusion and metabolism.
- The skull has a fixed volume with 3 main components: brain, blood, and cerebrospinal fluid (CSF).
- Four CT imaging features allow quick perfusion estimation: symmetry, cisterns, gray matter-white matter differentiation, and ventricles.
- Cranial pathology may be considered according to lobe (frontal, temporal, parietal, occipital, cerebellum) or cranial fossa (anterior, middle, posterior).
- Spinal lesions may be considered by level (craniocervical junction, cervical, thoracic, lumbar, sacral) and column (anterior, middle, and posterior).
- The posterior fossa is the "Manhattan" of the brain, with a lot of critical function and valuable real estate in a tiny space.
- Two important questions must be answered regarding any spinal column abnormality: (1) Does it compromise neural elements? (2) Is it stable?
- There are 5 types of hemorrhage in the central nervous system: (1) epidural hematoma, (2) subdural hematoma, (3) subarachnoid hemorrhage (SAH), (4) intracranial hemorrhage (ICH), and (5) intraventricular hemorrhage.
- Epidural hemorrhage is hemorrhage occurring between bone and dura.

Continued

Disclosure: The authors have no conflicts of interest.
[a] Department of Neurosurgery, Mount Sinai School of Medicine, One Gustave Levy Place, Box 1136, New York, NY 10029, USA; [b] Department of Anesthesiology, Mount Sinai School of Medicine, One Gustave Levy Place, Box 1010, New York, NY 10029, USA
* Corresponding author.
E-mail address: Irene.osborn@mssm.edu

Anesthesiology Clin 30 (2012) 149–173
http://dx.doi.org/10.1016/j.anclin.2012.06.003   anesthesiology.theclinics.com
1932-2275/12/$ – see front matter © 2012 Elsevier Inc. All rights reserved.

Continued

- Subdural hemorrhage is hemorrhage occurring between the dura and brain.
- The most common SAH is traumatic; the most devastating SAH is aneurysmal.
- Intracerebral hemorrhage is hemorrhage occurring within the brain parenchyma.
- Intraventricular hemorrhage is rarely isolated, is most often seen in association with SAH or ICH, and when present, significantly worsens prognosis.
- Intracranial masses may be broadly categorized as supratentorial or infratentorial and as extra-axial or intra-axial.
- Extra-axial masses involving the convexities are typically benign, quick, and relatively simple to remove. Skull-base extra-axial masses, although also histologically benign, represent some of the greatest surgical and anesthetic challenges.
- Infratentorial masses typically become problematic at a much smaller size than supratentorial masses.
- Hydrocephalus occurs for 1 of 3 reasons: (1) CSF production is increased, (2) CSF flow is compromised, or (3) CSF absorption is decreased.

INTRODUCTION

In central nervous system (CNS) pathology, as in real estate, the top 3 things to consider are: (1) location, (2) location, and (3) location. Neuroimaging provides critical information about the location, type, severity, and timing of CNS abnormalities. Familiarity with contemporary neuroimaging techniques and the abnormalities they reveal helps the anesthesiologist to anticipate challenges and provide optimal management and care. Neuroimaging guides patient care with important information regarding pathologic location, type, severity, and timing (**Table 1**). Safe and effective anesthetic and critical care management entails precise manipulation of CNS components revealed by neuroimaging.

IMAGING MODALITIES
Fluoroscopy and Radiography

Fluoroscopy and plain radiography are rarely used for cranial cases, owing to poor visualization of soft tissues.[1] These modalities are best for imaging bone and foreign bodies, and are frequently used for spine cases. These techniques have the advantages of being inexpensive, widely available, and rapid. Disadvantages include ionizing radiation and poor soft-tissue visualization.

Computed Tomography

Computed tomography (CT) produces cross-sectional images in which the attenuation degree or absorption coefficient of tissue is measured in Hounsfield Units (HU) and converted to grayscale. The cross-sectional images may be reformatted as needed to produce 3-dimensional images. Denser or higher absorption tissues (such as bone) have higher HU values and appear brighter on CT. Less dense or lower absorption tissues such as cerebrospinal fluid (CSF) have lower HU values and appear dark on CT (**Fig. 1, Table 2**).

Noncontrast CT has the advantages of availability, speed, and affordability. It is often the first neuroimaging modality obtained in the acute or emergency setting. Noncontrast CT is excellent for assessing acute hemorrhage and bone lesions such as fractures. Portable CT scanners are becoming more commonplace in the operating

Table 1
Neuroimaging provides critical information about the location, type, severity, and timing of central nervous system pathology

Pathology	Cranial Location	Spinal Location	Type	Severity	Timing	Imaging Modality
Hemorrhage	Frontal Temporal Parietal Occipital Posterior fossa	Cervical Thoracic Lumbosacral	EDH, SDH, ICH, SAH, IVH	Volume Modified Fisher Scale Shift	Acute Subacute Chronic	CT, MRI, angiography
Bone lesion	Facial Calvarial skull base	Craniocervical Cervical Thoracic Lumbosacral	Fracture, bony tumor, infection	Compression Neural impingement Stability	Acute Subacute Chronic	Fluorography, radiography, CT, MRI (spine)
Infarction	Anterior cerebral Middle cerebral Posterior cerebral Vertebrobasilar Watershed	Anterior spinal Adamkiewicz	Occlusive, ischemic, embolic	Volume	Acute Subacute Chronic	CT, MRI, angiography, SPECT, fMRI
Edema	Frontal Temporal Parietal Occipital Posterior fossa	Cervical Thoracic Lumbar	Neoplastic, vascular, infectious, inflammatory, traumatic	Volume Local Diffuse	Acute Chronic	CT, MRI, SPECT, fMRI
Mass lesion	Frontal Temporal Parietal Occipital Posterior fossa	Neoplastic, Vascular, Infectious, Traumatic	Neoplastic, vascular, infectious, traumatic	Volume Intra-axial Extra-axial	Acute Chronic	CT, MRI, angiography, ultrasonography
Hydrocephalus	Lateral Third Fourth External	Syringomyelia	Obstructive, communicating, post-hemorrhagic, postinfectious, NPH, ex vacuo	Intracranial pressure Ventricular size Transependymal flow	Acute Chronic	CT, MRI, ultrasonography

Abbreviations: CT, computed tomography; EDH, epidural hematoma; fMRI, functional magnetic resonance imaging; ICH, intracranial hemorrhage; IVH, intraventricular hemorrhage; MRI, magnetic resonance imaging; NPH, normal pressure hydrocephalus; SAH, subarachnoid hemorrhage; SDH, subdural hematoma; SPECT, single-photon emission computed tomography.

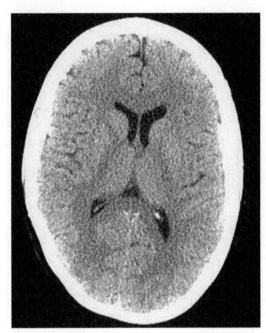

Fig. 1. Normal axial CT without contrast.

room (OR) and intensive care unit (ICU), and greatly facilitate intraoperative and critical care assessment monitoring and decision making.[2]

Contrast-enhanced CT involves injection of intravenous iodinated contrast dye, and is useful for imaging vascular structures (CT angiography) and abnormalities such as aneurysms and arteriovenous malformations (AVMs), as well as hypermetabolic lesions such as tumors and abscesses that readily take up the contrast dye.[3] Reconstructed 3-dimensional images are particularly useful for evaluation of skull-base and vascular lesions as well as spine fractures and deformity.

Disadvantages of CT include relatively poor visualization of posterior fossa structures, spinal cord, early ischemia or infarction, and subacute blood. The imaging modality also exposes the patient to ionizing radiation.[3]

Table 2
Imaging attenuation of various CNS structures on CT

Tissue	Density (HU)	CT Appearance
Bone	300–1000	Bright
Acute blood	60–80	Bright
Intervertebral disk	50–55	Light gray
White matter	40–50	Light gray
Gray matter	35–45	Gray
Cerebrospinal fluid	0	Dark
Fat	−20 to −50	Dark
Air	−300 to −1000	Very dark

Anesthetic considerations for CT:

- Usually shorter in duration than magnetic resonance imaging (MRI)
- Patient must be able to lie supine
- Considerable radiation exposure
- Procedure may be interrupted for patient interaction/care with resumption of scanning.

Magnetic Resonance Imaging

MRI uses radiofrequency pulses within a strong magnetic field to elicit characteristic tissue radiofrequency signals, which are digitized and converted to a grayscale image. Variations in the radiofrequency pulses can be used to create sequences for improved tissue visualization. T1-weighted images reveal excellent soft-tissue visualization and T2-weighted images reveal excellent fluid visualization. MR angiography and venography provide visualization of vascular structures and lesions without iodinated contrast. Diffusion-weighted and perfusion-weighted sequences can be particularly useful in the assessment of stroke and cerebrovascular lesions.[4] Contrast enhancement is obtained with intravenous gadolinium. Advantages of MRI include increased soft-tissue resolution and visualization of bone, and no risk of radiation exposure. Disadvantages include: (1) inability to visualize structures adjacent to metallic implants such as spinal fixation hardware, because of artifact; (2) inability to safely obtain an MRI scan in some patients such as those with ferromagnetic implants, pacemakers, or foreign bodies; (3) the time-consuming nature of the scan; and (4) limited availability.[5]

Hematomas, particularly large intracerebral hematomas, may not follow the imaging characteristics of blood noted above, and additional factors such as hemodilution, edema, and clotting may be important. Also, as an intracerebral hematoma resolves there may be rim enhancement such that a subacute infarction may mimic a neoplasm.[6]

Regarding anesthetic considerations for MRI, the excellent resolution of MR can be severely degraded by any patient movement. In addition, the required intense magnetic fields create unique problems with the use of physiologic monitors, standard anesthesia machines, and ventilators. MRI-compatible machines and monitors are currently available for the most complex anesthetic cases. Other considerations include[7]:

- Magnetic field disables conventional monitoring equipment
- Radiofrequency interference and risk of burns to patient
- Hazards of ferromagnetic projectiles
- Patient distance/inaccessibility
- Prolonged studies
- Distance from OR/postanesthesia care unit.

Angiography

Angiography uses intra-arterial contrast to visualize vasculature and vascular lesions (**Fig. 2**). Conventional angiography provides excellent visualization of intracranial vascular structures, and permits contemporaneous endovascular interventions. Disadvantages include its invasiveness, exposure to ionizing radiation, time-consuming nature, and expense. CT angiography and MR angiography provide noninvasive alternatives to conventional angiography, with capabilities for 3-dimensional reconstruction.[8] A

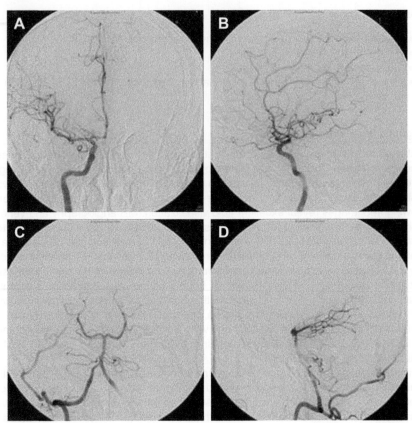

Fig. 2. Normal cerebral angiogram. (*A*) Anteroposterior (AP) right carotid injection, (*B*) lateral right carotid injection, (*C*) AP right vertebral injection, (*D*) lateral right vertebral injection.

detailed description of angiographic considerations is provided in an article elsewhere in this issue.

Functional Imaging

Positron emission tomography (PET) and single-photon emission CT (SPECT) are CT variations that involve intravenous administration of a radionucleotide. SPECT gives a higher-resolution image, and is especially useful for localizing function and determining the relationship of various abnormalities to eloquent regions of the brain in particular individuals. Functional MRI (fMRI) uses differences in the radiofrequency signals between oxygenated and deoxygenated blood to measure blood flow to a given region of the brain.[9] To date, fMRI has proved more useful in brain mapping research than in clinical applications. These modalities are not often used to evaluate acute injury.

Ultrasonography

Ultrasound imaging involves sound waves of frequencies above the range of human hearing, typically between 2 and 18 MHz, to visualize neural or vascular structures.

It is particularly useful for the rapid intraoperative or perioperative assessment of the ventricles or cystic lesions, and for assessment and percutaneous access of vascular structures such as the cervical carotid arteries.[10] However, it may be technically difficult and operator dependent, requiring expert interpretation.

CEREBRAL AND SPINAL METABOLISM
Perfusion and Imaging

The skeletal structures supporting and protecting the CNS are essentially a fixed-volume "container" with 3 constituents: neural elements, CSF, and blood. The container accommodates pathologic additions or subtractions with changes in pressure or constituent volume. In other words, if a mass enters the skull or spinal column, either the intracranial pressure (ICP) increases or a constituent must exit or shrink.[11] Pressure increases can cause direct injury, which can be very important in some locations such as the posterior fossa. Most commonly, ICP increases wreak havoc by decreasing perfusion. The only intracranial or intraspinal constituent capable of hasty independent exit is intravascular blood, so acute neuropathology often compromises perfusion by decreasing blood flow. Unfortunately, some treatments for elevated ICP, such as hyperventilation, also decrease perfusion. Moreover, prolonged hyperventilation impairs autoregulation. Knowing when and how long to hyperventilate a patient with intracranial abnormality and increased ICP requires a judgment call or quick risk-benefit analysis of perfusion. This analysis must often be made without the luxury of a perfusion MRI, PET, or SPECT study.[12]

Four imaging features of the brain on CT or MRI can be used to rapidly assess the degree to which a given intracranial process affects perfusion: symmetry, cisterns or subarachnoid spaces, gray matter–white matter differentiation, and ventricles. These features can be appreciated on the normal CT scan shown in **Fig. 1**.

1. *Symmetry: Symmetry is good.* The CNS should be bilaterally symmetric. Although a lack of symmetry is not always pathologic, as a general rule, the less the symmetry, the greater is the severity of a given abnormality. Midline shift of the brain from one side to the other is easily measured, and when greater than 5 mm is an indication for surgical intervention.[13] Significant midline shift may result in subfalcine herniation and compress the anterior cerebral arteries and their branches against the falx cerebri. In the setting of trauma or other acute process, this arterial compression decreases perfusion to territories supplied by the anterior cerebral arteries, often adding infarct to injury (**Fig. 3**).
2. *Cisterns and subarachnoid spaces: Cisterns should be open. Closed cisterns or cisterns filled with blood (subarachnoid hemorrhage [SAH]) are bad.* The basilar cisterns and subarachnoid spaces should be open, roughly symmetric, and filled with CSF. Because the cerebral vessels run in the cisterns and subarachnoid spaces, a process that compresses or compromises the cisterns and/or subarachnoid spaces is a process that compromises the cerebral, spinal, or radicular vessels, and therefore may compromise perfusion. For example, uncal herniation will produce obliteration of ipsilateral basal cisterns just before taking out the arteries they contain, namely the internal carotid, posterior communicating, posterior cerebral, and basilar arteries (see **Fig. 2**). In the setting of acute uncal herniation, aggressive hyperventilation that produces a global moderate decrease in perfusion but avoids this vascular occlusion gives the surgeon time to address the underlying pathology, and may save a brain.[14]
3. *Gray-white junction: Gray matter and white matter should be distinct.* Obliteration of the gray-white junction is frequently seen in processes that affect the brain on

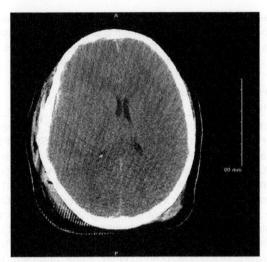

Fig. 3. Axial slice from a head CT showing few or apparently minor abnormalities of scalp swelling and contusion greater on the right than on the left, and a very thin acute right subdural hematoma (SDH) (compare with **Fig. 1**). The scan reveals: (1) asymmetry with approximately 5 mm midline shift, (2) obliteration of the subarachnoid spaces with loss of visible sulci (and basilar cisterns not seen on this slice), (3) decrease or loss of the gray-white junction over the right convexity, and (4) ventricular compression on the right with overall decreased ventricular size. Glasgow Coma Scale score in this trauma patient was 3, and on placement of an extraventricular drain (EVD), the intracranial pressure was 42 mm Hg and brain tissue oxygen partial pressure was 8 mm Hg (prefer >20 mm Hg).

a cellular level. These processes, such as diffuse axonal injury or early ischemia, may not obviously alter the gross structural anatomy of the brain, but may signal decreased perfusion. The most common scenario where this proves important is in the young acute multisystem trauma patient for whom there is no neurologic examination and the CT looks "normal" at first glance, but there is diffuse mild blurring of the gray-white junction. Early neurosurgical involvement and ventriculostomy placement in such patients sometimes reveals elevated ICP, quickly relieved by CSF drainage.[15] This action may avoid the scenario of a subsequently "brain-dead" patient following a massive acute trauma life support effort. In addition, habitual checking of the gray-white junction makes it more difficult to miss other lesions with approximately the same imaging density of brain, such as a subacute subdural hematoma (SDH).[16]

4. *Ventricles: Ventricles should be bilaterally symmetric, proportional to each other, and proportional to the subarachnoid spaces. They should contain only CSF and choroid plexus and be without periventricular edema. If a ventriculostomy catheter is present, the tip should optimally be at the foramen of Monro.* Although certain features such as bifrontal index greater than 30%, visible temporal horns, or rounding of the third ventricle have been suggested as ways to gauge normal ventricular size, they are unreliable.[17] Ventricular size alone is a poor indicator of ICP or perfusion, as changes may be physiologic, such as enlargement with aging. Certain pathologic conditions, such as pseudotumor cerebri, may produce enlarged ventricles. However, when taken together with features 1 to 3, assessment of the ventricles is very useful (see **Fig. 3**).

FUNCTIONAL NEUROANATOMY
Cranial Anatomy

Frontal lobes and anterior cranial fossa

The large frontal lobes sit within the anterior cranial fossa, are separated by the falx cerebri, and are shielded anteriorly and superiorly by the frontal bones and, to some extent, the face and sinuses. Functions of this portion of the brain include capabilities such as judgment and intuition. Structures entering and exiting the skull via the anterior cranial fossa include the olfactory nerves and anterior cerebral arteries. Patients with frontal lobe abnormality may not display focal or cranial nerve deficits, but have significant impairment in activities of daily living. Slow-growing frontal lobe lesions such as meningiomas may reach impressive size before presenting because of these features (**Fig. 4**).[18] Posteriorly, where the frontal lobe meets the parietal lobe, is the precentral gyrus, which is the home of the motor strip and controls contralateral movement. Inferiorly, areas critical for speech are located at the junction of the temporal and frontal lobes.

Temporal lobes and middle cranial fossa

The temporal lobes sit within the middle cranial fossae and are involved primarily in speech and memory. Because of relatively small temporal lobe size and the temporal lobe relationship with the internal carotid arteries and cranial nerves 2 to 8, temporal lobe lesions often produce cranial nerve palsies and become symptomatic at a much smaller size than frontal or anterior cranial fossa lesions. Similar to lesions of the cerebellum and posterior cranial fossa, lesions of the temporal lobes and middle cranial fossa can quickly compromise major vessels supplying blood to the brain, namely the internal carotid arteries.

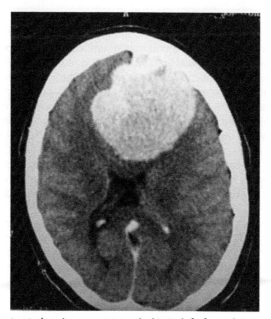

Fig. 4. CT with contrast showing an extremely large left frontal extra-axial mass, which proved to be an olfactory groove meningioma. Note deformation of the ventricles posteriorly with shift.

Parietal lobes

The parietal lobes are quite large, and intimate with the calvarium rather than the skull base. These lobes float posterior to the frontal lobes, above the temporal lobes, and anterior to the occipital lobes. The parietal lobes are involved with opposite-side sensation, movement, and visual association. As with frontal lobe lesions, lesions of the parietal lobes can reach impressive size before becoming symptomatic. The parietal lobes are indeed not closely associated with the circle of Willis or the skull base and cranial nerves.

Occipital lobes and the tentorium

The occipital lobes lie posterior and inferior to the temporal and parietal lobes, and on top of the tentorium, or dural membrane roof of the posterior fossa. The occipital lobes are involved in vision, visual association, and recognition. Because of the relationship of the posterior cerebral artery blood supply to the tentorium, the occipital lobes are vulnerable to cerebral hypoperfusion states and to increases in ICP.[19,20]

Cerebellum, Brainstem, and Posterior Fossa

This part of the brain is concerned with movement and vital processes as well as the lower cranial nerves, which are critical to airway maintenance and swallowing as well as autonomic functions. Because of these features, the unique arrangement of the vertebrobasilar circulation (see **Fig. 2**C), and the small size with the overlying tentorium, even benign posterior fossa lesions can be problematic. Any posterior fossa lesion larger than 2.5 cm deserves surgical consideration, and the anesthesiologist might secure the airway early and maintain it longer in patients with posterior fossa abnormality. An alert patient with intact cardiopulmonary system but with posterior fossa lesions may rapidly clinically deteriorate.

Spinal Anatomy

Cervical spine

The cervical nerve roots and spinal cord control arm movement and sensation. The cervical spinal cord also controls thoracic and lumbosacral function. For anesthetic purposes, the upper cervical spinal cord (above C3) is really an extension of the brainstem, and fractures, dislocations, or other abnormalities in this region may affect airway protection and maintenance as dramatically as posterior fossa lesions.[21] From C3 to C7, lesions will typically present either with upper extremity radiculopathies or with myelopathies. The spinal cord is supplied by 3 spinal arteries: 1 anterior, supplying 70% of the spinal cord, and 2 posterior, supplying only 30% of the cord tissue. The central gray matter is supplied almost entirely by the anterior spinal artery, and is also the region of the spinal cord with the highest metabolic demands. As such, it is therefore most vulnerable to ischemia. In cervical spine trauma, central cord syndrome is a common occurrence, with upper extremity distal paresis and dysautonomia.[22]

Surgical approaches to the cervical spine may involve direct manipulation of the trachea and esophagus, or indirect pressure and swelling that require airway protection and maintenance. As a general rule, cervical spine procedures longer than 6 hours in duration or with greater than 600 mL estimated blood loss deserve extreme caution with immediate postoperative extubation.[23]

Thoracic spine

The thoracic spinal cord and nerve roots are involved with truncal sensation and some core musculature. The thoracic spinal cord also controls lumbosacral function and is involved in visceral and autonomic regulation. Whereas the anterior spinal artery in the cervical spine derives from multiple radicular arteries, in the thoracic spinal cord the supply is via the solitary artery of Adamkiewicz. This lone artery usually arises from the 9th through the 12th intercostal arteries, but is quite variable, and if injury to the spinal column or other process affects this vessel, such an injury can result in severe multilevel infarction with paraplegia, typically with sensory sparing. Adamkiewicz infarctions are also seen in abdominal aortic aneurysm resections and cardiovascular procedures. Like the ischemic brain, the ischemic spinal cord swells and intraspinal pressure increases, causing ischemia. An intraoperative lumbar drain may be used as a safety valve in such procedures. Lumbar drains may also be efficacious in this regard for patients undergoing anterior thoracic spinal procedures.[24]

Lumbosacral spine

The lumbosacral nerve roots control the legs, perineum, and the genitalia. The spinal cord usually ends around L1 in adults. Thus, only upper lumbar or lumbosacral lesions produce myelopathies. Below this area, abnormalities produce radiculopathies. Anesthetic considerations in the lumbosacral spine include airway maintenance in the prone position, as most of these cases are performed posteriorly. It is important to be aware of cervical spine pathology and limitations when positioning these patients for surgery, as injury may occur from lack of vigilance regarding positional spinal cord or nerve root compression.[25]

Spinal columns

When considering the stability of spinal lesions, it is useful to consider the spine according to anterior, middle, and posterior columns. As a general rule, a lesion or fracture involving 2 or more columns is unstable. The anterior column comprises the anterior two-thirds of the vertebral body, the middle column the posterior third and the pedicles, and the posterior column the facet joints and posterior elements.

Spinal lesions

Although the bony spine protects the spinal cord and nerve roots, because of the small spaces involved and the eloquence of spinal tissues, spine fractures often directly compromise neural elements. Neural compromise is an indication for surgical decompression. The most common spine lesions resulting in neural element compromise are fractures, disk injuries, and ligamentous injuries, although tumor and infection may also result in neural compromise (**Fig. 5**). Differentiation between tumor involving the vertebrae and infection may be difficult in the spinal column. As a general rule, infection crosses the disk space whereas tumor does not. Stability is best assessed by the 3-column model previously discussed. CT and MRI are the best modalities for assessing spinal lesions: CT for bone, MRI for neural elements.[26] T2-weighted MRI is particularly useful in assessing spinal neural elements in acute injury (**Table 3**).

Cervical lesions

Particular anesthetic challenges with cervical spine fractures involve securing and maintaining the airway when the neck must be kept in neutral position. These patients may benefit from awake fiberoptic intubation. As previously discussed, cervical spine lesions may produce significant dysautonomia, particularly in patients with craniocervical junction spinal cord and lower medullary injuries (**Fig. 6**). Intra-axial spinal cord lesions resulting from acute neural element compromise fall into 3 categories from a prognostic standpoint, as shown in **Table 3**. For lesion types 1 and 3 of the cervical spine, prolonged airway protection is often required, making consideration of early tracheostomy a good idea.[27]

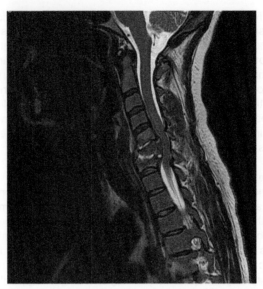

Fig. 5. T2-weighted MRI of the cervical spine showing lesion involving the C5-C7 vertebral bodies with compression of the cervical spinal cord. Infection crosses the disk space, tumor does not.

Thoracic lesions

Stability is important in the thoracic spine from a surgical standpoint. As the thoracic spine is effectively buttressed by the rib cage, maintaining neutral alignment and positioning is simpler than in the more flexible cervical and lumbar regions. Cervicothoracic and thoracolumbar junction injuries (so-called transition segment injuries) are the exception, as these injuries are subject to greater stresses at the transition between the relative flexible cervical or lumbar spine and the relatively stiff thoracic spine (**Fig. 7**).[28–31]

Table 3
Imaging characteristics of acute spinal cord injuries

Classification	T2-Weighted MRI Appearance	CT Appearance	Pathology	Degree	Prognosis
Type 1	Central hypodensity with rim hyperdensity	Hyperdensity, hemorrhage or contusion within the cord	Deoxyhemoglobin with rim methemoglobin	Severe cord dysfunction, often ascending levels	Little or no neurologic recovery
Type 2	Uniform hyperdensity	Isodense or hypodensity	Edema	Variable, often severe initially	Good to excellent
Type 3	Isodense centrally with rim hyperdensity	Isodense	Hemorrhage and edema	Variable, often severe initially	Variable

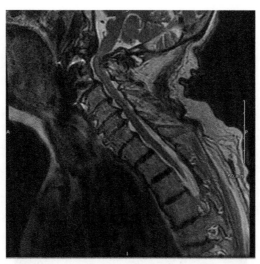

Fig. 6. T2-weighted MRI of the cervical spine showing severe craniocervical stenosis in a patient who suffered a fall 9 months earlier and sustained an odontoid fracture. The patient was diagnosed with Parkinson disease with progressive spastic quadriparesis and dysautonomia.

Neural element compromise is similar to that of the cervical spine, although lateral lesions affecting only the thoracic nerve roots may not require surgical intervention. With regard to thoracic spinal cord lesions, vascular anatomy is particularly important, and preoperative angiographic studies may be very helpful. Many procedures involving the thoracic and lumbar spine entail extensive blood loss, which can threaten spinal cord perfusion. In addition, the arterial supply of the anterior or motor region of the thoracic spinal cord has few or no collaterals.

Lumbosacral lesions

Because the spinal cord in adults ends at approximately L1, the spinal cord is usually relatively spared by lumbosacral abnormalities. However, because the load-bearing role of the lumbosacral spine is greater, stability issues are more common. Thus, although lumbosacral abnormalities may be of lesser acuity, they are much more common. Injuries often involve disk herniation, compression fractures, and stenosis.

IMAGING PATHOLOGY
Hemorrhage

The diagnosis and delineation of hemorrhage in the brain requires understanding of neuroanatomy and appropriate imaging modalities. Patient observation is also essential (**Fig. 8**).

Epidural Hematoma

Epidural hematoma (EDH) constitutes hemorrhage occurring between bone and dura, and is limited in its spread over the brain by dural attachments at the suture lines, but may cross the midline. EDHs are typically biconvex or lens-shaped on axial CT or MRI. EDHs are often seen in association with a frontal or temporal skull fracture and laceration of a dural artery such as the middle meningeal artery, and can expand very rapidly (**Fig. 9**). Cranial EDHs are usually traumatic, but the trauma may be mild and

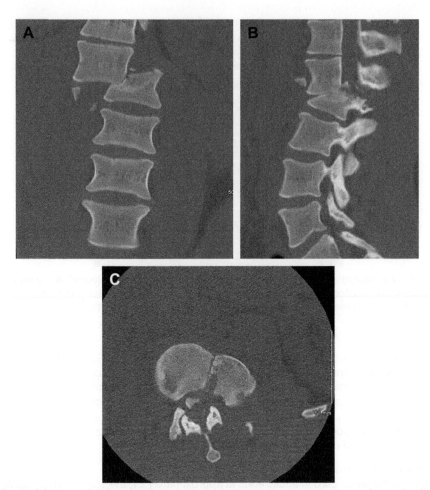

Fig. 7. (*A*) Coronal, (*B*) sagittal, and (*C*) axial CT images showing severe thoracolumbar (T12–L1) fracture dislocation.

involve only a brief or no loss of consciousness. EDHs are characterized by a lucid interval after the injury during which the patient is intact, but then progress very rapidly to coma and death. The patient should have surgical evacuation immediately, and often have excellent postoperative recoveries after rapid intervention.

Subdural Hematoma

There are 2 broad categories of SDHs from an anesthetic standpoint. First, the acute SDH in the comatose trauma patient, which should be treated much as an EDH with rapid surgical intervention. Second, the subacute or chronic SDH in older patients, which should be dealt with more deliberately and with careful attention to the axiom "treat the patient, not the scan." SDHs have a convex or moon-shaped appearance on axial CT or MRI (**Fig. 10**). Unlike EDHs, SDHs cross suture lines and spread out over the surface of the brain, but do not cross the midline. SDHs are typically seen over the convexities in older patients because the brain shrinks with age, and pulls away from the inner table of the skull as it does so, enlarging the subdural space and stretching the bridging veins on the cortical surface. In this situation of "a small fish

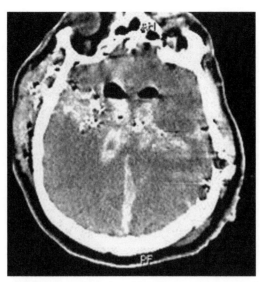

Fig. 8. Multicompartmental hemorrhage resulting from a gunshot to the head. This image also shows skull fractures and intracranial foreign bodies.

in a big bowl" (small brain in a big skull), even minor trauma can produce hemorrhage. Antiplatelet agents or anticoagulants increase the likelihood of a large SDH. SDHs virtually always involve some trauma, but the trauma may be very minor and there is often no history of trauma because of associated memory loss or unsteadiness from compression of the underlying brain in subacute or chronic SDH. Interhemispheric and tentorial SDHs seldom require surgical intervention.

SDHs are judged according to their size, degree of mass effect or shift, and clinical effects. In general, anything more than 1 cm in thickness or with greater than 5 mm of

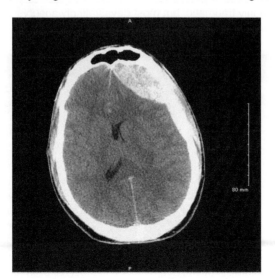

Fig. 9. Axial CT image of a left frontal epidural hematoma in a 24-year-old man who tripped and fell on his way home while intoxicated. The patient was brought in by friends, but awake and combative; he felt fine and wanted to go home.

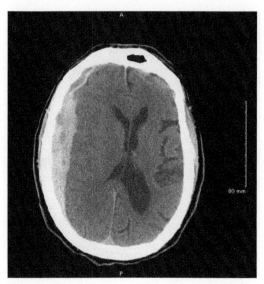

Fig. 10. Axial noncontrast CT showing a very large (>20 mm thick) right-convexity acute SDH with compression of the underlying cortex, mass effect on the right lateral ventricle, and midline shift of more than 15 mm.

midline shift usually merits operative intervention (**Fig. 11**). Chronic SDHs deserve a methodical approach, with great care to optimize any underlying medical conditions. Acute SDHs are treated similarly to EDHs, with the caveat that these patients often will require long-term postoperative intubation and ventilation with days or weeks in the ICU.

Subarachnoid Hemorrhage

SAH is most commonly traumatic, but most devastatingly aneurysmal. Differentiation of traumatic and aneurysmal SAH can be difficult, and the pattern of hemorrhage is

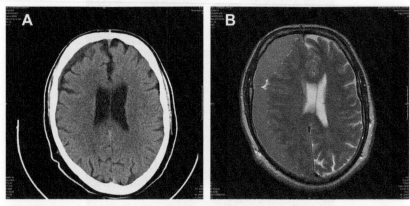

Fig. 11. (A) Initial scan showing thin right frontal subdural hygroma in a 66-year-old woman who was in a motor vehicle accident, hospitalized and observed overnight, then discharged home. (B) MRI in the same patient 3 weeks after the accident when the patient returned for follow-up and was noted to have mild left-sided weakness. Note the visible frontal bridging vein and associated small hyperacute (white on T2) hemorrhage at its base.

revealing but not diagnostic. SAHs may appear innocent because they have little direct neural element of compromise, but the ensuing effects on brain physiology can be devastating. The after-effects of SAH include hydrocephalus, edema, and vasospasm. SAHs can also cause rapid-onset cardiac dysfunction (wall-motion abnormalities, myocardial infarction) and pulmonary dysfunction (edema, acute respiratory distress syndrome), which present further challenges in patient management.[32]

Between 1% and 8% of the population has intracranial aneurysms, and these usually present with SAH. From an anesthetic standpoint, aneurysms are important in 3 ways: first and foremost for their ability to produce hemorrhage within the brain, most notably SAH, but also intraventricular hemorrhage (IVH) and intracerebral hemorrhage (ICH). The constellation of problems resulting from aneurysmal SAH are as complex and devastating as those of any brain lesion. Second, they may grow large enough to produce mass effect on surrounding structures, acting much like a tumor. Third, their treatment, be it surgical or endovascular, requires urgent care.

Like aneurysms, AVMs are most problematic when they result in hemorrhage or produce mass effect on the surrounding tissues. Unlike aneurysms, AVMs usually present with seizures or neurologic deficits from mass effect instead of a devastating SAH.

Intracerebral Hemorrhage

Intracerebral hemorrhage most commonly involves traumatic contusions or hemorrhagic infarctions, but may also result from hemorrhage into or around another lesion such as a tumor or AVM (**Fig. 12**). ICH represents 10% to 15% of first-ever strokes, with a 30-day mortality rate of 35% to 50%.[33] Hemorrhagic stroke represents 20% of all infarctions occurring in ischemic brain on reperfusion. Lobar hemorrhages coming to the surface with clinical deterioration often merit surgical intervention, although the utility and patient population in which this is most advantageous remains

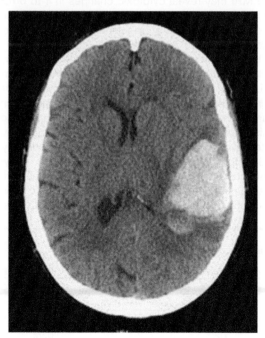

Fig. 12. Axial noncontrast CT showing a large right temporal parietal intracerebral hemorrhage (ICH).

under investigation. Unlike the other types of CNS hemorrhage, ICH always entails some brain or spinal cord destruction.[34] Also unlike other brain hemorrhagic lesions, ICHs have lower ambient oxygen levels and therefore "age" or evolve more rapidly on scans (**Table 4**). Hemorrhage into other lesions such as tumors may be difficult to distinguish from hemorrhagic infarction. The neoplasms most commonly associated with IVH are high-grade gliomas (glioblastoma multiforme) and certain metastases (melanoma, renal cell carcinoma).

Intraventricular Hemorrhage

IVH is hemorrhage within the ventricular system (**Fig. 13**). SAH and IVH differ from other hemorrhagic lesions in that the bleeding occurs in and mixes with CSF. Intraventricular hemorrhage is associated with hydrocephalus and with dysautonomia. The hydrocephalus resulting from IVH is often successfully treated with ventriculostomy, but keeping the ventriculostomy functional may be particularly challenging, as blood tends to clot the catheter. Use of intraventricular tissue plasminogen activator (tPA) for IVH is currently under investigation.[35] Although tPA may resolve problems with hydrocephalus and lessen the time ventriculostomy is required, it does little to treat the dysautonomia associated with IVH. Dysautonomia is most frequently associated with IVH in the third and fourth ventricles. This fact may represent particular challenges to the anesthesiologist intraoperatively, with cardiorespiratory, metabolic, infectious sequelae.

Ischemia and Edema

Ischemic infarctions represent the majority of acute strokes, occurring in 80% of all infarctions. MRI is much more sensitive than CT for detecting acute ischemia. Diffusion-weighted MRI may reveal cytotoxic changes in 4 to 6 hours, whereas CT changes are not seen until at least 12 hours (**Fig. 14**). Because distinguishing between cytotoxic and other kinds of edema on regular MR sequences is difficult, diffusion-weighted sequences should be obtained when acute infarction is suspected. In younger patients ischemic infarctions are often embolic, whereas in older patients they are most commonly occlusive (atherosclerotic). The most common vascular territory for infarction is that of the middle cerebral artery, followed by the vertebrobasilar system, the posterior cerebral artery, and the anterior cerebral artery territories.[36]

Edema and infarction have a similar hypodense or dark appearance on CT, and are often difficult to distinguish except by pattern. Edema associated with neoplasms or hydrocephalus often favors white matter. Periventricular hypodensity occurs in hydrocephalus when CSF is forced through the ependymal lining into the white matter interstitium. Arterial infarctions typically involve a distinct arterial territory, but venous infarctions may have unpredictable patterns and closely mimic edema. Edema associated with trauma tends to be more diffuse and subtle, and may best be evaluated by

Table 4
Imaging characteristics of blood on MRI and CT

Hemorrhage	Timing	T1 MRI	T2 MRI	CT	Blood Product
Hyperacute	<12 h	Dark to isodense	Bright	Bright	Oxyhemoglobin
Acute	12–48 h	Dark to isodense	Very dark	Bright	Deoxyhemoglobin
Subacute	48 h–2 wk	Bright	Isodense to bright	Isodense	Methemoglobin
Chronic	>2 wk	Dark	Very dark	Dark	Hemosiderin

Dark, bright, and isodense are relative to cerebral gray matter.

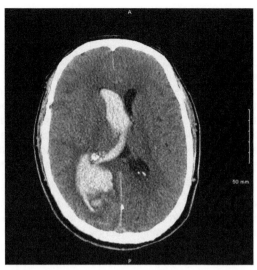

Fig. 13. Intraventricular hemorrhage associated with left occipital ICH.

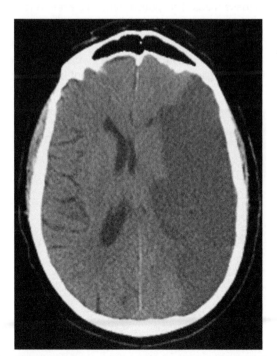

Fig. 14. Noncontrast CT showing left middle cerebral artery territory infarction. Note hypodensity of the infracted brain with mass effect on the left lateral ventricle and more than 5-mm midline shift.

assessment of the cisterns and subarachnoid spaces as well as gray-white differentiation (**Fig. 15**).

Mass Lesions

Mass lesions in the CNS involve many different causes (see **Table 1**). Excluding the hemorrhages and vascular lesions already reviewed, mass lesions of concern to the anesthesiologist are commonly neoplastic or infectious. Clinically useful characteristics of mass lesions that guide surgical and anesthetic management include location, particularly with regard to whether the mass is intra-axial or extra-axial and supratentorial versus infratentorial.[37] Extra-axial masses are external to or outside of the pial membrane that invests the brain, spinal cord, and the proximal portions of the nerve root.

Extra-axial masses

Meningiomas represent 15% of all intracranial tumors in adults, and are the most common histologically benign brain tumor in adults and the most common extra-axial tumor in adults. Meningiomas commonly enhance brightly and uniformly. Heterogeneity in extra-axial lesions is atypical. These slowly expanding lesions may reach an impressive size before becoming symptomatic (see **Fig. 4**). In the spine, both gradually evolving myelopathies and radiculopathies may be associated with large, slowly evolving extra-axial spine lesions such as meningiomas (**Fig. 16**).

When meningiomas or other lesions involve the skull base, resection may be lengthy and may result in large skull-base defects and cranial nerve palsies that often complicate intraoperative and perioperative management. **Fig. 17** shows extensive pneumocephalus following bag-mask ventilation after extubation following surgical resection of an anterior cranial fossa mass. This patient required a return to the OR for evacuation of the pneumocephalus and repeat skull-base repair.[38]

Intra-axial masses

In adults, the most common intra-axial masses are metastases and gliomas, the latter most often being malignant gliomas. Rim enhancement is most typical of intra-axial

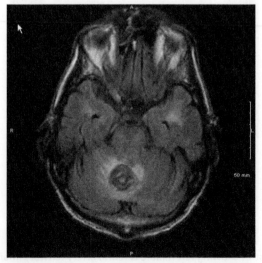

Fig. 15. MRI showing cerebellar mass with surrounding edema. Note also the visible temporal horns with periventricular hypodensity, suggestive of obstructive hydrocephalus.

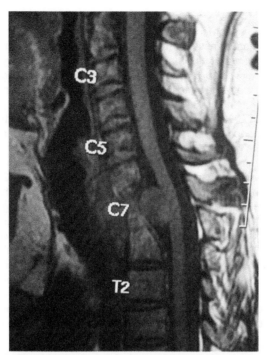

Fig. 16. T1-weighted noncontrast MRI of the cervical spine. Large extra-axial intradural mass at C7 with both spinal cord compression and vertebral body erosion, which proved to be a meningioma.

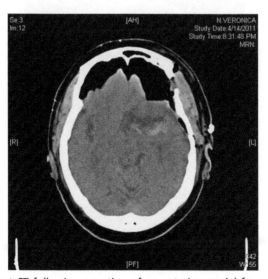

Fig. 17. Noncontrast CT following resection of an anterior cranial fossa mass in a patient who received bag-mask ventilation following extubation and was showing severe pneumo-cephalus. Note compression of the frontal lobes by trapped intracranial air.

neoplasms, although abscesses may have the same pattern of enhancement and appearance. Rim enhancement usually indicates a rapidly growing lesion with central necrosis, a bad characteristic for both intra-axial and extra-axial masses. Rim-enhancing lesions with irregular margins are more typically primary, whereas meta-static lesions typically have regular margins. Lack of enhancement for intra-axial lesions is generally better prognostically than extensive enhancement, with nonen-hancing or weakly enhancing lesions being lower grade and slower growing.

Gliomas represent 20% of all intracranial tumors in adults, and are the most common primary intra-axial neoplasm. Gliomas invade both gray and white matter, but typically originate in the white matter and follow white matter tracts as they increase in size.[5] Low-grade astrocytomas appear as poorly marginated low-density masses on CT, iso-intense or hypointense on T1-weighted MRI, and hyperintense on T2-weighted MRI.

Unfortunately, the most common glioma diagnosed in adults is the high-grade glioma or glioblastoma multiforme (GBM). This neoplasm is extremely aggressive and may double or triple in size in a few weeks. Although imaging characteristics are variable, GBM typically is irregular, inhomogeneous, and poorly marginated, with bright rim enhancement on CT and MRI (**Fig. 18**). On MRI, increased signal on T1-weighted images within the tumor may indicate subacute hemorrhage related to tumor invasion.[6]

Because they are very aggressive tumors often with extensive edema, necrosis, and hemorrhage, these tumors are associated with increased ICP and reduced cerebral perfusion pressures.[39] Particular attention must be paid to cerebral perfusion and hemodynamic stability in patients undergoing surgery for resection of these lesions.

Supratentorial Versus Infratentorial Masses

Specific anesthetic concerns are an increase in ICP and possible risk of herniation. Infratentorial masses may be associated with occult hemorrhage into the adjacent

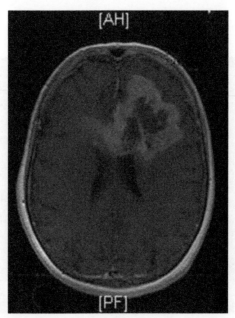

Fig. 18. Axial T1-weighted MRI with contrast showing a left frontal, irregular, rim-enhancing mass that proved to be glioblastoma multiforme. Note irregular extension of the enhancement across the corpus callosum and into the right frontal lobe.

brain or the CSF, thus close cerebral perfusion pressure monitoring, decreasing ICP, and close attention to changes in neuromonitoring are anesthetic goals.

Hydrocephalus

Because ventricular enlargement may occur in conjunction with aging or atrophy (hydrocephalus ex vacuo), and hydrocephalus does not always produce marked ventricular enlargement, diagnosing hydrocephalus can be challenging. Hydrocephalus may result from increased CSF production, blocked flow, or decreased absorption.

The synonymous terms obstructive and noncommunicating hydrocephalus refer to blockage of CSF flow within the ventricular system: from its production in the choroid plexus to its outlet at the fourth ventricular foramina of Magendie and Lushka. For example, obstruction of the foramen of Monro by a large suprasellar mass produces noncommunicating or obstructive hydrocephalus of the lateral ventricles (**Fig. 19**). So-called communicating hydrocephalus refers to blockage of CSF flow outside or distal to the ventricles, as in post-hemorrhagic or postmeningitic hydrocephalus, although SAH or meningitis may also produce an acute obstructive hydrocephalus. Hydrocephalus also occurs in conjunction with other neurologic syndromes such as Chiari malformations.

Normal pressure hydrocephalus is likely a form of communicating hydrocephalus, although the exact mechanism or cause of this condition is unknown. Patients with this condition do not have elevated ICP, but typically have markedly enlarged ventricles out of proportion to the degree of cerebral atrophy.[40] So-called external hydrocephalus is accumulation of CSF in the subdural spaces rather than the ventricles. Imaging characteristics, and quite possibly etiology, are similar to those of chronic SDHs.

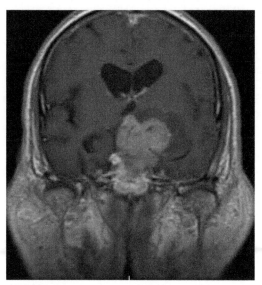

Fig. 19. Coronal T1-weighted MRI showing large sellar and suprasellar mass with cystic component, mass effect, deformation of the third ventricle, and marked enlargement of the lateral ventricles, consistent with obstructive hydrocephalus.

SUMMARY

Neuroimaging is essential in the management of neurologic disease, and it is important for the anesthesiologist to understand and interpret these modalities. Dynamic interdisciplinary communications between neurosurgeons, critical care physicians, and anesthesiologists undoubtedly result in better clinical management and outcome for patients.

REFERENCES

1. Lloyd DA, Carty H, Patterson M, et al. Predictive value of skull radiography for intracranial injury in children with blunt head injury. Lancet 1997;349:821–4.
2. McGunn M, Stuart M, Neal R, et al. Physician utilization of a portable computed tomography scanner in the intensive care unit. Crit Care Med 2000;28:3808–13.
3. Wintermark M, Reichart M, Thiran JP, et al. Prognostic accuracy of cerebral blood flow measurement by perfusion computed tomography, at the time of emergency room admission, in acute stroke patients. Ann Neurol 2002;51:417.
4. Schaefer PW, Grant PE, Gonzalez RG. Diffusion-weighted MR imaging of the brain. Radiology 2000;219:331–45.
5. Sawyer-Glover AM, Shellock FG. Pre-MRI procedure screening: recommendations and safety considerations for biomedical implants and devices. J Magn Reson Imaging 2000;12:92–106.
6. Gomori J, Grossman R. Mechanisms responsible for the MR appearance and evolution of intracranial hemorrhage. Radiographics 1988;8:427–40.
7. Metzner J, Posner KL, Domino KB. The risk and safety of anesthesia at remote locations: the US closed claims analysis. Curr Opin Anaesthesiol 2009;22:502–8.
8. Wilms G, Bosmans H, Demaerel P, et al. Magnetic resonance angiography of the intracranial vessels. Eur J Radiol 2001;38:10–8.
9. Ogawa S, Lee TM, Kar AR. Brain magnetic resonance imaging with contrast dependent on blood oxygenation. Proc Natl Acad Sci U S A 1990;87:9868.
10. Ivanov M, Wilkins S, Poeata I. Intraoperative ultrasound in neurosurgery—a practical guide. Br J Neurosurg 2010;24:510–7.
11. Mokri B. The Monroe-Kellie hypothesis: applications in CSF volume depletion. Neurology 2001;56(12):46–8.
12. Rosner MJ, Daughton S. Cerebral perfusion pressure management in head injury. J Trauma 1990;30:933–40.
13. Valadka AB, Gopinath SP, Robertson CS. Midline shift after severe head injury: pathophysiologic implications. J Trauma 2000;49:1–8.
14. Yuh EL, Gean AD, Manley GT, et al. Computer-aided assessment of head computed tomography (CT) studies in patients with suspected traumatic brain injury. J Neurotrauma 2008;25:1163–72.
15. Kim JJ, Gean AD. Imaging for the diagnosis and management of traumatic brain injury. Neurotherapeutics 2011;8:39–53.
16. Huisman TA, Sorensen AG, Hergan K, et al. Diffusion-weighted imaging for the evaluation of diffuse axonal injury in closed head injury. J Comput Assist Tomogr 2003;27:5–11.
17. Refaee EE, Baldauf J, Schroeder HW. Bilateral occlusion of the foramina of Monro after third ventriculostomy. J Neurosurg 2012;116:1333–6.
18. Niiro M, Yatsushiro K, Nakamura K. Natural history of elderly patients with asymptomatic meningiomas. J Neurol Neurosurg Psychiatry 2000;68:25–8.
19. Khetpal V, Donohue SP. Cortical visual impairment. Etiology, associated findings and prognosis in a tertiary care setting. J AAPOS 2007;11:235–9.

20. Zhou LJ, DU G, Mao Y, et al. Diagnosis and surgical treatment of brainstem hemangioblastomas. Surg Neurol 2005;63:307–15.
21. Crosby ET. Considerations for airway management for cervical spine surgery in adults. Anesthesiol Clin 2007;25:511–33.
22. Aito S, D'Andrea M, Wergenhagen L. Neurological and functional outcome in traumatic central cord syndrome. Spinal Cord 2007;45:292–7.
23. Epstein NE, Hollingsworth R, Nardi D, et al. Can airway problems following multi-level anterior cervical surgery be avoided? J Neurosurg 2001;94:185.
24. Weidauer S, Nichtweiss M, Lanfermann H. Spinal cord infarction: MR imaging and clinical features in 16 cases. Neuroradiology 2002;44:851–7.
25. Hindman BJ, Palecek JP, Posner KL, et al. Cervical spinal cord, root, and bony spine injuries: a closed claims analysis. Anesthesiology 2011;114:782–95.
26. Hong SH, Choi JY, Lee JW, et al. MR imaging assessment of the spine: Infection or an imitation? Radiographics 2009;29:599–612.
27. Crosby ET. Airway management in adults after cervical spine trauma. Anesthesiology 2006;104:1293–318.
28. Gillet P. The fate of the adjacent motion segments after lumbar fusion. J Spinal Disord Tech 2003;4:338–45.
29. Siddiqui FM, Bekker SV, Qureshi AI. Neuroimaging of hemorrhage and vascular defects. Neurotherapeutics 2011;8:28–38.
30. Kiswell CS, Wintermark CS. Imaging of intracranial haemorrhage. Lancet Neurol 2008;7:257–67.
31. Kloss BT, Lagace RA. Acute-on-chronic subdural hematoma. Int J Emerg Med 2010;3:511–2.
32. Bederson JB, Connoly ES, Batjer HH, et al. Guidelines for the management of subarachnoid hemorrhage. Stroke 2009;40:1–32.
33. Broderick JP, Brott T, Tomsick T, et al. Intracerebral hemorrhage more than twice as common as subarachnoid hemorrhage. J Neurosurg 1993;78:188–91.
34. Rincon F, Mayer SA. Clinical review: critical care management of spontaneous intracerebral hemorrhage. Crit Care 2008;12:237.
35. Nyquist P, Handey DF. The use of intraventricular thrombolytics in intraventricular hemorrhage. J Neurol Sci 2007;261:84.
36. Acciarresi M, Caso V, Venti M, et al. First-ever stroke and outcome in patients admitted to Perugia Stroke Unit: predictors for death, dependency, and recurrence of stroke within the first three months. Clin Exp Hypertens 2006;28:287–94.
37. Hakyemez B, Erdogan C, Bolca N, et al. Evaluation of different cerebral mass lesions by perfusion-weighted MR imaging. J Magn Reson Imaging 2006;24:817–24.
38. Perrin RG, Bernstein M. Tension pneumoventricle after placement of a ventriculo-peritoneal shunt: a novel treatment strategy. J Neurosurg 2005;102:386–8.
39. Park JK, Hodges T, Arko L, et al. Scale to predict survival after surgery for recurrent glioblastoma multiforme. J Clin Oncol 2010;28:3838–43.
40. Bradley WG. Normal pressure hydrocephalus: new concepts on etiology and diagnosis. AJNR Am J Neuroradiol 2000;21:1586–90.

Anesthetic Management of Patients with Acute Stroke

Alana M. Flexman, MD, FRCPC[a],*, Anne L. Donovan, MD[b],
Adrian W. Gelb, MBChB, FRCPC[b]

KEYWORDS

- Stroke • Thrombolysis • Anesthesia • Clinical outcome

KEY POINTS

- Both acute hemorrhagic stroke and ischemic stroke are important sources of morbidity and mortality throughout the world.
- Current therapies for acute ischemic stroke include intravenous thrombolysis and endovascular procedures such as intra-arterial thrombolysis and mechanical clot extraction.
- Patients with acute ischemic stroke must be assessed and treated rapidly to minimize time to brain reperfusion.
- Both hypertension and hypotension are associated with poor outcome in patients with ischemic and hemorrhagic stroke, but the optimal hemodynamic parameters are not clear.
- Although general anesthesia in patients with acute stroke has been associated with worse neurologic outcomes, current evidence is inadequate to guide the choice of anesthesia, and prospective data are urgently needed.

INTRODUCTION

Stroke is the third leading cause of death in the United States and throughout much of the developed world and the leading cause of disability worldwide.[1,2] The World Health Organization defines stroke as "rapidly developing clinical signs of focal (or global) disturbance of cerebral function, with symptoms lasting 24 hours or longer or leading to death, with no apparent cause other than of vascular origin."[3] Stroke may be ischemic or hemorrhagic in etiology; acute ischemic strokes account for

Funding Sources: None.

Conflict of Interest: None.

[a] Department of Anesthesiology, Pharmacology and Therapeutics, Vancouver General Hospital, University of British Columbia, J Pattison Pavilion North, Room 3300, 910 West 10th Avenue, Vancouver, British Columbia V5Z 1M9, Canada; [b] Department of Anesthesia and Perioperative Care, University of California, San Francisco, 521 Parnassus Avenue, Room C-450, San Francisco, CA 94143-0648, USA

* Corresponding author.

E-mail address: alana.flexman@vch.ca

Anesthesiology Clin 30 (2012) 175–190

doi:10.1016/j.anclin.2012.04.002

85% to 95% of first-ever strokes, and they are associated with a mortality rate of 16%.[2,4] Patients with a spontaneous intracerebral hemorrhage (ICH) fare worse, with a mortality rate of 42%, and only 20% are functionally independent at 6 months.[2,5,6]

The anesthesiologist may be involved in multiple aspects of the care of patients with acute stroke including stabilization in the emergency department, the interventional neuroradiology suite, the operating room, and the neurointensive care unit. As the volume of intracranial endovascular procedures, including treatments for acute ischemic stroke are the fastest growing component of operative neurosurgery,[7] anesthesiologists will be presented with these patients more frequently in the future. It is critical that anesthesia practitioners have an approach to the clinical assessment, treatment, and anesthetic management for patients with acute stroke. This article reviews the pathophysiology, assessment, and treatment options for acute ischemic stroke and discusses the evidence supporting the anesthetic management of patients with acute stroke, including type of anesthesia and hemodynamic goals. The primary focus will be on acute ischemic stroke, with a lesser emphasis on acute hemorrhagic stroke.

PATHOPHYSIOLOGY OF ACUTE STROKE

Research delineating the pathophysiology of acute ischemic stroke has been based on a model of large vessel occlusion, most commonly the middle cerebral artery. A sudden interruption of cerebral blood flow produces a gradient of hypoperfusion characterized by an ischemic core surrounded by zones of penumbra and oligemia.[8] The ischemic core is an area of severe hypoperfusion resulting in irreversible cell death, while the penumbra and oligemic zones represent potentially salvageable tissue and therapeutic targets for thrombolysis. The penumbra is characterized by impaired autoregulation and increased oxygen extraction, while the oligemic compartments exhibit milder hypoperfusion and are not normally vulnerable to infarction. While these are considered areas of reversible ischemia, further insults such as hypotension and increased intracranial pressure should be strenuously avoided, as they may promote recruitment of these areas into the ischemic core.

In contrast, ICH may be primary or secondary in origin. The vast majority of spontaneous or primary intracranial hemorrhage results from rupture of small penetrating arteries and arterioles damaged by chronic arterial hypertension or amyloid angiopathy.[9] Secondary ICH may result from several factors including coagulopathy, arteriovenous malformation, intracranial tumor, hemorrhagic conversion of ischemic infarct, and cocaine abuse.[10] ICH progresses dynamically through the initial hemorrhage phase, followed by hematoma expansion and finally peri-hematoma edema. Hematoma expansion often results in early neurologic deterioration, and hematoma volume is predictive of mortality.[9]

ASSESSMENT OF PATIENTS WITH ACUTE STROKE FOR ANESTHESIA

The assessment of patients with suspected or diagnosed acute stroke is guided by the anesthetic considerations. Both ischemic stroke and hemorrhagic stroke constitute medical emergencies, and they are not reliably distinguished clinically but rather through radiographic imaging.[11] These patients must be efficiently evaluated due to the narrow therapeutic window in ischemic stroke and potential for rapid deterioration in hemorrhagic stroke. Compared with the normal rate of neuron loss in brain aging, the ischemic brain ages 3.6 years for each hour without therapy.[12]

Given the relative urgency in determining the etiology of stroke symptoms and therefore the appropriate treatment, recommendations have been made by the American Heart Association regarding the initial management of patients with suspected ischemic stroke and spontaneous intracerebral hemorrhage.[4,13] Several of these recommendations are relevant to the preanesthetic evaluation.

History

History of patients with suspected or confirmed acute stroke should focus on identifying the nature and duration of symptoms and possible underlying etiology. The timing of onset of symptoms is critical in the management of acute ischemic stroke and may be the single most important piece of historical information.[13] The windows for acute intravenous thrombolysis and intra-arterial thrombolysis are less than 3 hours and 6 hours from onset of symptoms, respectively (**Table 1**). Patients should be questioned for the presence of common risk factors for ischemic stroke such as hypertension, diabetes, and smoking, as well as risk factors for hemorrhagic stroke,

Table 1	
Indications for treatment of acute ischemic stroke	
Non-neurointerventional Treatments of Acute Ischemic Stroke	
Intravenous rtPA	Diagnosis of ischemic stroke causing measurable neurologic deficit
	Symptoms should not be minor and isolated nor clearing spontaneously
	Symptoms should not be suggestive of subarachnoid hemorrhage
	Onset of symptoms <3 h before beginning treatment
Aspirin 325 mg orally	Recommended within 24–48 h after stroke onset for most patients but is not a substitute for intravenous rtPA
Intracranial Endovascular Neurointerventional Treatments	
Intra-arterial thrombolysis	Major stroke <6 h duration due to occlusion of the middle cerebral artery
	Consider for patients who have contraindications to the use of intravenous thrombolysis (eg, recent surgery)
	The availability of intra-arterial thrombolysis should not generally preclude the intravenous administration of rtPA in otherwise eligible patients
	Requires experienced stroke center with immediate access to cerebral angiography and qualified interventionalists
Mechanical clot extraction	The Concentric Merci device can be useful for extraction of intra-arterial thrombi in appropriately selected patients, the utility in improving outcomes after stroke is unclear
	The usefulness of other endovascular devices is not yet established, but they may be beneficial

Data from Adams HP Jr, del Zoppo G, Alberts MJ, et al. Guidelines for the early management of adults with ischemic stroke: a guideline from the American Heart Association/American Stroke Association Stroke Council, Clinical Cardiology Council, Cardiovascular Radiology and Intervention Council, and the Atherosclerotic Peripheral Vascular Disease and Quality of Care Outcomes in Research Interdisciplinary Working Groups: the American Academy of Neurology affirms the value of this guideline as an educational tool for neurologists. Stroke 2007;38(5):1655–711; and Meyers PM, Schumacher HC, Higashida RT, et al. Indications for the performance of intracranial endovascular neurointerventional procedures: a scientific statement from the American Heart Association Council on Cardiovascular Radiology and Intervention, Stroke Council, Council on Cardiovascular Surgery and Anesthesia, Interdisciplinary Council on Peripheral Vascular Disease, and Interdisciplinary Council on Quality of Care and Outcomes Research. Circulation 2009;119(16):2235–49.

including hypertension, alcohol abuse, and oral anticoagulation.[9,14] Potential contra-indications to intravenous thrombolysis such as recent surgery or bleeding should be elicited to help guide management strategy. Finally, a history or symptoms sugges-tive of cardiovascular conditions such as arrhythmia and myocardial ischemia should be elicited, as they are relatively common in this population.

Physical Examination

Physical examination should focus on the patient's vital signs and neurologic status. The clinician should carefully assess the patient's vital signs, noting any significant hyper- or hypotension that may predispose the patient to further decompensation or neurologic injury. Neurologic assessment is often facilitated by standardized scales or scores such as the National Institutes of Health Stroke Scale (NIHSS) and should focus on level of consciousness, focal neurologic deficits, and speech abnormali-ties.[13] Cardiac and respiratory examinations should focus on ruling out unstable cardiovascular conditions such as arrhythmias, myocardial ischemia, and congestive heart failure. Finally, the patient should be assessed to determine his or her ability to cooperate and suitability for local or general anesthesia if he or she is scheduled to undergo neurointerventional treatments for acute ischemic stroke.

Investigations

While all patients with suspected stroke should be investigated to determine the under-lying etiology of the neurologic symptoms, which influences management strategy, unnecessary tests should be avoided. Nevertheless, all patients should have complete blood count including platelet count, coagulation profile, electrolytes, and blood glucose. Identification of an underlying coagulopathy or hypoglycemia may preclude thrombolysis or suggest another etiology for stroke symptoms. In addition, an electro-cardiogram and cardiac enzymes should be done to exclude cardiac complications such as ischemia and arrhythmia. A chest radiograph is no longer routinely recommen-ded unless aspiration or neurogenic pulmonary edema is suspected. Similarly, exami-nation of the cerebrospinal fluid is not done unless clinically indicated.

Some form of brain imaging is indicated in all patients with suspected stroke before initiating treatment, such as thrombolysis. A noncontrast computed tomography (CT) scan of the brain is sufficient to identify most cases of intracranial hemorrhage or nonvascular causes of neurologic symptoms.[13] Furthermore, specific findings on CT such as early signs of brain injury and the dense artery sign have been associated with increased complications from thrombolysis and a worse prognosis.[13] Magnetic resonance imaging (MRI) includes diffusion- and perfusion-weighted imaging and may be able to detect relatively small areas of ischemia and regions that are difficult to visualize using standard CT imaging. MRI perfusion studies may be able to identify potentially salvageable areas of the brain in the penumbra while avoiding ionizing radi-ation. Despite these advantages, MRI is impractical in many centers owing to the cost and the time constraints during assessment of acute stroke.[13]

TREATMENT OF ACUTE ISCHEMIC STROKE
Avoiding Secondary Neurologic Injury

Secondary neurologic injury should be avoided in patients with acute ischemic stroke. Hypoxia should be avoided in all patients with suspected or confirmed stroke and supplemental oxygen provided if required to maintain oxygen saturation to greater than 92%.[13] Neither hyperbaric nor supplemental oxygen is recommended in patients with normal oxygen levels, as no benefit has been demonstrated in clinical trials.[13]

Similarly, avoidance of hyperglycemia is recommended during acute stroke, yet up to a third of patients have elevations in blood glucose on presentation.[13] Higher blood glucose levels are associated with worse functional outcome in patients with acute ischemic stroke.[15] Despite this association, a randomized trial comparing euglycemia (blood glucose 4–7 mmol/L) with hyperglycemia failed to demonstrate improved outcome with euglycemia after acute stroke, although this study was underpowered.[16] To date, it is unclear whether hyperglycemia is in itself detrimental or merely a marker for stroke severity.[8]

Technique—Best Practices

Intravenous and intra-arterial thrombolysis

Several therapies have been developed to dissolve or remove clot from the intracranial vessels in acute ischemic stroke. These therapies include intravenous thrombolysis and endovascular techniques such as intra-arterial thrombolysis and mechanical clot extraction (see **Table 1**). Currently, recombinant tissue plasminogen activator (rtPA) is the only recommended drug for intravenous thrombolysis. Intravenous thrombolysis with rtPA within 3 hours of stroke onset increases the likelihood of complete or nearly complete neurologic recovery 3 months after stroke.[17] Treatment with rtPA has not been associated with increased mortality at 3 or 12 months when compared with placebo despite an increased risk of intracranial hemorrhage (approximately 6%). Meticulous blood pressure control before and following thrombolysis is essential to minimize the risk of intracranial hemorrhage. Currently guidelines recommend maintaining blood pressure less than 180/105 mm Hg for at least 24 hours after thrombolysis (**Table 2**). Other uncommon but potentially life-threatening complications of thrombolysis relevant to the anesthesia practitioner include anaphylaxis and angioedema of the airway.[18]

Endovascular therapy for acute ischemic stroke includes both selective thrombolysis into the occluded vessel and techniques for mechanical extraction of clot. A recent meta-analysis of the efficacy of intra-arterial thrombolysis for acute ischemic stroke found an increased recanalization rate and increased likelihood of good clinical

Table 2	
Guidelines for treating elevated blood pressure in acute ischemic stroke	
Eligible for intravenous rtPA	Blood pressure must be lowered and stabilized to a systolic blood pressure ≤185 mm Hg and diastolic blood pressure ≤110 mm Hg before lytic therapy is started
	Maintain blood pressure below 180/105 mm Hg for at least 24 h after intravenous rtPA
Eligible for intra-arterial thrombolysis	Same guidelines as for patients eligible for intravenous rtPA
Not eligible for intravenous rtPA	Antihypertensive medications should be withheld until systolic blood pressure >220 mm Hg and diastolic blood pressure >120 mm Hg
	Suggested goal is to lower blood pressure by approximately 15% in the first 24 h after onset of stroke

Data from Adams HP Jr, del Zoppo G, Alberts MJ, et al. Guidelines for the early management of adults with ischemic stroke: a guideline from the American Heart Association/American Stroke Association Stroke Council, Clinical Cardiology Council, Cardiovascular Radiology and Intervention Council, and the Atherosclerotic Peripheral Vascular Disease and Quality of Care Outcomes in Research Interdisciplinary Working Groups: the American Academy of Neurology affirms the value of this guideline as an educational tool for neurologists. Stroke 2007;38(5):1655–711.

outcomes in acute ischemic stroke.[19] Although this modality of treatment may be associated with a delay to treatment, some patients may specifically benefit from this procedure such as those with proximal vessel occlusion, severe neurologic deficits, and presentation between 3 and 6 hours after stroke onset.[13] In addition, as intra-arterial thrombolysis involves selective injection of thrombolytic drugs directly into intracranial vessels at lower doses than the intravenous route, this technique may be appropriate in patients who have contraindications to intravenous thrombolysis such as recent surgery.[20] Several devices to mechanically extract intra-arterial thrombi are used in conjunction with intra-arterial thrombolysis and may increase efficacy in patients with a high clot burden.[20]

Decompressive craniectomy

Decompressive craniectomy has been studied in several major trials in the past decade. Large infarctions of the supratentorial compartment as well as the cerebellum may result in severe swelling, increased intracranial pressure, herniation, and compression of the brainstem.[1] This phenomenon may occur several days after stroke onset and is associated with a mortality rate of 80%.[21,22] Removal of part of the skull may release pressure on the swollen brain and prevent secondary ischemic injury; however, controversy surrounding the potential for increased survivors with poor functional outcome exists.[23] Several large, randomized clinical trials have demonstrated that early decompressive craniectomy after malignant infarction of the middle cerebral artery brain territory in patients less than 60 years of age reduces mortality by more than half and increases favorable outcome in survivors.[24,25] The efficacy of this technique in older patients and optimal patient selection have not been established; however, some of these uncertainties may be addressed by ongoing clinical trials.[26]

HEMODYNAMIC MANAGEMENT OF PATIENTS WITH ACUTE STROKE
Patients with Acute Ischemic Stroke

The optimal hemodynamic management of patients with acute ischemic stroke remains controversial. A U-shaped relationship between systolic blood pressure during the first 24 hours after stroke and both mortality and poor neurologic outcome has been reported. The most favorable outcomes occurred with systolic blood pressures of 150 and 180 mm Hg in 2 studies.[27,28] Furthermore, systolic blood pressure variability independently predicted worse stroke outcome in patients without recanalization after intravenous thrombolysis in another study, suggesting that blood pressure reductions are detrimental during ongoing ischemia.[29] A large randomized, placebo-controlled trial evaluating the effect of candesartan in blood pressure reduction after acute stroke did not show a benefit, and suggested a higher risk of poor outcome in patients treated with candesartan.[30,31] Another recent retrospective study found that a systolic blood pressure less than 140 mm Hg was an independent predictor of poor neurologic outcome in patients undergoing endovascular therapy for acute stroke.[32] Regardless, severe hypertension must often be avoided, as blood pressure above 185/110 mm Hg is a contraindication to thrombolysis.[13] Overall, the precise hemodynamic goals for patients with acute stroke remain elusive, but excessive hypotension and hypertension should be avoided. A summary of the American Heart Association/American Stroke Association guidelines for blood pressure control after ischemic stroke is provided in **Table 2**.

Given the consistent association between low blood pressure and poor outcome after stroke, the augmentation of blood pressure with vasopressor medications has been studied in acute ischemic stroke. The evidence supporting this practice is weak and consists of a few small studies with variable outcomes. Overall, this practice may be associated with theoretical harm, and the routine use of vasopressors is not recommended in current guidelines.[13]

Patients with Acute Intracranial Hemorrhage

Elevated blood pressure is associated with intracranial hematoma expansion and poor outcome after ICH; however, the clinical treatment thresholds are not yet defined. One study suggested that systolic blood pressure greater than 140 to 150 mm Hg may be associated with a twofold increase in death or dependency,[33] yet aggressive reductions in blood pressure and cerebral perfusion pressure may be poorly tolerated in these patients. A randomized controlled trial is underway to examine the effect of escalating systolic blood pressure reduction goals using intravenous nicardipine, and preliminary results suggest that this technique is associated with an improvement in favorable outcomes and is well-tolerated.[34] The American Heart Association/American Stroke Association guidelines for the treatment of elevated blood pressure in spontaneous ICH are provided in **Table 3**.

Choice of Antihypertensive Agents

The literature is similarly limited in guiding the optimal choice of antihypertensive agents in patients with acute stroke. Whether 1 antihypertensive agent is preferable over another is currently unknown. A list of commonly used intravenous antihypertensive medications is provided in **Table 4** for practical purposes.

ANESTHETIC NEUROPROTECTION

Effective neuroprotective agents have long been sought during times of ischemic injury to prevent and attenuate neurologic injury. Most intravenous and inhalational anesthetic agents have demonstrated neuroprotective effects in animal models of focal and global brain ischemia, yet these effects have not translated into clinical trials in traumatic brain injury, aneurysm surgery, or acute stroke.[35] Most recently, a posthoc analysis of the Intraoperative Hypothermia for Aneurysm Surgery (IHAST) study

Table 3	
Guidelines for treating elevated blood pressure in spontaneous intracerebral hemorrhage	
Patient Parameters	**Suggested Recommendation**
Systolic blood pressure >200 or MAP >150 mm Hg	Consider aggressive reduction of blood pressure with continuous intravenous infusion, frequent blood pressure monitoring every 5 min
Systolic blood pressure >180 or MAP >130 mm Hg with elevated ICP	Consider monitoring ICP and reducing blood pressure using intermittent or continuous intravenous medications to keep CPP >60–80 mm Hg
Systolic blood pressure >180 or MAP >130 without elevated ICP	Consider modest reduction in blood pressure (eg, MAP of 110 mm Hg or target blood pressure 160/90 mm Hg) using intermittent or continuous intravenous medications to control blood pressure and clinical re-examine the patient every 15 min

Abbreviations: CPP, cerebral perfusion pressure; ICP, intracranial pressure; MAP, mean arterial blood pressure.

Data from Broderick J, Connolly S, Feldmann E, et al. Guidelines for the management of spontaneous intracerebral hemorrhage in adults: 2007 update: a guideline from the American Heart Association/American Stroke Association Stroke Council, High Blood Pressure Research Council, and the Quality of Care and Outcomes in Research Interdisciplinary Working Group. Circulation 2007; 116(16):e391–413.

Table 4
Common intravenous medications used to control elevated blood pressure

Drug	Intravenous Bolus Dose	Intravenous Infusion Dose
Labetalol	5–20 mg every 15 min	2–8 mg/min (maximum 300 mg/d)
Hydralazine	5–20 mg every 30 min	1.5 to 5 µg/kg/min
Esmolol	250 µg/kg loading dose	25–300 µg/kg/min
Nicardipine	NA	5–15 mg/h
Nitroprusside	NA	0.1–10 µg/kg/min
Nitroglycerin	NA	20–400 µg/min
Enalapril	0.625–1.25 mg intravenously every 6 h	NA

Abbreviations: kg, kilogram; mg, milligrams; min, minutes; NA, not applicable; µg, micrograms.

Data from Broderick J, Connolly S, Feldmann E, et al. Guidelines for the management of spontaneous intracerebral hemorrhage in adults: 2007 update: a guideline from the American Heart Association/American Stroke Association Stroke Council, High Blood Pressure Research Council, and the Quality of Care and Outcomes in Research Interdisciplinary Working Group. Circulation 2007;116(16):e391–413; and Adams HP Jr, del Zoppo G, Alberts MJ, et al. Guidelines for the early management of adults with ischemic stroke: a guideline from the American Heart Association/American Stroke Association Stroke Council, Clinical Cardiology Council, Cardiovascular Radiology and Intervention Council, and the Atherosclerotic Peripheral Vascular Disease and Quality of Care Outcomes in Research Interdisciplinary Working Groups: the American Academy of Neurology affirms the value of this guideline as an educational tool for neurologists. Stroke 2007;38(5):1655–711.

data failed to demonstrate an improvement in neurologic outcomes with supplemental protective drug.[36] While a detailed review of the literature on anesthetic neuroprotection is beyond the scope of this article, several recent review papers summarize the topic nicely.[35,37] Overall, no convincing evidence exists to guide the choice of anesthetic agent to provide neuroprotection.

Hypothermia

Hypothermia has been investigated extensively as a potential neuroprotectant. While animal studies have consistently demonstrated the benefits of therapeutic hypothermia in minimizing brain infarction in experimental models, these effects have not translated into clinical practice. Although therapeutic hypothermia was demonstrated to improve neurologic outcome in select survivors of cardiac arrest due to ventricular fibrillation, this technique has failed to show a consistent improvement in outcome in other human models. Hypothermia has not been shown to confer clear benefit as a neuroprotective strategy in traumatic brain injury, intracranial aneurysm clipping, and acute stroke.[38–40]

Fever

Nevertheless, fever has been associated with worse neurologic outcome in ischemic stroke and should be strictly avoided in these patients. Its harmful effects likely result from an increase in metabolic demand, free radical formation, and release of neurotransmitters.[41]

GENERAL VERSUS LOCAL ANESTHESIA FOR PATIENTS UNDERGOING ENDOVASCULAR TREATMENT FOR ACUTE ISCHEMIC STROKE
General Considerations

Patients with acute stroke who undergo neurointerventional procedures may require anesthesia. Both local and general anesthesia may be considered, and a full discussion of the relative risks and benefits of both will be discussed. Regardless of the chosen anesthetic technique, these patients must be managed efficiently to minimize time delay to treatment. In addition, invasive blood pressure monitoring in the radial or femoral artery is recommended to avoid significant hypo- or hypertension. The procedure should not be delayed to obtain these monitors, however, as invasive blood pressure monitoring may be temporarily achieved through the femoral access port inserted by the interventional radiologists. A summary of the important clinical considerations is provided in **Box 1**.

General Vs Local Anesthesia

Several retrospective studies have suggested that general anesthesia may be associated with poorer outcomes than local anesthesia in patients undergoing endovascular treatment of acute stroke.[32,42–44] Whether local anesthesia is superior to general anesthesia in this patient population is contentious, as recent evidence has generated significant discussion about the potential influence of anesthesia on neurologic outcome. The relative advantages and disadvantages of general and local anesthesia will be discussed, as well as a review of the available evidence.

In a recent survey of anesthesia and sedation practices among neurointerventionalists performing endovascular therapy for acute stroke, general anesthesia was the most frequently used and preferred modality.[45] Despite this, many disadvantages of general anesthesia were cited, including potential time delay, lack of anesthesia provider availability, risk of cerebral ischemia due to hypoperfusion, and potential anesthetic neurotoxicity. Nevertheless, general anesthesia was perceived to have

---

Box 1
Practical anesthetic considerations for patients with acute ischemic stroke undergoing endovascular therapy

Minimize time to thrombolysis

    Efficient preanesthetic evaluation

    Minimize delays for anesthetic procedures

Prevent secondary neurologic injury

    Avoid significant hypo- or hypertension

    Consider invasive blood pressure monitoring if minimal delay

    Avoid hyperthermia, hyperglycemia, and hypoxia

Potential neurologic complications

    Seizures

    Hemorrhagic transformation of infarct

    Malignant brain edema

Potential non-neurologic complications

    Airway obstruction

    Aspiration

    Arrhythmias and myocardial ischemia

    Pneumonia

    Neurogenic pulmonary edema

    Pulmonary embolism

the advantages of a motionless patient, increased safety, and faster procedural time. An overview of the advantages and disadvantages of general anesthesia and local anesthesia are seen in **Table 5**. Regardless of preference or evidence supporting local anesthesia or sedation, some patients will require general anesthesia due to factors such as altered level of consciousness, poor cooperation, and inadequate airway protection. For this reason, the mechanisms through which general anesthesia influences patient outcome, if at all, must be identified.

Associated Outcomes

Recent retrospective studies have examined the association between type of anesthesia and outcomes after acute ischemic stroke (**Table 6**).[32,42–44] All of these studies retrospectively reviewed data from patients with acute ischemic stroke presenting for endovascular therapy. Associations between type of anesthesia administered (general or sedation) and outcomes were determined. To varying degrees, all 4 studies found an association between increased sedation or general anesthesia and poor functional outcome and increased mortality. However, in all 4 studies, patients who received general anesthesia or heavy sedation had more severe strokes as documented by higher NIHSS scores. These findings are not surprising in light of the fact that a poor baseline neurologic status correlated with both a worse prognosis and a higher likelihood of requiring a general anesthetic. However, this association between general anesthesia and worse outcome persists despite controlling for baseline stroke severity in several of the studies.[32,43,44] Finally, Davis and colleagues[32] showed that a systolic blood pressure less than 140 mm Hg was an independent predictor for poor neurologic outcome, which may partially explain the poor outcomes seen with general anesthesia.

These studies provide additional information about potential advantages and disadvantages of general anesthesia other than neurologic outcome. Nichols and colleagues showed a higher rate of pneumonia and sepsis in patients receiving heavy sedation or

Table 5
Potential advantages of general versus local anesthesia for endovascular management of acute ischemic stroke

General Anesthesia	Local Anesthesia with Sedation
Advantages	
Motionless patient	Ongoing neurologic assessment
Control of oxygenation and ventilation	Potentially less hypotension
Increased patient comfort	Less time delay to reperfusion depending on anesthesia availability
Theoretical anesthetic neuroprotection	
Disadvantages	
Unable to perform neurologic assessment	Risk of hypercarbia and hypoxia with increasing sedation
Reliant on anesthesia availability	Aspiration in unprotected airway
Increased hypotension	Not appropriate for patients with significant deficits
Possibly increased risk of pneumonia	Patient discomfort during lengthy procedure
Possible anesthetic neurotoxicity	May require urgent conversion to general anesthesia
Possible poorer neurologic outcomes (controversial)	

Table 6
The effect of local anesthesia versus general anesthesia for endovascular treatment of acute ischemic stroke: a summary of the evidence

Trial	Study Design	Population	Categories of Anesthesia	Variables Controlled for in Statistical Model	Outcome(s)	Relative Risk (RR) or Odds Ratio (OR) (CI95)
Davis et al,[32] 2012	Retrospective cohort study	AIS N = 96	LA GA	Baseline NIHSS Comorbidities Hypotension Blood glucose None	Modified Rankin score <3 at 3 mo Death	LA: RR 3.2 (1.5–6.8) P = .002 GA: RR 2.3 (1.1–3.7) P = .039
Nichols et al,[44] 2010	Retrospective cohort study	Moderate-to-severe AIS treated with combined intravenous/intra-arterial thrombolysis N = 75	No sedation Mild sedation Heavy sedation Pharmacologic paralysis	Baseline NIHSS Male gender Baseline NIHSS Baseline systolic blood pressure Baseline glucose	Modified Rankin Score <3 at 3 mo Death	Mild or no sedation: OR 5.7 (1.8–17.8) P<.01 Heavy sedation or paralysis: OR 5.0 (1.3–18.7), P = .02
Jumaa et al,[43] 2010	Retrospective cohort study	AIS (MCA occlusion) N = 126	Intubated Nonintubated	Baseline NIHSS Successful recanalization Age Age	Modified Rankin Score <3 at 3–6 mos Death	Nonintubated: OR 3.06, P = .042 Nonintubated: OR 0.32, P =.011
Abou-Chebl et al,[42] 2010	Retrospective cohort study	Anterior circulation AIS N = 980	General anesthesia Concious sedation	Baseline NIHSS Age TIMI 0/1 recanalization Symptomatic ICH Asymptomatic ICH Carotid terminus occlusion Stent placement Baseline NIHSS Age TIMI 0/1 recanalization Symptomatic ICH Carotid terminus occlusion	Modified Rankin score >=3 at 3 mo Death	GA: 2.33 (1.67–3.25), P = .0001 GA: OR 1.68 (1.23–2.30), P = .0001

Abbreviations: AIS, acute ischemic stroke; CI95, 95% confidence interval; GA, general anesthesia; ICH, intracranial hemorrhage; LA, local anesthesia; MCA, middle cerebral artery; TIMI, thrombolysis in myocardial infarction.

paralysis, and Jumaa and colleagues[43,44] found longer intensive care unit stays among intubated patients, although in both studies, the higher baseline NIHSS scores likely predisposed these patients to these complications regardless of anesthetic technique. The rate of intraprocedural and access site complications did not significantly nor consistently differ between type of sedation in several studies.[43,44] While many neuro-interventionalists are concerned about potential time delays with general anesthesia,[45] the time to thrombolysis was either reduced[43] or equivalent[32,42,44] with general anesthesia and heavy sedation. Several of the patients in 1 study[43] required urgent intubation during the procedure for vomiting, agitation, and altered level of consciousness, demonstrating some of the risks of local anesthesia and sedation.

The association between general anesthesia and poor clinical outcome in acute stroke seen in these studies has generated speculation that general anesthesia causes poor clinical outcome. While the results of these studies are interesting, they must be interpreted with caution due to several important limitations. First, all of these studies are limited by their retrospective design, small sample sizes, and large confidence intervals. All are confounded by the multitude of factors that may influence clinical outcome. The baseline NIHSS score was controlled in statistical models, but many other unmeasured factors may be associated with the likelihood of receiving general anesthesia. **Table 6** illustrates the considerable variation in the measured confounders among retrospective studies comparing local and general anesthesia. All of these studies are subject to confounding despite statistical modeling, as receiving general anesthesia is clearly a marker for poor baseline status due to inability to cooperate. Finally, these trials tell little about the effect of different anesthetic agents on neurologic outcome.

There are several studies examining the effect of anesthetic modality on the incidence of stroke in different populations, and these trials offer additional insight into the controversy involving stroke patients. Several animal studies on acute stroke have compared the effect of general anesthesia with the awake state and found reduced infarct size and neurologic deficit in the group receiving general anesthesia.[46–48] Human data are more controversial. Evidence is accumulating that general anesthesia may be neurotoxic in children and associated with poorer neurocognitive development.[49] Similarly, inhalational anesthesia may result in more postoperative cognitive dysfunction in elderly patients than a regional technique alone.[50] A recent retrospective study found an elevated risk of stroke in preeclamptic women undergoing cesarian section under general anesthesia when compared with patients receiving spinal or epidural anesthesia.[51] There are numerous confounding variables that may explain these results; however, these studies highlight how little is known about the effect of mode of anesthesia in patients at risk for stroke. Finally, a well-designed prospective randomized trial showed equivalent outcomes including stroke between general and local anesthesia for carotid endarterectomy in patients with carotid stenosis despite being possibly underpowered.[52] The results of this study do not support the hypothesis that general anesthesia is detrimental to patients at risk for stroke, and indicate that data from retrospective studies should be interpreted with caution. Overall, the optimal mode of anesthesia to prevent or reduce brain ischemia or cognitive dysfunction is not clear and is likely one factor among many that determine neurologic outcome.

SUMMARY

Stroke is a major cause of death and disability throughout the world. Anesthesiologists are likely to encounter patients with stroke in many contexts, including the emergency department, interventional radiology suit,e and operating room, and they must be aware of the anesthetic considerations for these patients. Given the rapid rate of neuronal death in ischemic stroke and potential for rapid deterioration in hemorrhagic stroke, patients with suspected stroke must be evaluated efficiently. Both intravenous thrombolysis and intra-arterial thrombolysis are effective treatments for acute ischemic stroke as are evolving endovascular techniques such as mechanical clot retrieval. Recent retrospective studies have found an association between general anesthesia and poor clinical outcome that has generated much discussion about the potential harms of anesthesia in this patient population. The results of these studies must be interpreted cautiously, however, given that general anesthesia is often given to patients with more severe strokes. Although anesthetic agents have not been shown to be neuroprotective in human models of brain ischemia, hypotension in acute stroke has been associated with poor outcome and should be avoided regardless of anesthetic technique. Overall, current evidence is inadequate to guide the choice of anesthesia in patients with acute stroke, and this decision must be based on individual patient factors until prospective trials are completed.

REFERENCES

1. Kollmar R, Schwab S. Ischaemic stroke: acute management, intensive care, and future perspectives. Br J Anaesth 2007;99(1):95–101.
2. Feigin VL, Lawes CM, Bennett DA, et al. Stroke epidemiology: a review of population-based studies of incidence, prevalence, and case–fatality in the late 20th century. Lancet Neurol 2003;2(1):43–53.
3. The World Health Organization MONICA Project (monitoring trends and determinants in cardiovascular disease): a major international collaboration. WHO MONICA Project Principal Investigators. J Clin Epidemiol 1988;41(2):105–14.
4. Broderick J, Connolly S, Feldmann E, et al. Guidelines for the management of spontaneous intracerebral hemorrhage in adults: 2007 update: a guideline from the American Heart Association/American Stroke Association Stroke Council, High Blood Pressure Research Council, and the Quality of Care and Outcomes in Research Interdisciplinary Working Group. Circulation 2007;116(16):e391–413.
5. Flaherty ML, Haverbusch M, Sekar P, et al. Long-term mortality after intracerebral hemorrhage. Neurology 2006;66(8):1182–6.
6. Bamford J, Sandercock P, Dennis M, et al. A prospective study of acute cerebrovascular disease in the community: the Oxfordshire Community Stroke Project–1981-86. 2. Incidence, case fatality rates and overall outcome at one year of cerebral infarction, primary intracerebral and subarachnoid haemorrhage. J Neurol Neurosurg Psychiatry 1990;53(1):16–22.
7. Hughey AB, Lesniak MS, Ansari SA, et al. What will anesthesiologists be anesthetizing? Trends in neurosurgical procedure usage. Anesth Analg 2010;110(6): 1686–97.
8. Moustafa RR, Baron JC. Pathophysiology of ischaemic stroke: insights from imaging, and implications for therapy and drug discovery. Br J Pharmacol 2008;153(Suppl 1):S44–54.
9. Elliott J, Smith M. The acute management of intracerebral hemorrhage: a clinical review. Anesth Analg 2010;110(5):1419–27.
10. Qureshi AI, Tuhrim S, Broderick JP, et al. Spontaneous intracerebral hemorrhage. N Engl J Med 2001;344(19):1450–60.
11. Goldstein LB, Simel DL. Is this patient having a stroke? JAMA 2005;293(19): 2391–402.

12. Saver JL. Time is brain-quantified. Stroke 2006;37(1):263–6.
13. Adams HP Jr, del Zoppo G, Alberts MJ, et al. Guidelines for the early management of adults with ischemic stroke: a guideline from the American Heart Association/American Stroke Association Stroke Council, Clinical Cardiology Council, Cardiovascular Radiology and Intervention Council, and the Atherosclerotic Peripheral Vascular Disease and Quality of Care Outcomes in Research Interdisciplinary Working Groups: the American Academy of Neurology affirms the value of this guideline as an educational tool for neurologists. Stroke 2007;38(5): 1655–711.
14. Hylek EM, Singer DE. Risk factors for intracranial hemorrhage in outpatients taking warfarin. Ann Intern Med 1994;120(11):897–902.
15. Baird TA, Parsons MW, Phanh T, et al. Persistent poststroke hyperglycemia is independently associated with infarct expansion and worse clinical outcome. Stroke 2003;34(9):2208–14.
16. Gray CS, Hildreth AJ, Sandercock PA, et al. Glucose-potassium-insulin infusions in the management of post-stroke hyperglycaemia: the UK Glucose Insulin in Stroke Trial (GIST-UK). Lancet Neurol 2007;6(5):397–406.
17. The National Institute of Neurological Disorders and Stroke rt-PA Stroke Study Group. Tissue plasminogen activator for acute ischemic stroke. N Engl J Med 1995;333(24):1581–7.
18. Hill MD, Barber PA, Takahashi J, et al. Anaphylactoid reactions and angioedema during alteplase treatment of acute ischemic stroke. CMAJ 2000;162(9):1281–4.
19. Lee M, Hong KS, Saver JL. Efficacy of intra-arterial fibrinolysis for acute ischemic stroke: meta-analysis of randomized controlled trials. Stroke 2010;41(5):932–7.
20. Meyers PM, Schumacher HC, Higashida RT, et al. Indications for the performance of intracranial endovascular neurointerventional procedures: a scientific statement from the American Heart Association Council on Cardiovascular Radiology and Intervention, Stroke Council, Council on Cardiovascular Surgery and Anesthesia, Interdisciplinary Council on Peripheral Vascular Disease, and Interdisciplinary Council on Quality of Care and Outcomes Research. Circulation 2009;119(16):2235–49.
21. Hacke W, Schwab S, Horn M, et al. 'Malignant' middle cerebral artery territory infarction: clinical course and prognostic signs. Arch Neurol 1996;53(4):309–15.
22. Ropper AH, Shafran B. Brain edema after stroke. Clinical syndrome and intracranial pressure. Arch Neurol 1984;41(1):26–9.
23. Lanzino G. Decompressive craniectomy for acute stroke: early is better. J Neurosurg 2008;109(2):285 [discussion: 286].
24. Juttler E, Schwab S, Schmiedek P, et al. Decompressive Surgery for the Treatment of Malignant Infarction of the Middle Cerebral Artery (DESTINY): a randomized, controlled trial. Stroke 2007;38(9):2518–25.
25. Vahedi K, Hofmeijer J, Juettler E, et al. Early decompressive surgery in malignant infarction of the middle cerebral artery: a pooled analysis of three randomised controlled trials. Lancet Neurol 2007;6(3):215–22.
26. Juttler E, Bosel J, Amiri H, et al. DESTINY II: DEcompressive Surgery for the Treatment of malignant INfarction of the middle cerebral arterY II. Int J Stroke 2011; 6(1):79–86.
27. Leonardi-Bee J, Bath PM, Phillips SJ, et al. Blood pressure and clinical outcomes in the International Stroke Trial. Stroke 2002;33(5):1315–20.
28. Castillo J, Leira R, Garcia MM, et al. Blood pressure decrease during the acute phase of ischemic stroke is associated with brain injury and poor stroke outcome. Stroke 2004;35(2):520–6.

29. Delgado-Mederos R, Ribo M, Rovira A, et al. Prognostic significance of blood pressure variability after thrombolysis in acute stroke. Neurology 2008;71(8): 552–8.

30. Sandset EC, Bath PM, Boysen G, et al. The angiotensin-receptor blocker candesartan for treatment of acute stroke (SCAST): a randomised, placebo-controlled, double-blind trial. Lancet 2011;377(9767):741–50.

31. Schrader J, Luders S, Kulschewski A, et al. The ACCESS Study: evaluation of Acute Candesartan Cilexetil Therapy in Stroke Survivors. Stroke 2003;34(7):1699–703.

32. Davis MJ, Menon BK, Baghirzada LB, et al. Anesthetic management and outcome in patients during endovascular therapy for acute stroke. Anesthesiology 2012;116(2):396–405.

33. Zhang Y, Reilly KH, Tong W, et al. Blood pressure and clinical outcome among patients with acute stroke in Inner Mongolia, China. J Hypertens 2008;26(7): 1446–52.

34. Qureshi AI, Palesch YY, Martin R, et al. Effect of systolic blood pressure reduction on hematoma expansion, perihematomal edema, and 3-month outcome among patients with intracerebral hemorrhage: results from the antihypertensive treatment of acute cerebral hemorrhage study. Arch Neurol 2010;67(5):570–6.

35. Head BP, Patel P. Anesthetics and brain protection. Curr Opin Anaesthesiol 2007; 20(5):395–9.

36. Hindman BJ, Bayman EO, Pfisterer WK, et al. No association between intraoperative hypothermia or supplemental protective drug and neurologic outcomes in patients undergoing temporary clipping during cerebral aneurysm surgery: findings from the Intraoperative Hypothermia for Aneurysm Surgery Trial. Anesthesiology 2010; 112(1):86–101.

37. Schifilliti D, Grasso G, Conti A, et al. Anaesthetic-related neuroprotection: intravenous or inhalational agents? CNS Drugs 2010;24(11):893–907.

38. Todd MM, Hindman BJ, Clarke WR, et al. Mild intraoperative hypothermia during surgery for intracranial aneurysm. N Engl J Med 2005;352(2):135–45.

39. Kollmar R, Schwab S. Hypothermia in focal ischemia: implications of experiments and experience. J Neurotrauma 2009;26(3):377–86.

40. Sydenham E, Roberts I, Alderson P. Hypothermia for traumatic head injury. Cochrane Database Syst Rev 2009;2:CD001048.

41. Hajat C, Hajat S, Sharma P. Effects of poststroke pyrexia on stroke outcome: a meta-analysis of studies in patients. Stroke 2000;31(2):410–4.

42. Abou-Chebl A, Lin R, Hussain MS, et al. Conscious sedation versus general anesthesia during endovascular therapy for acute anterior circulation stroke: preliminary results from a retrospective, multicenter study. Stroke 2010;41(6):1175–9.

43. Jumaa MA, Zhang F, Ruiz-Ares G, et al. Comparison of safety and clinical and radiographic outcomes in endovascular acute stroke therapy for proximal middle cerebral artery occlusion with intubation and general anesthesia versus the nonintubated state. Stroke 2010;41(6):1180–4.

44. Nichols C, Carrozzella J, Yeatts S, et al. Is periprocedural sedation during acute stroke therapy associated with poorer functional outcomes? J Neurointerv Surg 2010;2(1):67–70.

45. McDonagh DL, Olson DM, Kalia JS, et al. Anesthesia and sedation practices among neurointerventionalists during acute ischemic stroke endovascular therapy. Front Neurol 2010;1:118.

46. Inoue S, Drummond JC, Davis DP, et al. Combination of isoflurane and caspase inhibition reduces cerebral injury in rats subjected to focal cerebral ischemia. Anesthesiology 2004;101(1):75–81.

47. Gelb AW, Bayona NA, Wilson JX, et al. Propofol anesthesia compared to awake reduces infarct size in rats. Anesthesiology 2002;96(5):1183–90.
48. Sakai H, Sheng H, Yates RB, et al. Isoflurane provides long-term protection against focal cerebral ischemia in the rat. Anesthesiology 2007;106(1):92–9 [discussion: 98–10].
49. Stratmann G. Review article: neurotoxicity of anesthetic drugs in the developing brain. Anesth Analg 2011;113(5):1170–9.
50. Zhang B, Tian M, Zhen Y, et al. The effects of isoflurane and desflurane on cognitive function in humans. Anesth Analg 2012;114(2):410–5.
51. Huang CJ, Fan YC, Tsai PS. Differential impacts of modes of anaesthesia on the risk of stroke among preeclamptic women who undergo Caesarean delivery: a population-based study. Br J Anaesth 2010;105(6):818–26.
52. Gough MJ, Bodenham A, Horrocks M, et al. GALA: an international multicentre randomised trial comparing general anaesthesia versus local anaesthesia for carotid surgery. Trials 2008;9:28.

Pediatric Epilepsy Surgery
Anesthetic Considerations

Jeffrey L. Koh, MD, MBA[a],*, Brian Egan, MD[b],
Terrence McGraw, MD[a]

KEYWORDS

- Pediatric epilepsy • Seizures • Epilepsy surgery • Pediatric anesthesiology

KEY POINTS

- In the past 15 years, the surgical options for the treatment of pediatric epilepsy have increased and clarification has evolved regarding the indications for particular surgical procedures.
- Epilepsy surgery may have an important role in the treatment of refractory epilepsy, resulting in improved seizure control and quality of life.
- Understanding of the potential effects of anesthetics on seizure threshold is important for the anesthesiologist caring for patients with seizures, as well as understanding of the effect of AED on anesthetic management of these patients.

INTRODUCTION

The most common treatment of recurrent seizures is pharmacologic with antiepileptic medication (AED). Approximately 70% of patients respond to AED management. Those who continue to have seizures are considered to have medically refractory epilepsy, and are at risk for adverse effects on quality of life, brain development, learning, language, and injury. Even if effective, AED management can also have negative effects on patients' quality of life. The negative impact of epilepsy on cognitive development may be especially important in young children, whose brain is in the most rapid state of development at the time of the highest incidence of seizures. The effect of AED management on the developing brain is also unknown and may put this population at risk for further negative cognitive development. For patients with refractory seizures, surgical intervention offers an important option that can result in rendering the patient either seizure free or in markedly decreasing the frequency of seizures.

[a] Department of Anesthesiology and Perioperative Medicine, Doernbecher Children's Hospital/Oregon Health and Sciences University, 3181 SW Sam Jackson Park Road, BTE-2, Portland, OR 97205, USA; [b] Division of Pediatric Anesthesiology, Department of Anesthesiology and Perioperative Medicine, Oregon Health and Sciences University, 3181 SW Sam Jackson Park Road, BTE-2, Portland, OR 97205, USA
* Corresponding author.
E-mail address: kohj@ohsu.edu

Anesthesiology Clin 30 (2012) 191–206
doi:10.1016/j.anclin.2012.05.001   anesthesiology.theclinics.com

This article reviews pediatric epilepsy and its management in children, focusing on surgical interventions with which anesthesiologists may be involved.

EPIDEMIOLOGY

Epilepsy is a common medical condition affecting 3% to 5% of the world's population, roughly 45 million people. The incidence of seizure disorders in the United States has been reported to be approximately 6 to 8 per 1000 people, with the highest incidence in young children and the elderly (more than 60 years of age).[1,2] Most commonly, there is no specific cause found for the onset of seizures, but causes such as stroke, head trauma, tumors, and infection can all have seizures associated with the underlying disease process.

Seizures in the Pediatric Population

In children, the incidence of new seizure onset is 1% to 2% per year, and plateaus in early childhood, with the highest incidence being in the first year of life. There is a gradual decline in incidence after 10 years of age.[2] Approximately 10% to 40% of these patients have seizures refractory to AEDs and may require surgical intervention. Although the early state of brain development may put these patients at higher risk for negative impacts on development by refractory seizures, the increased neuroplasticity of the developing brain may also make them better candidates for aggressive surgical management.[3,4] In the last 2 decades, surgical intervention for epilepsy has been performed earlier and more frequently, with improved results.[5]

An exhaustive review of epilepsy syndromes is beyond the scope of this article; however, a brief summary is given to provide background for the anesthesiologist caring for these children.

Epileptic disorders are defined by the International League Against Epilepsy (ILAE), which classifies seizures according to presumed location and cause.[6] Most children with epileptic disorders (63%) have partial (focal) seizures, indicating that the epileptic foci come from a localized area of the brain. Generalized epilepsy occurs in approximately 12% of patients, indicating either multiple epileptic foci or generalization of seizure activity, and 26% are classified as undetermined (either focal or generalized).[7] The cause of many seizure disorders (49%) is cryptogenic with a presumed, but not identifiable, lesion. The rest are either idiopathic or associated with an identifiable lesion (eg, tumor).

The clinical course for different seizure types varies. The more severe disorders, such as myoclonic epilepsy of infancy, have an onset in the first year of life and can be difficult to treat. In contrast, idiopathic generalized epilepsy, benign rolandic epilepsy, and febrile seizures tend to have a good prognosis for remission (**Table 1**).[2]

Most children (60%–90%) respond to medical management and become either seizure free or have a significant decrease in the number of seizures. In one review, 79% of patients were in remission on 2-year follow-up, and 59% were in remission and off medication.[7]

Medically refractory epilepsy is usually defined as inadequate seizure control with at least 2 AEDs at maximally tolerated doses over 18 months to 2 years. Patients who have adequate seizure control but suffer unacceptable AED side effects are also considered medically refractory. There is considerable discussion regarding other factors, such as the definition of AED failure, acceptable minimum seizure frequency, and duration of unresponsiveness to medication.[2]

There have been certain anatomic and physiologic abnormalities that have been associated with refractory seizures, including cortical malformation, abnormal neuronal migration, and abnormal cortical organization. Certain syndromes, such as Rasmussen

Table 1
Common seizure disorders by age

Neonate	Infant
Benign neonatal convulsions	Febrile seizures
Benign neonatal familial convulsions	Early infantile epileptic encephalopathy
Miscellaneous neonatal seizures	Early myoclonic encephalopathy
	Infantile spasms (West syndrome)
	Benign myoclonic epilepsy of infancy
	Severe myoclonic epilepsy of infancy
	Benign partial epilepsy of infancy
	Benign infantile familial convulsions
	Symptomatic/cryptogenic partial epilepsies

Toddler/Preschool	School Age and Adolescence
Epilepsy with myoclonic absences	Childhood absence epilepsy
Lennox-Gastaut syndrome	Benign partial epilepsy with centrotemporal spikes
Epilepsy with myoclonic-astatic seizures (Doose syndrome)	Benign occipital epilepsy
Acquired epileptic aphasia (Landau-Kleffner syndrome)	Reflex epilepsies (eg, photosensitive)
Epilepsy with continuous spike-waves during slow wave sleep	Juvenile absence epilepsy
Epilepsy with gelastic seizures and hypothalamic hamartoma	Autosomal dominant nocturnal frontal lobe epilepsy
Symptomatic/cryptogenic partial epilepsies	Symptomatic/cryptogenic partial epilepsies

syndrome, West syndrome, and Sturge-Weber syndrome, have been associated with a higher risk of medical intractability. In addition, patients with onset of seizures at less than 1 year of age may be at higher risk for medical intractability, although some recent reports suggest that age of onset is not an accurate predictor of prognosis.[2]

A major concern for children with epilepsy is how seizures and/or AEDs might affect cognitive and social development. This question is difficult to answer because many patients with intractable seizures have associated diagnoses that may affect their developmental level independently of seizures. Nevertheless, there is increasing evidence that prolonged or repeated seizures do have an impact on brain function and development.

As noted earlier, children in the first few months of life have a high incidence of new-onset seizure disorders, which may, in part, be because the immature brain seems to be more susceptible to seizures with a lower seizure threshold.[4] Although infrequent, uncomplicated seizures may have little long-term effect on the brain, refractory seizures can affect cognitive and social development in patients, with infants being at highest risk. Animal studies suggest that, ,although there is less seizure-related cell death in immature animals, the immature animals still display impaired cognitive development and impaired learning. This finding may be caused by other changes that have been shown to occur in the glutamate and γ-aminobutyric acid (GABA) systems.[4] Cognitive impairment and learning disabilities are often present in infants and children with seizures, especially those with refractory seizure disorders.[8] These problems are most likely multifactorial in origin, with various causes including repeated seizures, underlying brain abnormalities, and AED toxicity. There is some evidence that those patients who have a good result from surgical intervention for refractory seizures also show improvement in cognitive and learning measurements.[9] Social development can also be negatively affected for children at all developmental stages if their seizures are poorly controlled and/or they suffer significant side effects from their AEDs. The potential negative cumulative impact of refractory seizures, the cognitive side effects of AEDs, and the effect on social development that can occur in young children all provide support for aggressive evaluation and possible surgical intervention for young patients with refractory seizure disorders.

ANTIEPILEPTIC DRUGS AND ANESTHESIA

Children presenting for epilepsy surgery have typically responded inadequately or adversely to various medical therapies. However, most present for surgery taking at least 1 AED. Because of this, it is important for the anesthesia provider to be familiar with AEDs, the effects of anesthetic medications on seizures, and the effects of the AEDs on the pharmacology of anesthetic medications.

Antiepileptic Drugs

Phenobarbital and phenytoin represented the mainstay of AEDs in the first half of the twentieth century. In the past 50 years, numerous new medications have been developed. The mechanism of action of these medications typically involves potentiation of GABA pathways or inhibition of ion channels (Na^+ or Ca^{2+}) within the central nervous system. In general, AEDs developed in the past 2 decades have fewer side effects and better safety profiles than older AEDs. However, although there exists a general consensus regarding choice of AED and seizure type, it is often difficult to predict which medication might be most suitable for a particular child. Profiles of AEDs are listed in **Table 2**.

Anesthesia and Seizure Thresholds

Many anesthetic agents have anticonvulsant properties. This property is desirable in most situations, in which it is hoped that seizure activity will be minimized or avoided. However, several medications have been shown to exhibit anticonvulsant and/or proconvulsant properties (**Table 3**). The property exhibited is generally dose dependent, and proconvulsant properties are not generally seen at the dosages that are used clinically. For example, sevoflurane is often used for inhalation induction without precipitating seizures in children with epilepsy. It is occasionally optimal (eg, cortical mapping, sedated electroencephalography [EEG]) to use anesthetic agents devoid of anticonvulsant properties. Dexmedetomidine has been successfully used in this setting.[10] Overall, seizures are uncommon while a patient is anesthetized, but they can been observed in patients who have severe refractory seizures or when patients are under light levels of general anesthesia.

AEDs and Anesthetic Pharmacology

The most commonly observed consequence of AEDs on anesthetics is resistance to the effects of nondepolarizing muscle relaxants (NDMR), which is classically observed with first-generation AEDs such as phenytoin, carbamazepine, and phenobarbital.[11–21] The effect on NDMRs is the result of several processes. At first, they inhibit the release of acetylcholine (ACh) quanta at the nerve terminal. Patients on AEDs, therefore, experience an acute increase in sensitivity to NDMRs. Over a few weeks, decreased ACh quanta results in an increase in ACh receptors. Along with induction of NDMR liver metabolism and increased release of acute phase reactant proteins (which bind some NDMR and change volume of distribution), this results in observed resistance to NDMRs. In addition, epileptic patients receiving AEDs may require higher

Table 2
Profiles of antiepileptic drugs

Drug	Mechanism of Action	Seizure Types Treated	Adverse Effects	Drug Interactions
Carbamazepine	Na^+ channel inhibition	Partial Tonic-clonic	Neurologic: dizziness, diplopia, ataxia, vertigo Non-neurologic: aplastic anemia, leukopenia, gastrointestinal irritation, hepatotoxicity, hyponatremia, skin rash	Enzyme substrate: CYP 3A4, 2C8 Enzyme inducer: CYP 1A2, 2B6, 2C8, 2C9, 2C19, 3A4 Enzyme inhibitor: none
Clonazepam (Klonopin)	Potentiate GABA receptor function	Absence Atypical absence Myoclonic	Neurologic: ataxia, sedation, lethargy Non-neurologic: anorexia	Enzyme substrate: CYP 3A4 Enzyme inducer: none Enzyme inhibitor: none
Ethosuximide	T-type Ca^{2+} channel inhibition in thalamus	Absence	Neurologic: ataxia, lethargy, headache Non-neurologic: gastrointestinal irritation, skin rash, bone marrow suppression	Enzyme substrate: CYP 3A4 Enzyme inducer: none Enzyme inhibitor: none
Felbamate (Felbatol)	NMDA receptor antagonist and increase GABA availability	Partial Lennox-Gastaut	Neurologic: insomnia, dizziness, sedation, headache Non-neurologic: aplastic anemia, hepatic failure, weight loss, gastrointestinal irritation	Enzyme substrate: CYP 2E1, 3A4 Enzyme inducer: CYP 3A4 Enzyme inhibitor: CYP 2C19
Gabapentin (Neurontin)	GABA analog for α-2 δ subunit	Partial	Neurologic: sedation, dizziness, ataxia, fatigue Non-neurologic: gastrointestinal irritation, weight gain, edema	Enzyme substrate: none Enzyme inducer: none Enzyme inhibitor: none
Lamotrigine (Lamictal)	Decrease glutamate release	Partial Tonic-clonic Atypical absence Myoclonic Lennox-Gastaut	Neurologic: dizziness, diplopia, sedation, ataxia, headache Non-neurologic: skin rash	Enzyme substrate: UGT1A4 Enzyme inducer: none Enzyme inhibitor: none

(continued on next page)

Table 2
(continued)

Drug	Mechanism of Action	Seizure Types Treated	Adverse Effects	Drug Interactions
Levetiracetam (Keppra)	Synaptic vesicle release modulation	Partial	Neurologic: sedation, fatigue, incoordination, psychosis Non-neurologic: anemia, leukopenia	Enzyme substrate: none Enzyme inducer: none Enzyme inhibitor: none
Oxcarbazepine (Trileptal)	Na$^+$ channel inhibition	Partial	Neurologic: fatigue, ataxia, dizziness, diplopia Non-neurologic: aplastic anemia, leukopenia, gastrointestinal irritation, hepatotoxicity, hyponatremia, skin rash	Enzyme substrate: CYP Enzyme inducer: CYP 3A4 Enzyme inhibitor: CYP 2C19
Phenobarbital	Potentiate GABA receptor function	Partial Tonic-clonic	Neurologic: sedation, ataxia, confusion, dizziness, decreased libido, depression Non-neurologic: skin rash, hepatotoxicity	Enzyme substrate: CYP 2C9, 2C19, 2E1 Enzyme inducer: CYP 1A2, 2A6, 2B6, 2C8, 2C9, 3A4 Enzyme inhibitor: none
Phenytoin (Dilantin)	Na$^+$ and Ca^{2+} channel inhibition	Partial Tonic-clonic	Neurologic: dizziness, diplopia, ataxia, confusion Non-neurologic: gingival hyperplasia, peripheral neuropathy, lymphadenopathy, hirsutism, osteomalacia, hepatotoxicity, facial coarsening, skin rash	Enzyme substrate: CYP 2C9, 2C19, 3A4 Enzyme inducer: CYP 2B6, 2C8, 2C9, 2C19, 3A4, and UDPGT Enzyme inhibitor: none
Pregabalin (Lyrica)	GABA analog for α-2 δ subunit	Partial	Neurologic: ataxia, somnolence, dizziness, blurred vision, diplopia Non-neurologic: peripheral edema, increased appetite	Enzyme substrate: none Enzyme inducer: none Enzyme inhibitor: none
Rufinamide (Banzel)	Na$^+$ channel inhibition	Lennox-Gastaut	Neurologic: headache, dizziness, fatigue, somnolence, convulsion, diplopia, tremor, nystagmus Non-neurologic: nausea, vomiting, nasopharyngitis, blurred vision	Enzyme substrate: CYP 3A4 Enzyme inducer: none Enzyme inhibitor: none

Drug	Mechanism	Seizure types	Side effects	Enzyme
Tiagabine (Gabitril)	Increase GABA availability	Partial; Tonic-clonic	Neurologic: confusion, sedation, depression, speech problems, paresthesias, psychosis. Non-neurologic: gastrointestinal irritation	Enzyme substrate: CYP 3A4; Enzyme inducer: none; Enzyme inhibitor: none
Topiramate (Topamax)	Na^+ channel inhibition	Partial; Tonic-clonic; Lennox-Gastaut	Neurologic: psychomotor slowing, sedation, speech problems, fatigue, paresthesias. Non-neurologic: kidney stones, glaucoma, weight loss, hypohydrosis	Enzyme substrate: none; Enzyme inducer: CYP 3A4; Enzyme inhibitor: CYP 2C19
Valproic acid (Depakote)	T-type Ca^{2+} channel inhibition in thalamus; Increase GABA availability	Partial; Tonic-clonic; Absence; Atypical absence; Myoclonic	Neurologic: ataxia, sedation, tremor. Non-neurologic: hepatotoxicity, thrombocytopenia, gastrointestinal irritation, weight gain, hyperammonemia	Enzyme substrate: UGT 1A6, 1A9, 2B7, β-oxidation; Enzyme inducer: CYP 2A6; Enzyme inhibitor: CYP 2C9, 2C19, 2D6, 3A4
Vigabatrin (Sabril)	Analog of GABA, inhibits GABA catabolism	Complex partial; infantile spasms	Neurologic: headache, fatigue, drowsiness, dizziness, tremor, agitation, visual field defects, abnormal vision, diplopia. Non-neurologic: nausea, vomiting, diarrhea, weight gain, skin rash	Enzyme substrate: none; Enzyme inducer: none; Enzyme inhibitor: none
Zonisamide (Zonegran)	Na^+ channel inhibition	Partial	Neurologic: sedation, dizziness, confusion, headache, psychosis. Non-neurologic: Anorexia, renal stones, hypohydrosis	Enzyme substrate: CYP 2C19, 3A4; Enzyme inducer: none; Enzyme inhibitor: none

Abbreviations: NMDA, N-methyl-D-aspartate; UDPGT, uridine diphosphate glucuronosyl density.
From US Department of Health & Human Services Agency for Research and Quality. Evaluation of effectiveness and safety of antiepileptic medications in patients with epilepsy. Available at: http://www.effectivehealthcare.ahrq.gov. Published online: July 1, 2010.

Table 3
Proconvulsant and anticonvulsant properties of anesthetic agents

Anesthetic	Proconvulsant	Anticonvulsant
Nitrous oxide	+	−
Halothane	+	++
Enflurane	+++	+
Isoflurane	++	+++
Sevoflurane	++	
Desflurane	−	
Thiopental	++	+++
Methohexital	+++	+++
Etomidate	+++	+++
Benzodiazepines		+++
Ketamine	++	+
Propofol	++	++
Opioids	+++	

Empty cells indicate without known [proconvulsant, anticonvulsant] effects.
Data from Gratrix AP, Enright SM. Epilepsy in anaesthesia and intensive care. Contin Educ Anaesth Crit Care Pain 2005;5(4):118–21.

doses of fentanyl to maintain a comparable depth of anesthesia.[22] The cause or causes of this resistance to opioids is unknown. Possibilities include changes in the number of receptors and/or alterations in drug metabolism.

EVALUATION OF THE PATIENT WITH REFRACTORY SEIZURES

Patients who are presenting for epilepsy surgery usually have an established diagnosis and at least some work-up. However, a review of the preoperative evaluation that occurs in these children is informative, especially because the anesthesiologist may become involved at this phase to provide sedation for imaging or other evaluation procedures that require a still and/or cooperative patient.[9,23]

A thorough history and physical examination is the important first step in evaluating these patients. Information about the age of onset of seizures, the progression, and description of the seizure activity itself can help identify or confirm the seizure type and location. It is also important to identify associated comorbidities that can be associated with syndromes or metabolic disease that may include seizures, as well as to develop an initial sense of cognitive level and impairment. Current or past AED use is also important in guiding decisions about future treatment.

Neuropsychology testing is essential in the preoperative evaluation of potential patients for epilepsy surgery. This mode of testing can determine the preoperative global cognitive function of the patient, as well as any focal deficits. This information can help predict the potential impact, if any, epilepsy surgery will have on cognitive function. Testing can also aid in the lateralization of language as well as other nonverbal functions. In addition, neuropsychology testing can provide further comparative information on the location of the seizure focus.

The EEG has been a standard for the evaluation of patients with seizures for years. EEG evaluation generally begins with the scalp EEG, which can confirm the presence of abnormal electrical activity and give a sense of localization of the seizure focus.

Video EEG on an inpatient unit has the additional benefit of documenting the frequency of ictal events, types of both ictal and interictal activity, and may provide further information about location of the focus. Invasive EEG monitoring is often used in pediatric patients to facilitate accurate localization of the seizure focus and definition of its relationship to areas of the brain crucial for language and motor activity (so-called eloquent areas). Its use is especially important for extratemporal seizures, which are more common in pediatric patients than temporal seizures. Most commonly, cortical grids are placed in the operating room as part of a staged resection (details of this staged procedure are discussed later in this article). In adults, depth electrodes can be placed and left for longer periods of time, which may be helpful when long-term monitoring is needed for better characterization of the seizure activity and location. Long-term monitoring is not commonly used in children.

The development of imaging technology such as magnetic resonance imaging (MRI), single photon emission-computed tomography (SPECT), and positron emission tomography (PET) has greatly improved the ability to localize the seizure focus and characterize its relationship to the functional areas of the brain. MRI is now a part of the routine work-up of new seizures given its ability to identify structural abnormalities of the brain. Specialized forms of MRI (eg, MRI angiography, functional MRI) may provide further anatomic information, and have been used to identify language lateralization in cooperative patients. The SPECT scan can be especially useful during the ictal period, because the seizure focus shows increased perfusion compared with the interictal period, when the focus shows hypoperfusion. Timing of the radionuclide at seizure onset is critical to obtain maximum benefit from this test. This timing requires close coordination with the anesthesia provider to sedate the patient (if needed) within the needed timeframe. The PET scan can further clarify the seizure location by showing an area of decreased metabolism at the seizure focus during the interictal period, when it is most commonly performed. Ictal PET scans show the seizure focus to be hypermetabolic. These 3 scans together may provide a clear picture of the seizure focus, allowing planning of the surgical resection by the multidisciplinary team. The importance of accurate data from these studies is also critical for the surgical procedure because the data can be entered into a navigation system for precise intraoperative localization.

A more recently developed noninvasive imaging technique is magnetoencephalography (MEG). MEG measures magnetic dipoles produced by electric currents in the brain. It can localize seizure foci with 90% concordance of invasive EEG monitoring using subdural electrodes. Information from this study, combined with MRI data, is also useful for localization of multiple foci, which can aid in guiding placement of invasive EEG monitoring grids. Use of MEG is not common and there are limited data in the literature regarding its use, especially in the pediatric population.

The Wada test consists of selective angiographic carotid arterial injection of amobarbital to determine language dominance. It is the most invasive test used in the evaluation of patients with refractory seizures. The Wada test is rarely used in children.

Sedation for Preoperative Testing

Although most preoperative tests used in the evaluation of the patient having seizures are noninvasive, they still require a cooperative patient who can remain still for prolonged periods of time. Given the importance of preoperative testing on the evaluation and surgical planning for these patients, it is common for sedation to be needed, especially in younger or cognitively impaired patients. The level of sedation can range from anxiolysis to deep sedation. A particularly challenging scenario involves the EEG in children unable to cooperate for lead placement, because most sedatives have some effect on the EEG tracing. One option is to provide propofol sedation for placement of the EEG leads, then allowing the propofol to wear off before starting to record data. Successful sedation for EEG has been reported using a variety of agents including chloral hydrate[24] and dexmedetomidine.[25] Deep sedation is more common for longer procedures such as MRIs and SPECT scans, and is often achieved using propofol as the primary sedative agent. Whatever agent is chosen, there should be clear communication with the neurologists or radiologist to ensure that the sedative agent does not interfere with testing or influence the results.

SURGERY

The choice of surgical intervention recommended for a given patient is largely dictated by the results of preoperative testing described earlier. Work-ups generally point to therapies aimed either at an epileptogenic focus or to the general seizure threshold. The most common surgical procedures performed in children are focal resection and vagal nerve stimulator (VNS) placement. Hemispheric resection has been used in specific circumstances of intractable seizures in patients with specific diagnosis such as cortical development malformations, infarction, infantile hemiplegia, and Sturge-Weber syndrome. Children with temporal lobe seizures associated with mesial temporal sclerosis (MTS) have a particularly good prognosis with surgery. In one study of children with MTS, 72% of children were seizure free following surgery, compared with 23% of those treated with AEDs.[26]

Preoperative Evaluation

As with all patients having surgery, the preoperative evaluation of the patient undergoing any type of epilepsy surgery is important. The basics of any preoperative evaluation should be included, such as history of any other significant chronic medical issues, prior anesthetic history (including any difficulty with seizures in the perioperative period), and allergies. Any recent acute illness should also be identified and the course explored, especially for those patients undergoing a more invasive procedure such as cortical resection. It may be prudent to postpone patients with recent acute illnesses, depending on the severity.

The anesthesiologist should understand the type of seizure disorder and the underlying cause, if known. As noted earlier, patients with refractory seizure disorders often have associated syndromes, genetic abnormalities, or metabolic problems that may include other organ systems. Characteristics and frequency of seizures should be documented and communicated to all team members, especially after surgery. Any recent change in seizure frequency or type should also be noted.

Current AED therapy is important to document and the anesthesiologist should understand whether the preoperative plan includes cessation of the AED to facilitate EEG monitoring and localization after grid placement. If the preoperative plan is to continue AED administration, the anesthesiologist can reinforce the acceptability of taking the AED at the appropriate time even if the patient is allowed nothing by mouth. Potential effects of current AED, as outlined earlier, should also be noted.

Patients currently being managed with a ketogenic diet should also be identified before surgery. The ketogenic diet is high in fat and low in protein and carbohydrates, and has been used for many years in patients with intractable seizures. Depending on how strict a diet protocol the patient is on, consideration should be given to the use of sugar-containing syrups for premedication, type of perioperative intravenous (IV) fluid, and monitoring of acid-base balance. Ichikawa and colleagues[27] reported the use of lactated ringers for fluid administration, thinking that this solution allowed better acid-base balance, preventing metabolic acidosis that can occur with ketosis. Overall, there are few data concerning anesthetic implications of patients who are on a keto-genic diet.

Routine preanesthetic physical examination, including airway examination, should be performed. In addition, it may be useful to discuss with the parents whether they think that their child will need a premedication before surgery. For cases that may include intraoperative electrophysiologic monitoring, it may be important to avoid the use of benzodiazepines before surgery. In this circumstance, the use of simple behavioral techniques, child life specialists, or a parent present during induction would be preferable. However, because intraoperative electrophysiologic monitoring is not a frequent tool used for many of the procedures described, use of premedication is often guided primarily by the patient's need.

SURGICAL PROCEDURES
Vagal Nerve Stimulation

The most common surgical intervention for intractable pediatric epilepsy is the place-ment of a VNS. The VNS is often an option when resection of the epileptic focus is not feasible. The first VNS was placed experimentally in humans in 1988. Since US Food and Drug Administration approval in 1997, VNSs have become a mainstay in the management of refractory seizures in both children and adults. A meta-analysis of multiple efficacy reports suggests that seizures are reduced by 50% or more (frequency and/or intensity) in approximately 50% of the patients receiving VNS implants.[28] Positive predictors of a favorable outcome include younger age of inser-tion and tuberous sclerosis.[29]

The mechanism of action of VNSs is not understood. It is presumed that vagal stim-ulation results in activation of nucleus tractus solitarius and other brainstem centers, which then promulgate signals that modulate cerebral neuronal excitability, either through activation of the limbic system, noradrenergic neurotransmitter systems, or generalized brainstem arousal systems.

The surgical technique consists of exposing the left vagus nerve in the region of the sternocleidomastoid muscle, attaching a stimulating electrode to the nerve, and attaching the electrode to a generator placed in the pectoralis fascia via a tunneled connection. The left vagus is used to minimize cardiac stimulation. Once in place, the generator is typically programmed to provide a pulse of electrical current (eg, 1–2 mA for 0.5 milliseconds), which is repeated continuously (eg, 20–30 Hz for 30 seconds every 5 minutes). In addition, magnets may be electively placed over the generator to provide either an extra pulse of current output or to inhibit current output. Anesthetic considerations for VNS placement have been published[30] and include those of AEDs and anesthesia in general (discussed earlier). In addition, the remote possibility of major vessel bleeding and tracheal impingement should be kept in mind.

Common postsurgical side effects include hoarseness and sore throat. Uncommon complications include cardiac bradyarrhythmias, facial muscle palsies, and exacerba-tion of obstructive sleep apnea. Following VNS placement, if patients require MRI, the VNS needs to be turned off during the MRI.

Focal Resection

The ideal surgical option is resection of the seizure foci when the seizure is unifocal and the focus is not in proximity to motor or language areas of the brain. Most commonly in children, the seizure focus is extratemporal in location compared with adults in whom the temporal location is most common. Although extratemporal resection has a lower rate of seizure cessation (48% vs 68%), an additional 35% of patients have substantial improvement in seizure control.[23]

The specifics of the focal resection technique is beyond the scope of this article. The procedure includes a craniotomy to expose the identified area of brain that includes the seizure focus. Often, this is done with stereotactic guidance to integrate the MRI and/or SPECT results for more accurate localization. In many cases, focal resection is a 2-stage procedure. In the first stage, the craniotomy is made and an EEG grid is place directly over the suspected area of brain. Closure is then performed with the EEG wires externalized to allow monitoring in the intensive care unit for approximately 48 hours. The second stage is sometimes delayed if there has not been adequate seizure activity for localization. Early return to the OR may be necessitated by onset of fever and concern for infection. The second stage involves reopening of the craniotomy, identification of the area to be resected, and resection.

In most cases, the initial procedure is performed during a routine general anesthetic. As noted earlier, premedication is commonly used but may be omitted if intraoperative EEG monitoring is used. Induction is commonly performed either with inhaled sevoflurane or propofol, depending on the age of the child. Two peripheral IVs are often placed, as well as an arterial line. The arterial line is placed to allow the anesthesia provider to assess beat-to-beat monitoring of blood pressure during brain manipulation, because an acute change may be an early sign of impending brain injury. For the second procedure, patency of IV lines and the arterial line (if still in place) should be confirmed. In most cases, the anesthetic can be maintained for both procedures using inhalational agent, opioid, and muscle relaxant. If intraoperative monitoring is to be used, total intravenous anesthetic may be required, as well as avoidance of muscle relaxant. Propofol infusion has been successfully used for intraoperative EEG monitoring, as has dexmedetomidine.[31] Communication should be maintained between the anesthesiologist and the monitoring personnel to ensure appropriate conditions for accurate monitoring results.

Although significant blood loss is unusual, it is prudent to have at least a type and screen available, although it is our practice to have a type and cross ready before surgery. If a significant amount of tissue is to be resected during the second phase, it may be appropriate to follow coagulation studies to identify the development of a coagulopathy. In addition, there is usually no contraindication to emergence and extubation immediately after either phase of this procedure. As with all neurosurgical procedures, this allows early examination by the neurosurgical team to identify any postoperative deficits. Postoperative computed tomography or MRI is often required within 24 hours.

Corpus Callosotomy

Similar to VNS placement, corpus callosotomy is an option for patients with intractable seizures who are not candidates for focal resection. In most cases, it is performed in children with tonic and atonic seizures that result in frequent drop attacks that can put the patient at risk for multiple injuries such as abrasions, lacerations, and fractures.[32] Corpus callosotomy is a palliative procedure, preventing propagation of the seizure across the brain, and is not meant to be curative. However, reports suggest that this procedure can result in an 80% to 100% reduction in generalized tonic-clonic and atonic seizures.[32,33] Although mental retardation is common in patients considered for this procedure, outcome seems to be better for those with less severe mental retardation and those with a more focal cerebral abnormality.

When initially described, the corpus callosotomy was performed as a complete resection. Because of the high incidence of the acute disconnection syndrome (mutism, left arm and leg apraxia, and confusion), current practice involves initially performing a limited anterior callosotomy. If results are inadequate, a second procedure can be performed months later to complete the callosotomy. In a report of 18 children undergoing corpus callosotomy by Nordgren,[33] 83% of children had an 80% reduction in seizures. In that report, the acute disconnection syndrome was not seen in any patients.

Overall, the anesthetic considerations for corpus callosotomy are similar to those already described. As noted earlier, patients undergoing corpus callosotomy may have associated cognitive impairment of varying degrees. Preoperative identification of the degree of impairment, methods of communication, and pain behaviors should be discussed with the family, because this facilitates appropriate postoperative care. It is also helpful to discuss the need for preoperative sedation with the parents, because it may not be clear to health care providers. Otherwise, routine anesthetic management used for craniotomy can be used. Intraoperative electrophysiologic monitoring is not usually needed for this procedure and is therefore not a consideration for the anesthetic.

Hemispheric Surgery

Hemispheric resection is the most aggressive surgical intervention, reserved for patients with intractable seizures caused by diffuse hemispheric disease. Basheer and colleagues[34] reported the results of hemispheric surgery in 24 patients over a 10-year period. Diagnosis included malformation of cortical development, infarction, infantile hemiplegia, Sturge-Weber syndrome, and Rasmussen encephalitis. Cerebral hemosiderosis was initially reported superficially as a common complication, which resulted in various modifications of the technique, including the development of peri-insular hemispherotomy, which has been reported to have lower morbidity and mortality. Other complications have included infection and hydrocephalus. Overall, seizure control is reported in the range of 43% to 79%.[9]

Anesthetic considerations for hemispheric surgery are similar to focal resection, with the exception of the high likelihood for transfusion. Basheer and colleagues[34] reported that most children in their series required transfusion of blood products. Therefore, preoperative coagulation studies, cessation of any medication that may affect coagulation, and type and crossmatching for blood products should be performed. Consideration could also be given to preoperative methods for maximizing blood volume, such as erythropoietin (EPO) administration. Although there are no reports of its use with hemispherectomy, tranexamic acid infusion has been used successfully for other cranial procedures,[35] and could be considered. After induction of anesthesia, adequate IV access should be ensured and consideration should be given to central line placement if peripheral access is difficult or blood loss is thought to be likely. Regular monitoring of hematocrit and coagulation should be performed during the procedure, and appropriate transfusion as needed. In addition, unlike patients who have resection of an isolated seizure focus, patients who undergo hemispherectomy frequently have delayed emergence from surgery and anesthesiology, and require transfer to the intensive care unit for weaning from mechanical ventilation.

Other Procedures

Several other surgical procedures have been developed to treat refractory seizures. One such procedure is multiple subpial transections (MST). MST has been used when the seizure focus is either in or near the eloquent cortex. MST involves disruption of peripheral cortical gray matter, in hopes of preserving deeper white matter function to modify the spread of seizure activity. In one review, MST resulted in 68% to 87% of patients having a 95% reduction in seizure frequency. Between 19% and 23% of these patients developed new neurologic deficits.[36] MST is occasionally performed in children.[37,38]

Another uncommon procedure is deep brain stimulation, which was originally described in the 1960s. There are some data to suggest that stimulation of the centro-median thalamic nucleus may reduce seizure frequency in certain patients with intractable seizures, but this remains controversial. Deep brain stimulation is occasionally used in children with intractable seizures who are not candidates for other surgical procedures, and in whom VNS insertion is ineffective or not feasible.[9,39]

SUMMARY

Despite advances in AED therapy, a significant number of pediatric patients with epilepsy have seizures that are not well controlled. In the past 15 years, the surgical options for the treatment of pediatric epilepsy have increased and clarification has evolved regarding the indications for particular surgical procedures. Surgical treatment has become an early therapy of choice in several circumstances. This evolution of surgical techniques, along with the advent of new and improved AEDs, has allowed a significant improvement in the quality of life for children with epilepsy, including improved cognitive function for many patients. It has also resulted in more children with epilepsy coming to surgery. It is therefore important that anesthesiologists caring for children be aware of these advances and the anesthetic implications.

REFERENCES

1. French JA, Pedley TA. Initial management of epilepsy. N Engl J Med 2008;359: 166–76.
2. Go C, Snead OC. Pharmacologically intractable epilepsy in children: diagnosis and preoperative evaluation. Neurosurg Focus 2008;25(3):E2.
3. Homes GL, Ben-Ari Y. Seizures in the developing brain: perhaps not so benign at all. Neuron 1998;21:1231–4.
4. Ben-Ari Y, Holmes GL. Effects of seizures on developmental processes in the immature brain. Lancet Neurol 2006;5:1055–63.
5. Schwartz TH, Jeha L, Tanner A, et al. Late seizures in patients initially seizure free after epilepsy surgery. Epilepsia 2006;47(3):567–73.
6. Duchowny M, Harvey AS. Pediatric epilepsy syndromes: an update and critical review. Epilepsia 1996;37(Suppl 1):S26–40.
7. Wilfong A. Epilepsy syndromes in children. UpToDate; 2012. Available at: http://www.uptodate.com/contents/epilepsy-syndromes-in-children. Accessed March 15, 2012.
8. Camfield P, Camfield C. Epileptic syndromes in childhood: clinical features, outcomes, and treatment. Epilepsia 2002;43(Suppl 3):27–32.
9. Noachtar S, Borggraefe I. Epilepsy surgery; a critical review. Epilepsy Behav 2009;15:66–72.
10. Mason KP, O'Mahony E, Zurakowski D, et al. Effects of dexmedetomidine sedation on the EEG in children. Paediatr Anaesth 2009;19:1175–83.
11. Ebrahim Z, Bulkley R, Roth S. Carbamazepine therapy and neuromuscular blockade with atracurium or vecuronium. Anesth Analg 1988;67:S55.

12. Ornstein E, Matteo R, Schwartz A, et al. The effect of phenytoin on the magnitude and duration of neuromuscular block following atracurium or vecuronium. Anesthesiology 1987;67:191–6.

13. Ornstein E, Matteo R, Young W, et al. Resistance to metocurine-induced neuromuscular blockade in patients receiving phenytoin. Anesthesiology 1985;63: 294–8.

14. Roth S, Ebrahim Z. Resistance to pancuronium in patients receiving carbamazepine. Anesthesiology 1987;66:691–3.

15. Tempelhoff R, Modica P, Jellish W, et al. Resistance to atracurium-induced neuromuscular blockade in patients with intractable seizure disorders treated with anticonvulsants. Anesth Analg 1990;71:665–9.

16. Liberman BA, Norman P, Hardy BG. Pancuronium–phenytoin interaction: a case of decreased duration of neuromuscular blockade. Int J Clin Pharmacol Ther Toxicol 1988;26:371–4.

17. Szenohradszky J, Caldwell JE, Sharma ML, et al. Interaction of rocuronium (ORG 9426) and phenytoin in a patient undergoing cadaver renal transplantation: a possible pharmacokinetic mechanism? Anesthesiology 1994;80:1167–70.

18. Ornstein E, Matteo R, Weinstein J, et al. Accelerated recovery from doxacurium-induced neuromuscular blockade in patients receiving chronic anticonvulsant therapy. J Clin Anesth 1991;3:108–11.

19. Hans P, Ledoux D, Bonhomme V, et al. Effect of anticonvulsant level on pipecuronium-induced neuromuscular blockade: preliminary results. J Neurosurg Anesthesiol 1995;7:254–8.

20. Spacek A, Neiger F, Katz R, et al. Chronic carbamazepine therapy and the duration of neuromuscular blockade (NB) by rocuronium [abstract]. J Neurosurg Anesthesiol 1995;7:319.

21. Fernandez-Candil J, Gambus PL, Troconiz IF, et al. Pharmacokinetic pharmacodynamic modeling of the influence of chronic phenytoin therapy on the rocuronium bromide response in patients undergoing brain surgery. [Recent report underscoring the continued presence of phenytoin-induced resistance to the newer neuromuscular blocking drugs]. Eur J Clin Pharmacol 2008;64: 795–806.

22. Tempelhoff R, Modica P, Spitznagel EJ. Anticonvulsant therapy increases fentanyl requirements during anaesthesia for craniotomy. Can J Anaesth 1990;37:327–32.

23. Centeno RS, Yacubian EM, Sakamoto AC, et al. Pre-surgical evaluation and surgical treatment in children with extratemporal epilepsy. Childs Nerv Syst 2006;22:945–59.

24. Olson DM, Sheehan MG, Thompson W, et al. Sedation of children for electroencephalograms. Pediatrics 2001;108:163–5.

25. McMorrow SP, Abramo TJ. Dexmedetomidine sedation. Pediatr Emerg Care 2012;28(3):292–6.

26. Kumlien E, Doss RC, Gates JR. Treatment outcome in patients with mesial temporal sclerosis. Seizure 2002;11(7):413–7.

27. Ichikawa J, Nishiyama K, Ozaki K, et al. Anesthetic management of a pediatric patient on a ketogenic diet. J Anesth 2006;20:135–7.

28. Englot DJ, Chang EF, Auguste KI. Vagus nerve stimulation for epilepsy: a meta-analysis of efficacy and predictors of response. J Neurosurg 2011;115(6): 1248–55.

29. Benifla M, Rutka JT, Logan W, et al. Vagal nerve stimulation for refractory epilepsy in children: indications and experience at The Hospital for Sick Children. Childs Nerv Syst 2006;22:1018–26.

30. Hatton KW, McLarney JT, Pittman T, et al. Vagal nerve stimulation: overview and implications for anesthesiologists. Anesth Analg 2006;103(5):1241–9.
31. Bekker A, Sturaitis MK. Dexmedetomidine for neurological surgery. Neurosurgery 2005;57(ONS Suppl 1):ONS-1–10.
32. Buchhalter JR, Jarrar RG. Therapeutics in pediatric epilepsy, part 2: epilepsy surgery and vagus nerve stimulation. Mayo Clin Proc 2003;78:371–8.
33. Nordgren RE, Reeves AG, Viguera AC, et al. Corpus callosotomy for intractable seizures in the pediatric age group. Arch Neurol 1991;48:364–72.
34. Basheer SN, Connolly MB, Lautzenhiser A, et al. Hemispheric surgery in children with refractory epilepsy: seizure outcome, complications, and adaptive function. Epilepsia 2007;48(1):133–40.
35. Goobie SM, Meier PM, Pereira LM, et al. Efficacy of tranexamic acid in pediatric craniosynostosis surgery: a double-blind, placebo-controlled trial. Anesthesiology 2011;114(4):862–71.
36. Spencer SS, Shcram J, Wyler A, et al. Multiple subpial transaction for intractable partial epilepsy: an international meta-analysis. Epilepsia 2002;43(2):141–5.
37. Hufnagel A, Zentner J, Fernandez G, et al. Multiple subpial transection for control of epileptic seizures: effectiveness and safety. Epilepsia 1997;38(6):678–88.
38. Tovar-Spinoza Z, Rutgar JT. Multiple subpial transections in children with refractory epilepsy. In: Cataltepe O, Jallo G, editors. Pediatric epilepsy surgery: preoperative assessment and surgical treatment in pediatric patients. New York: Thieme Publishers; 2010. p. 268–71.
39. Kossoff EH, Jallo G. Cortical and deep brain stimulation. In: Cataltepe O, Jallo G, editors. Pediatric epilepsy surgery: preoperative assessment and surgical treatment in pediatric patients. New York: Thieme Publishers; 2010. p. 290–2.

Anesthetic Neurotoxicity

Ansgar M. Brambrink, MD, PhD[a],*, Andrea Orfanakis, MD[a],
Jeffrey R. Kirsch, MD[b]

KEYWORDS

- Anesthetics • Neurotoxicity • Developing brain • Aging brain

KEY POINTS

- Anesthetic agents cause apoptosis of neurons and glia cells and impair neurogenesis in animal models of both the developing and elderly brain.
- There is no evidence from clinical research that could guide a change in clinical practice for either the young or the elderly population, and results from experimental studies require clinical verification before they may be considered relevant in humans. Mechanisms of injury include excitatory neurotransmission, loss of calcium homeostasis, inflammation, and modulation of trophic factors.
- Anesthetic exposure to the developing brain in animal models has shown long-term behavioral, developmental, and cognitive deficits.
- Retrospective analysis of anesthetic exposure in the pediatric population suggests the possibility for behavioral and developmental injury but the causal nature remains uncertain.
- Anesthetic exposure to the elderly brain may cause cognitive dysfunction, which presents early and is temporary.
- Several researchers argue that exposure of the aging brain to anesthesia is not a cause of permanent injury but may unmask existing cognitive disease.

INTRODUCTION

Anesthesiologists have developed a safe perioperative environment to provide anesthesia and analgesia and enable surgical intervention. Although perioperative outcomes are outstanding in many respects, there is increasing concern that both the young and the aged brain might be vulnerable to deleterious effects by many contemporary anesthetic agents.

Strong evidence comes from animal studies that exposure to sedation and anesthesia induces morphologic injury to brain cells and neurocognitive deficits.[1–3] In contrast, the available evidence of potential correlates in humans is ambiguous.[4–6]

[a] Department of Anesthesiology and Perioperative Medicine, Oregon Health and Science University, 3181 SW Sam Jackson Park Road, UHS-2, Portland, OR 97239-3098, USA;
[b] Department of Anesthesiology and Perioperative Medicine, Oregon Health and Science University, 3181 SW Sam Jackson Park Road, KPV 5A; Portland, OR 97239-3098, USA
* Corresponding author.
E-mail address: brambrin@ohsu.edu

Anesthesiology Clin 30 (2012) 207–228
http://dx.doi.org/10.1016/j.anclin.2012.06.002
1932-2275/12/$ – see front matter © 2012 Published by Elsevier Inc.
anesthesiology.theclinics.com

For practical decisions, health care provider and patients are left with a dilemma, because most currently available anesthetics cause harm in animal models and no valid alternatives are available.

The available data do not allow definite conclusions about the relevance of the phenomenon in humans, and therefore no practice changes are currently warranted.

However, concern (at least for the potential toxicity of anesthetics in young children[7]) has led to a consortium between government and scientific organizations that is tasked with guiding the discussions between professionals and society about research and development in this field (see also http://www.smarttots.org).[8,9]

This article explores current data regarding anesthesia-induced brain injury to the developing brain as well as postanesthetic cognitive dysfunction in the aged nervous system, in both animal models and human observational studies.

The Developing Brain

Infants experience pain and stress in response to surgery. Providing adequate analgesia and sedation during surgery or other painful interventions reduces the risk that these individuals will go on to develop hyperalgesia,[10] brain development alterations,[11] and behavioral challenges.[12–14] Nevertheless, the interventions that are available to treat pain, provide sedation, and maintain anesthesia, may cause brain toxicity in human fetuses and infants with prolonged exposure. Thus, there is debate regarding the risk/benefit relationship of administering anesthetics in newborns.[15]

Experimental evidence for anesthetic toxicity in the developing brain

Strong evidence suggests that anesthetic drugs currently used in humans can cause widespread neuroapoptosis in immature mice, rats, pigs, guinea pigs, and nonhuman primates.[1,2] This injury occurs in developing animal brains at doses and durations that are clinically relevant and associated with long-term neurocognitive deficits present weeks and months following the exposure (**Tables 1** and **2**).

Potential mechanisms Most anesthetics interact with γ-aminobutyric acid (GABA$_A$), and/or N-methyl-D-aspartate (NMDA) glutamate receptors. Recent research in this field has evolved from reports of deleterious effects in young rodent brains that had been exposed to NMDA receptor blocking drugs or to ethanol, which both blocks NMDA receptors and activates GABA$_A$ receptors.[16,17] Since these early reports, similar deleterious effects have been reported after exposure to ketamine,[18,19] midazolam,[18,19] propofol,[20] isoflurane,[21–23] sevoflurane,[22–25] desflurane,[23,26] chloral hydrate,[27] and antiepileptic drugs including those that block voltage-gated sodium channels.[28] Studies that tested the combinations of NMDA antagonistic drugs and GABA$_A$-mimetic drugs during 1 exposure showed even potentiated neuroapoptotic effects.[18,19,29]

The morphology and temporal manifestation of anesthesia-induced cell death is consistent with programmed cell death (apoptosis) and involves mechanisms that are characteristic for apoptotic cell death induced by other injury mechanisms.[16–18,30–32] However, little is known about the specific cellular cascades by which anesthetics induce apoptosis in the developing brain. One line of evidence suggests that exposure to anesthetics upregulates cell death–promoting signaling like Bax,[33] p53,[34] and hypoxia inducible factor-1a,[35] and, at the same time, downregulates prosurvival signaling cascades like phosphorylated extracellular signal–regulated protein kinase (pERK),[36–38] Bclx$_L$,[38,39] and Bcl-2.[34,38,40,41] Anesthesia-induced cell death seems to involve mitochondrial injury that results in leakage of cytochrome c into the cytosol,[33,34,38–41] and may trigger intracellular changes culminating in activation of caspase-3.[19,33,42,43] Other reports describe

Table 1
Most recent experimental data (rodents) of anesthetic toxicity in the developing brain

Authors	Animal Species	Anesthetics Tested	Results/Conclusion	Evidence for Toxicity
Kodama et al,[26] 2011	Mouse	Desflurane, isoflurane, or sevoflurane	Desflurane associated with greater degree of apoptosis compared with isoflurane or sevoflurane; impaired memory only found with desflurane exposure	Positive
Zhu et al,[72] 2010	Rat	Isoflurane	Repeated exposure to isoflurane associated with memory deficit and reduction in hippocampal stem cell number	Positive
Zhou et al,[64] 2011	Rat	Nitrous oxide/isoflurane	Exposure associated with increased apoptosis	Positive
De Roo et al,[68] 2009	Rat	Midazolam, propofol, ketamine	Exposure increases dendritic spine density	Negative
Briner et al,[70] 2011	Rat	Propofol	Exposure very early decreased dendritic spine density; exposure early increased spine density and synapse number	Positive/negative
Briner et al,[69] 2010	Rat	Isoflurane, sevoflurane, desflurane	Exposure increased dendritic spine density; no appreciable cell death	Negative
Stratmann et al,[71] 2009	Rat	Isoflurane	Exposure very early impaired memory but exposure in adulthood improved memory	Positive
Jiang et al,[35] 2012	Rat	Isoflurane	Exposure impaired learning and memory	Positive
Yon et al,[39] 2006	Rat	Isoflurane	Exposure at 7 d old but not after 14 d increased apoptosis	Positive
Zou et al,[53] 2008	Rat	Isoflurane/nitrous oxide	Exposure of both volatile agents in combination increased apoptosis but not with the single agent	Positive

Table 2
Experimental evidence (non-human primates [NHP]) of anesthetic toxicity in the developing brain

Authors	Animal Species	Anesthetics Tested	Results/Conclusion	Evidence for Toxicity
Slikker et al,[77] 2007	Monkey	Ketamine	Increased neuronal cell death	Positive
Zou et al,[66] 2009	Monkey	Ketamine	Increased neurodegeneration	Positive
Brambrink et al,[79] 2010	Monkey	Isoflurane	Increased neuroapoptosis	Positive
Brambrink et al,[78] 2012	Monkey	Isoflurane/ketamine	Triggers neuronal and glial apoptosis	Positive
Paule et al,[84] 2011	Monkey	Ketamine	Permanent cognitive deficit	Positive
Brambrink et al,[65] 2012	Monkey	Isoflurane	Apoptosis of oligodendrocytes	Positive
Zou et al,[81] 2011	Monkey	Isoflurane/nitrous oxide	Neuronal apoptosis and necrosis in the 2-gas group but not in either single-gas group	Positive

brain-derived neurotrophic factor (BDNF) –dependent[33,42,44] and death receptor–dependent pathways[45,46] leading to cell destruction. In addition, some investigators suggest that exposure of the developing brain to anesthetics results in an excitotoxic injury.[47–49] The specific timing of ion-transporter protein expression during ontogenetic development results in cellular chloride gradients that are different from those of adults. According to this concept, excitation of the neuronal circuitry results when $GABA_A$ receptors are acutely (over)activated by anesthetics during early development (ie, earlier than the second postnatal week).[50–52]

These observations suggest promising strategies to protect the developing animal brain from anesthesia-induced injury. For example, successful experimental neuroprotection from anesthesia-induced brain injury has been shown using lithium (blocks the reduction of pERK concentration[38]), melatonin (mitochondria membrane stabilizer[39]), xenon (increases Bcl-2 and reduces cytochrome c release and p53 activation[34,40]), dexmedetomidine (reverses Bcl-2 and pERK reduction[38,41]), or L-carnitine (an antioxidant[53]). The experimental blockade of neuronal chloride uptake, the driving force for the proposed $GABA_A$ receptor–mediated depolarization of immature neurons, using bumetanide[54] was neuroprotective in the laboratory. Neuroprotection similarly resulted when anesthesia exposure–associated signaling via the p75 neurotrophin receptor of uncleaved proBDNF was blocked using receptor-specific inhibitors.[55,56] Because anesthesia-induced cell death is apoptotic and therefore requires the execution of specific cellular programs, coadministration of hypothermia, which reduces cell metabolism, was tested for its neuroprotective potential and was shown to completely suppress neuroapoptosis following isoflurane and ketamine exposure.[1] Although these results are preliminary, the therapeutic relevance lies in hypothermia being more commonly used as a therapeutic means to improve outcome after cardiac arrest and hypoxic-ischemic injury in human neonates.

For most of the interventions discussed earlier, it still is uncertain whether they would also ameliorate the neurobehavioral outcomes that have been observed following anesthesia exposure at young age or merely postpone the initiation of the process. Exceptions are dexmedetomidine, which, when coadministered with isoflurane on postnatal day 7, reduced neuronal apoptosis and abolished the memory impairment that was observed in further matured rats that were exposed on postnatal day 7 to isoflurane alone.[41] Beneficial effects were similarly reported after coadministration of erythropoietin to anesthetized mice, which ameliorated both isoflurane-induced neurodegeneration and subsequent learning deficits.[57] Most recent preliminary data suggest that dexmedetomidine provided for 12 hours as the only sedative agent to pregnant rhesus monkeys at gestation age 120 days does not result in significant neuroapoptosis (caspase-3, terminal deoxynucleotide transferase-mediated dUTP nick-end labeling [TUNEL]) in the brain of the fetus 6 hours later, compared with ketamine anesthesia, which induced measurable neuronal injury in the same model.[58]

A conceptual problem of all experimental research in this area is that anesthesia effects to the developing brain have always been evaluated in the absence of noxious stimulation. This limitation has raised concerns that the experimental conditions do not adequately reflect the interaction of anesthesia and surgical stimulation in the clinical environment and therefore the results are not relevant for the human condition. Liu and colleagues[59] recently reported experimental data from a study addressing this issue. Ketamine anesthesia in the presence of continuous sensory stimulation secondary to intraplantar formalin injections resulted in less neuroapoptosis compared with the effects of ketamine in animals that were not injected, confirming the concept that constant peripheral noxious stimulation has the potential to attenuate the neurotoxic potential of ketamine in the neonatal rat brain.[58] Future research is necessary to determine whether the same intervention would also differentially affect the long-term functional outcome after ketamine in this rodent model. It also remains to be shown what the morphologic and functional consequences of general anesthesia are for the developing brain when simultaneously exposed to classic surgical procedures, such as bowel, brain, or heart surgery.

A treatment strategy was recently suggested for anesthesia-induced cognitive decline in developing rodents.[60] Anesthesia-exposed rats (sevoflurane for 4 hours on postnatal day 7) released into an enriched environment starting at 28 days after the exposure had better cognitive function 4 weeks later compared with anesthetized animals that remained in the deprived standard laboratory environment. The neurocognitive capacity of control animals that spent the 4 weeks in the enriched environment also improved, and, at 8 weeks, both the anesthesia-exposed animals and the control animals performed similarly.[60] It is not clear what process was targeted in these experiments and how the results could be applied clinically, because children are already exposed daily to an enriched environment compared with that of rodents in a standard laboratory setting.

Regions/cell types affected Neuroapoptosis affects all brain regions, but is more pronounced in regions that receive and integrate sensory information through both visual and auditory association pathways, which are critical for normal neurocognitive function. In fetal brains of nonhuman primates that were exposed to anesthetics in utero, we observed thalamus and basal ganglia injury, mirroring observations in human children[61–63] exposed in utero to alcohol or antiepileptic drugs. Although anesthetic exposure seems to affect glutamatergic, GABAergic, and dopaminergic neurons in the young, it exclusively spares cholinergic neurons in the basal forebrain.[64]

Exposure to anesthetics does not only affect neurons but also glia cells, as we recently observed in immature nonhuman primate brains. This injury involves young oligodendroglia that undergo apoptosis in larger numbers following exposure to anesthetics,[65,66] as they do after exposure to alcohol.[67] Oligodendrocytes myelinate axons that interconnect neurons throughout the developing brain, and the deletion of these cells may have neurobehavioral consequences that would be additive to those of anesthesia-induced neuroapoptosis.[66] It also remains unclear whether the window of oligodendroglial vulnerability to anesthetic exposure parallels that of neurons or is further extended, given the ongoing myelination in later childhood.

Exposure to anesthetics also affects neuronal dendrites and synapsis. For example, the number of immature dendritic spines and synapses was reduced in developing murine brain exposed to isoflurane, which is assumed to be mediated via anesthetic-induced p75 receptor signaling.[55,56] Other studies show that isoflurane, sevoflurane, desflurane, and propofol uniformly reduced synaptic spine density in newborn rodents but not in rodents that were 16 to 25 days old.[68-70]

Equally concerning is that exposure to anesthetics also seems to affect proliferation and differentiation of newborn neurons. Even more importantly, the impairment of neurogenesis, particularly after multiple anesthetic exposures, seems persistent and associated with long-term neurocognitive deficits that became progressively more severe with advancing age.[71,72] These results echo findings in neonatal rodents treated with ethanol[73] or various sedatives and anticonvulsants[74] that, later in life, showed a permanent reduction in the number of dentate hippocampal neurons and persistent neurocognitive deficits.

Window of vulnerability In the developing brain, anesthetics seem to be particularly deleterious during the period of rapid synaptogenesis, the so-called brain growth spurt.[16,18] However, the timing varies between species and is considered for rodents to occur in the early postnatal period, whereas in humans synaptogenesis continuous from about midgestation to several years after birth[75,76] and therefore vulnerability to anesthetics in humans may extend beyond infancy. In addition, it is possible that the window of vulnerability varies for certain subgroups of brain cells.

Retrospective studies in humans suggest an increased risk for neurobehavioral deficits when anesthesia is provided to patients less than the age of 1 to 4 years. Studies on nonhuman primates have high translational relevance as long as it is taken into consideration that neurodevelopmental milestones are reached at slightly different ontogenetic times. For instance, a third trimester rhesus fetus corresponds approximately with a human neonate, whereas a rhesus infant 5 or 6 days old is approximately equivalent to a 6-month old human infant.[75,76] Based on these considerations, data from nonhuman primates from our own laboratory and that of others support the concerns for an extended period of vulnerability. For example, ketamine anesthesia in the pregnant rhesus macaques induced fetal neuroapoptosis in the beginning of the third trimester,[77,78] and, in infants of the same species that were 5 to 6 days old, general anesthesia using isoflurane,[65,79] ketamine,[66,77,78,80] or nitrous oxide plus isoflurane[81] resulted in widespread apoptotic cell death. We also observed that isoflurane induced more severe damage in the neonatal than the fetal brain, whereas, with ketamine exposure, the relationship was reversed,[78,80] indicating that vulnerability to a certain drug likely also depends on the developmental age at the time of exposure to that particular anesthetic agent. Thus, we suggest that human outcome research should include children who were exposed to anesthesia in utero or as premature infants.

Besides age at exposure, peak vulnerability likely varies for the different cell type (neurons, glia, and stem cells), and also depends on the drug or drug combinations and the doses applied. It remains unclear whether one or the other, or even a combination of the mechanisms mentioned earlier, leads to the neurobehavior deficits in humans, because they have been observed at a later age in rodents[18,24,29,60,72,82,83] and in nonhuman primates.[84]

Clinical evidence for anesthetic toxicity in the developing brain

Although early laboratory observations of neurotoxic effects of anesthetics were fundamentally challenged,[85–87] more recent epidemiologic studies suggest that the experimental observations may have relevance in the human (**Table 3**). Although mostly large and reasonably well controlled, the data from these retrospective studies provide an inconclusive picture.[4,5] Nevertheless, several reports suggest an increased risk for neurobehavioral disturbances following anesthesia exposure during the first years of life and suggest age at exposure, number of exposures, and total duration of anesthesia as potentially important variables.

In a large cohort of children enrolled in the NY Medicaid system, the exposure to anesthesia before age 3 years more than doubled the risk for behavioral disorders during later childhood compared with a matched control group of children who were not exposed. The risk was even higher in those children who were exposed twice or more during the first 3 years of life.[88] A subsequent analysis of a birth cohort of siblings from the same database suggests a 60% greater risk of being diagnosed with behavioral disorders for children who were exposed to surgery under general anesthesia compared with siblings who were not exposed to surgery or anesthetic agents.[89]

An analysis of a county-wide database (Mayo Clinic) revealed that the risk for learning disabilities was not increased when young children (<age 4 years) received a single general anesthetic. Children exposed to 2 or more anesthetics (median duration 75 minutes) before the age of 2 years (independent of comorbidities) had a 2-fold higher hazard ratio for the development of learning disabilities, and anesthesia durations beyond 2 hours were associated with the highest risk.[90,91] Results based on the same database suggest that repeated anesthesia exposure before age 2 years, independently of comorbidities, doubles the risk for the diagnosis of attention-deficit/hyperactivity disorder until age 19 years.[92] Others, although relying on smaller sample sizes, found that anesthesia before 1 year of age was particularly concerning. For example, in one study anesthesia exposure dose dependently increased the risk to score very low in school achievement tests compared with the population norm,[93] and, in another study, exposure as an infant increased the risk to develop neurocognitive impairments compared with children who were older at the time of anesthesia exposure.[94] However, these results are in contrast with findings from some population studies. For example, a large national database failed to identify evidence for impaired academic achievement in children who were exposed to 1 short anesthetic (30–60 minutes) as an infant.[95] Another nationwide study on monozygotic twins showed that, in those twin pairs in which 1 twin was exposed to anesthesia and the other twin was not, the academic achievements were similar between the two.[96]

These studies suggest that the phenomenon of anesthetic-induced brain injury in early development may also exist in the human and suggests the need for further prospective clinical studies. In particular, these studies report only associations and, because of their inherent methodological limitations as well as their limited focus, a causal relationship in the human cannot be proven. Two large, multicenter, randomized clinical trials are underway to further clarify the relationship.[97–100]

Methodological concerns involve the data quality, because all studies used observational data that were collected for other purposes, and some even included information from parental interviews. It is also a concern that the anesthesia data used for associations involving current neurocognitive status reflect clinical practice that dates back several decades. Since then, many anesthetic practices have changed significantly, including the choice of drugs and standard of care for monitoring during anesthesia (eg, quantitative measurements of anesthetic gases; capnometry/capnography; pulse oximetry).

Table 3
Retrospective clinical data of anesthetic toxicity in the developing brain

Authors	Study Design	Type of Exposure	Results/Conclusion	Evidence for Toxicity
DiMaggio et al,[88] 2009	Retrospective analysis of patients on NY Medicaid	Exposure to surgery before 3 y of age	Increased incidence of developmental or behavioral disorder	Positive association
DiMaggio et al,[89] 2011	Retrospective analysis of state Medicaid program participants	Children exposed to surgery before 3 y of age compared with their siblings not exposed to surgery	Increased incidence of developmental or behavioral disorder compared with siblings without surgical event	Positive
Wilder et al,[90] 2009	Population-based retrospective birth cohort	Children exposed to anesthesia and surgery before 4 y of age	Single exposure to anesthesia was not associated with learning disability but 2 or more exposures was a risk factor	Positive
Hansen et al,[95] 2011	Retrospective analysis	Children exposed to inguinal hernia repair and anesthesia within 1 y of life	No association with reduction in academic performance as teenagers if exposed to a single anesthetic and surgery	Negative
Bartels et al,[96] 2009	Retrospective analysis of monozygotic twins	Children exposed to anesthesia before age 3 y and between 3 and 12 y of age	Exposure to anesthesia before age 3 y associated with lower educational achievement, although unexposed co-twin did not differ from the twin sibling, eliminating a causal relationship	Negative

Several investigations are limited to subjects exposed only briefly or once to anesthetic drugs. There are other concerns about study-specific biases resulting from selective and non–population-based databases (eg, Medicare recipients), the absence of information about the indication for anesthesia, the drugs used, the number of exposures and duration of the anesthetic, and a lack of control for other confounders like socioeconomic status or family conditions. Several researchers reanalyzed existing databases and were able to use more information to further clarify the role of putative confounders such as duration of exposure, combination of drugs, and developmental age at exposure. Until data from these and other relevant research projects become available, it will remain a matter of debate whether the experimental data reflect what happens in the developing human brain under various anesthesia exposure conditions.

The Aging Brain

Anesthesia and surgery may also pose risks to the aging brain.[3,6] The elderly population is at risk for neurocognitive dysfunction following hospitalization for injury and illness without exposure to surgery and anesthesia. This risk is most clearly seen in the clinical state of delirium. Advanced age is an independent risk factor for development of delirium. Delirium poses significant risk for an increase in morbidity and mortality associated with hospitalization incurring increased hospital days, increased ventilator days, increased mortality, and an increase in posthospitalization cognitive impairment.[101] Sedation has been linked to an increase in delirium but it is not known whether this causal association can be broadened to include the pharmacologic agents most common in anesthesia.

Although the recognition and diagnosis of delirium has been well studied, including standardization of diagnostic tools and algorithms, the more subtle diagnosis of cognitive dysfunction, specifically postoperative cognitive dysfunction (POCD), lacks commonly accepted means with which to identify and treat in the perioperative period, and some investigators propose that it frequently goes unrecognized and therefore is likely underreported.[102] Neuropsychological testing is the most sensitive method to diagnose cognitive impairment or dysfunction. Patients rarely, if ever, arrive for surgery having previously completed this analysis. Should it be attempted immediately after surgery, neuropsychological testing could be clouded by comorbid conditions such as pain, immobility, administered pharmacologic agents, and the possibility of hospital-acquired delirium.[103]

Clinical evidence for anesthetic toxicity in the aging brain

Despite the limitations posed, several groups have attempted this analysis and evaluated patients' neurocognitive function in the weeks, months, and years following a surgical and anesthetic event (**Table 4**). Two broad categories exist in this area of study: the cardiac and the noncardiac surgical populations.

Post–cardiac surgery cognitive dysfunction has been the center of attention for many years. In particular, multiple studies have been designed to evaluate the degree of risk associated with cardiopulmonary bypass (ie, on-pump vs off-pump coronary artery bypass).[104] Several small studies have identified cardiopulmonary bypass as a strong risk factor for cognitive dysfunction.[105] A larger study completed through the Veteran's Affairs medical centers showed no difference in neuropsychological testing at 1 year when comparing on-pump with off-pump coronary artery bypass patient groups.[106] Despite the lack of evidence to clearly associate cardiopulmonary bypass with neurologic injury, these studies have shown an increased risk for cognitive dysfunction following cardiac surgery both in the early and late postoperative

Table 4
Observational clinical studies of anesthetic toxicity in the aged brain

Authors	Study Design	Results/Conclusion	Evidence for Toxicity
Diegeler et al,[104] 2000	Off-pump vs conventional coronary bypass	Neurocognitive impairment associated with cardiopulmonary bypass	Positive but confounded by cardiopulmonary bypass
Shroyer et al,[106] 2009	On-pump vs off-pump coronary artery bypass surgery	No difference between groups in neurocognitive testing at 1 y	Negative for association with cardiopulmonary bypass
Moller et al,[107] 1998	Observational study of incidence of postoperative cognitive dysfunction	Age is the greatest risk factor for late cognitive dysfunction	Positive
Williams-Russo et al,[108] 1995	Comparison of epidural vs general anesthesia for orthopedic surgery	No difference between groups in incidence of short-term or long-term postoperative cognitive dysfunction	Negative
Evered et al,[109] 2011	Retrospective analysis of regional, general anesthesia, cardiac, and noncardiac surgery	POCD is not associated with type of surgery or type of anesthetic	Negative
Heyer et al,[124] 2002	Incidence of POCD following endarterectomy vs spinal surgery	Cognitive dysfunction at 30 d noted only in endarterectomy group	Positive association with surgery but not anesthesia
Avidan,[111] 2009	Observational study of patients with and without dementia exposed to illness or noncardiac surgery	Anesthesia and surgery do not increase incidence of long-term POCD or alter trajectory of baseline disease	Negative
Monk et al,[125] 2008	Observational study of cognitive dysfunction in noncardiac surgery	Age is a significant risk factor for cognitive dysfunction following noncardiac surgery. POCD associated with increase in mortality	Positive
Mracek et al,[126] 2012	General vs local anesthesia for carotid endarterectomy	General anesthesia impaired cognitive function immediately after surgery, but not greater than 1 wk	Negative long term
An et al,[127] 2011	Incidence of POCD in deep vs light total IV anesthetic for neurosurgery	Decreased incidence of POCD in patients exposed to deep vs light anesthetic	Negative
Jankowski et al,[128] 2011	Cognitive function and incidence of postoperative delirium in an elderly population	Postoperative delirium did not predict long-term cognitive decline	Negative long term

stages. However, if previously suspected hypoxemic and embolic events associated with cardiopulmonary bypass are not the clear culprit, it remains unclear what the reasons are that lead to the postoperative deficit after cardiac surgery. Potential mechanism include the induction of a systemic disease state such as poor cardiac output, direct effects of the surgical intervention that result in upregulation of inflammation, or the exposure to anesthetic agents.

Patients who had not had cardiac surgery have less frequently been subjects of systematic clinical studies regarding POCD. The most well known is the International Study of Post-Operative Cognitive Dysfunction (ISPOCD) investigation. ISPOCD was originally designed to study hypotension and hypoxemia as causes of injury, and found age to be the strongest risk factor for late-appearing cognitive dysfunction. Repeat operation, lower education level, infection, and respiratory failure seemed to be risk factors for early cognitive dysfunction. This well-powered study suggests that POCD in noncardiac surgery is a real and present danger and urges further investigation into methods to risk stratify, mitigate, and treat this perioperative complication.[107]

However, similar to the situation in the young, it remains a challenge to design adequate studies that could identify the injurious factor as either surgery or anesthesia or the individual patient.

One way to explore this question further is to proceed with a design that explores neurocognitive deficits in a setting of surgery that can be conducted equally well under general or regional anesthesia.

Williams-Russo and colleagues[108] found no difference in change from baseline cognitive function between 2 groups randomized to epidural versus general anesthesia for total knee replacement surgery with a median age 69 years. The study was well powered to detect a difference in neuropsychological testing and identified a 5% incidence of long-term POCD in the overall group. Age again seemed to be a risk factor for POCD. However, no control group was exposed to either anesthetic without surgery, which made it impossible to evaluate surgery or anesthesia as an independent risk factor for POCD in this data set.

Evered and colleagues[109] expanded on these observations when they evaluated type of anesthetic, invasive degree of surgical procedure, and preoperative cognitive function as independent risk factors for POCD. Increase in early POCD was greater in the cardiac surgery group but, at 3 months after surgery, group differences had disappeared. The investigators concluded that POCD incidence at 3 months was independent of type of surgery or anesthetic.

Others have called into question the general role of anesthesia or surgery in the development of persistent cognitive dysfunction, and instead consider POCD a factor of the patient's baseline functional status, proposing that exposure to anesthesia or surgery does not accelerate the course of mental disease that is already present.

Avidan and Evers[110] argue that POCD is overdiagnosed and that most patients recover full function in the long term. In contrast, those who do exhibit permanent disability are showing the normal trajectory of their native disease state, which is independent of anesthesia or surgery according to this group's analysis.[111]

Several population-based studies have been performed to detect the incidence of cognitive dysfunction in age-matched cohorts exposed to surgery versus no surgery. Such endeavor can be difficult because multiple variables in health status and illness make matching and analysis nearly impossible to determine the causal nature of the exposure.

Avidan and colleagues[111] attempted this analysis to support their theory that the normal trajectory of dementia is both misunderstood and difficult to diagnose before surgery, and that neuropsychological testing in prior postoperative exposure studies overestimated the incidence of POCD and its association with long-term cognitive decline. Avidan and Evers[110] followed 575 patients who either had no evidence of dementia or mild or very mild dementia. Patients were followed after exposure to surgery, illness, or no events. A percentage of the group without evidence of dementia did go on to develop dementia but this was not different among those exposed to illness, surgery, or no event. Those with a diagnosis of dementia at day 0 did decline more rapidly than their no-dementia counterparts but their trajectory was not accelerated by exposure to illness or surgery compared with the control group. The investigators concluded that surgery and anesthesia do not accelerate progression to dementia or increase incidence of persistent cognitive dysfunction. This well-designed study has two relevant limitations that warrant mentioning. First, to diagnose POCD, it is important to complete neuropsychological testing within weeks or months of the surgical or illness event, and then to repeat testing within the year. Participants in this study were evaluated yearly. Second, POCD was considered insignificant if it was temporal rather than permanent. Even if the effect is temporary, POCD can be a significant hindrance to inpatient recovery, to a patient's quality of life, and to the ability to return to baseline, and is therefore worthy of investigation to both avoid and treat. Nevertheless, data in this important field of clinical research continue to accumulate and remain both controversial and contradictory.

Experimental evidence for anesthetic toxicity in the aged brain

The laboratory allows in-depth analysis of the extent and mechanism of potential toxic effects of anesthetics on the aging brain by modeling what manifests clinically as POCD in the human. The mechanistic concepts currently receiving the greatest levels of interest to explain detrimental effects of anesthetics on the adult brain include direct toxic effects involving glutamate receptor function and intracellular calcium regulation (excitotoxic injury), alteration of protein integrity and degradation leading to protein deposits similar to those seen in Alzheimer disease (neurodegenerative process), and activation of inflammatory cascades attacking exiting neuronal circuits and neuroplasticity of hippocampal stem cells (immunomodulative mechanism). Experimental models to investigate toxic effects of anesthetics to the aging brain have been developed predominantly in rats, mice, and in ex vivo and in vitro cultures, mostly to explore potential mechanisms. **Table 5** summarizes selected experimental studies that evaluate effects of anesthesia on learning and memory in aged animals, in some cases in combination with an exploration of histologic and biochemical end points. Representative reports that highlight the currently controversial discussion about potential pathomechanisms are discussed in more detail below.

Mawhinney and colleagues[112] exposed aged rats (18 months old) to 4 hours of inhalational anesthetic (nitrous oxide and isoflurane) and evaluated for learning and memory at 2 weeks and 3 months. The animals exposed to anesthesia showed spatial memory impairment at these time points, whereas animals that were not exposed (controls) were not impaired. Analysis of hippocampal and neocortical protein lysates showed altered (increased) expression of the NMDA receptor subunit NR2B and a reduction in extracellular signal-regulated kinase (ERK) 1/2 in the anesthesia-exposed rats, suggesting that disruption of NMDA receptor–mediated signaling pathways in the hippocampus and cortex may lead to the spatial learning deficits observed.

Another potential mechanism is closely related to the excitotoxic pathway outlined earlier but involves the disruption of the cytosolic calcium homeostasis that is well known to damage neurons in other types of brain injury.[113,114] In vitro models of neuronal exposure to isoflurane support the theory that inhalational anesthetics may affect the intracellular calcium regulation via activation of endoplasmic reticular

Table 5
Experimental data of anesthetic toxicity in the aged brain

Authors	Animal Species	Anesthetics Tested	Results/Conclusion	Evidence for Toxicity
Wang et al,[129] 2012	Rats	Isoflurane	Exposure associated with impaired learning and memory	Positive
Lin et al,[130] 2012	Rats	Isoflurane	Exposure associated with impaired learning and memory, although no permanent neuropathologic changes noted	Positive
Mawhinney et al,[112] 2012	Rats	Isoflurane	Exposure associated with impaired spatial memory and altered protein expression in NMDA receptor–mediated pathway	Positive
Liu et al,[119] 2012	Rats	Isoflurane	Exposure associated with impaired spatial memory but no appreciable increase in biomarkers of Alzheimer disease	Positive
Stratman et al,[122] 2010	Rats	Isoflurane	No effect on cell death, hippocampal neurogenesis, or long-term cognitive outcome	Negative
Callaway et al,[131] 2012	Rats	Isoflurane	No effect on memory of middle-aged rats	Negative
Culley et al,[132] 2004	Rats	Isoflurane/nitrous oxide	Long-term impairment of spatial memory associated with exposure	Positive

calcium release receptors leading to dangerously high levels of cytosolic calcium and subsequent mitochondrial dysfunction and injury.[115]

Although in vitro models suggested this mechanism, only evidence from ex vivo experiments has so far confirmed this pathway as potentially relevant for anesthesia-induced injury to adult neurons. An example is the work of Zhan and colleagues,[116] who noted an increase in intracellular calcium in hippocampal slices of aging rats following exposure to isoflurane. Whether or not intracellular calcium-level dysregulation is a relevant independent mechanism that results in injury leading to cognitive deficit in the aged brain after exposure to anesthesia requires further investigation involving appropriate in vivo models that assess functional outcome following mechanistic interventions targeting the proposed mechanism.

Loss of protein integrity and protein degradation are processes that may lead to cell death and cognitive dysfunction, as seen in Alzheimer disease. Researchers were intrigued and began to explore this mechanism of injury to explain anesthesia-induced cognitive deficits in the aged brain. Xie and colleagues[117] were able to show that rats exposed to isoflurane developed an increase in caspase activation and Alzheimer disease–associated protein aggregation in neurons 24 hours after a clinically relevant dose of inhalational anesthetic. Perucho and colleagues[118] showed that repetitive isoflurane anesthesia (twice a week for 3 months) results in increased mortality, long-lasting neurobehavioral deficits, increased proapoptotic proteins and neuroapoptosis in the hippocampus, reduced astroglial and increased microglial responses, increased A-β aggregates and high-molecular-weight peptides, abnormal chaperone responses, and reduced autophagy in mice transgenic for Alzheimer disease but not in wild-type mice. The data led the investigators to conclude that anesthesia-induced neurodegeneration and its behavioral consequences in the adult seems restricted to the susceptible brain but does not affect the healthy nervous system. Liu and colleagues[119] explored the same concept, focusing on volatile agent neurotoxicity through deposition of hyperphosphorylated tau proteins and amyloid plaques and their respective functional consequences. They noted spatial memory impairment in aged rats exposed to isoflurane several days after exposure but, in contrast with the two groups mentioned earlier, did not find concomitant increases in amyloid β and tau phosphorylation. Protein degradation may present in the early period following exposure of adult neurons to volatile anesthetics, but whether these molecular changes are the source of POCD in the elderly requires further investigation.

Inflammation has been suggested as a pathway to various neurodegenerative insults including Alzheimer disease and Huntington disease. However, neuroinflammation is potentially detrimental outside the development of Alzheimer disease and may be a pathway to injury of its own. Wu and colleagues[120] examined mouse brain tissues following exposure to isoflurane and noted increases in messenger RNA and protein expression of such markers as tumor necrosis factor α, interleukin (IL)-6, and IL-1β. They also noted increased levels of inflammation in transgenic Alzheimer disease mice compared with wild-type mice, suggesting the propensity of isoflurane to accelerate an existing neurodegenerative process. However, the role of surgery in the development of inflammation cannot be ignored this context. Rosczyk and colleagues[121] studied mice of varying ages following minor surgery, with learning and memory tasks as well as histologic analysis for markers of inflammation. Adult mice did not seem to decline in memory or learning and histologically did not show an increase in neuroinflammation. However, aged mice did show slight neurocognitive decline as well as an increase in hippocampal cytokine levels consistent with neuroinflammation. The question then remains whether anesthesia, surgery, or both contribute to the inflammatory process and in what manner can either be changed to mitigate injury.

Some experimental data question whether a single anesthetic exposure can effectively injure the aged brain and induce measureable long-term neurocognitive deficit. Stratmann and colleagues[122] exposed aged rats (16 months old) to isoflurane and assessed functional status and histopathology at 4 months. At that time, anesthesia-exposed animals showed no evidence for ongoing cell death, impaired hippocampal neurogenesis, or long-term cognitive impairment, and were not different from the nonexposed control animals.

Based on the controversial evidence presented earlier, more clinical and experimental work is needed before definite conclusions can be drawn about incidence, presentation, and potential mechanisms of postoperative cognitive impairment in humans, and to determine whether anesthesia or surgery can cause persistent neurologic decline or precipitate dementia in the elderly.

SUMMARY

Concerns for toxic effects of anesthesia to the brains of the young and the elderly are mounting. However, although the experimental evidence for such effects in the developing brain is strong, the phenomenon is still disputed in the aged brain.

For the developing brain, anesthetic neurotoxicity has been described in a variety of different mammal species, including nonhuman primates, and several pathomechanisms have been proposed. Nevertheless, knowledge of the underlying mechanisms is still scarce and debate continues as to whether human infants and children are also at risk for anesthetic neurotoxicity. The only currently available clinical evidence comes from retrospective studies and suggests an association between exposure to anesthesia at young age (<3 years of age) and neurobehavioral disturbances during later development, but the same data do not show whether this is a causal relationship.

In contrast, the phenomenon of postoperative cognitive deterioration in elderly patients remains controversial. Time course, severity, and whether or not it persists long term are under debate. Some investigators argue that there is little clinical evidence to support a link between surgery or anesthesia and dementia.

There is no evidence from clinical research that could guide a change in clinical practice for both patient groups, and results from experimental studies require clinical verification before they may be recommended. Moreover, even if clinical evidence were available to fundamentally challenge current perioperative practice and show that anesthetics render dose-dependent neurotoxic effects on the developing and on the aged brain, the lack of alternatives to the current practice would pose a challenge to the health care system. Changes in drug selection, dosage, and duration may then be acutely considered if no pharmacologic tools are available that allow the provision of anesthesia without neurotoxic effects to the young or the elderly.

Meanwhile, it is imperative to conduct well-designed human trials to determine the clinical risk, to identify key confounding variables, and to support relevant translational research that focuses on prevention of anesthetic neurotoxicity, on noninvasive diagnosis of injury,[123] on postexposure treatment, and on pharmacologic innovation to successfully tackle this critical issue.

REFERENCES

1. Creeley CE, Olney JW. The young: neuroapoptosis induced by anesthetics and what to do about it [review]. Anesth Analg 2010;110:442–8.
2. Stratmann G. Neurotoxicity of anesthetic drugs in the developing brain [review]. Anesth Analg 2011;113:1170–9.

3. Hudson AE, Hemmings HC. Are anaesthetics toxic to the brain? [review]. Br J Anaesth 2011;107:30–7.
4. Sun L. Early childhood general anaesthesia exposure and neurocognitive development [review]. Br J Anaesth 2010;105(Suppl 1):i61–8.
5. Hughes CG, Pandharipande PP. The effects of perioperative and intensive care unit sedation on brain organ dysfunction [review]. Anesth Analg 2011;112:1212–7.
6. Monk TG, Price CC. Postoperative cognitive disorders [review]. Curr Opin Crit Care 2011;17:376–81.
7. Kuehn BM. FDA considers data on potential risks of anesthesia use in infants, children. JAMA 2011;305:1749–50, 1753.
8. Jevtovic-Todorovic V. Pediatric anesthesia neurotoxicity: an overview of the 2011 SmartTots panel. Anesth Analg 2011;113:965–8.
9. Ramsay JG, Rappaport BA. SmartTots: a multidisciplinary effort to determine anesthetic safety in young children. Anesth Analg 2011;113(5):963–4.
10. Ruda MA, Ling QD, Hohmann AG, et al. Altered nociceptive neuronal circuits after neonatal peripheral inflammation. Science 2000;289:628–31.
11. Anand KJ, Scalzo FM. Can adverse neonatal experiences alter brain development and subsequent behavior. Biol Neonate 2000;77:69–82.
12. Simons SH, van Dijk M, Anand KJS, et al. Do we still hurt newborn babies? A prospective study of procedural pain and analgesia in neonates. Arch Pediatr Adolesc Med 2003;157:1058–64.
13. Bouza H. The impact of pain in the immature brain. J Matern Fetal Neonatal Med 2009;22:722–32.
14. Huang W, Deprest J, Missant C, et al. Management of fetal pain during invasive fetal procedures: a review. Acta Anaesthesiol Belg 2004;55:119–23.
15. Davidson AJ. Neurotoxicity and the need for anesthesia in the newborn: does the emperor have no clothes? Anesthesiology 2012;116:507–9.
16. Ikonomidou C, Bosch F, Miksa M, et al. Blockade of NMDA receptors and apoptotic neurodegeneration in the developing brain. Science 1999;283:70–4.
17. Ikonomidou C, Bittigau P, Ishimaru MJ, et al. Ethanol-induced apoptotic neurodegeneration and fetal alcohol syndrome. Science 2000;287:1056–60.
18. Jevtovic-Todorovic V, Hartman RE, Izumi Y, et al. Early exposure to common anesthetic agents causes widespread neurodegeneration in the developing rat brain and persistent learning deficits. J Neurosci 2003;23:876–82.
19. Young C, Jevtovic-Todorovic V, Qin YQ, et al. Potential of ketamine and midazolam, individually or in combination, to induce apoptotic neurodegeneration in the infant mouse brain. Br J Pharmacol 2005;146:189–97.
20. Cattano D, Young C, Olney JW. Sub-anesthetic doses of propofol induce neuroapoptosis in the infant mouse brain. Anesth Analg 2008;106:1712–4.
21. Johnson SA, Young C, Olney JW. Isoflurane-induced neuroapoptosis in the developing brain of non-hypoglycemic mice. J Neurosurg Anesthesiol 2008; 20:21–8.
22. Liang G, Ward C, Peng J, et al. Isoflurane causes greater neurodegeneration than an equivalent exposure of sevoflurane in the developing brain of neonatal mice. Anesthesiology 2010;112:1325–34.
23. Istaphanous GK, Howard J, Nan X, et al. Comparison of the neuroapoptotic properties of equipotent anesthetic concentrations of desflurane, isoflurane, or sevoflurane in neonatal mice. Anesthesiology 2011;114:578–87.
24. Zhang X, Xue Z, Sun A. Subclinical concentration of sevoflurane potentiates neuronal apoptosis in the developing C57BL/6 mouse brain. Neurosci Lett 2008;447:109–14.

25. Satomoto M, Satoh Y, Terui K, et al. Neonatal exposure to sevoflurane induces abnormal social behaviors and deficits in fear conditioning in mice. Anesthesiology 2009;110:628–37.

26. Kodama M, Satoh Y, Otsubo Y, et al. Neonatal desflurane exposure induces more robust neuroapoptosis than do isoflurane and sevoflurane and impairs working memory. Anesthesiology 2011;115:979–91.

27. Cattano D, Straiko MM, Olney JW. Chloral hydrate induces and lithium prevents neuroapoptosis in the infant mouse brain. Am Soc Anesthesiol Annual Meeting 2008; #A315 published online. Available at: http://www.asaabstracts.com. Accessed June 20, 2012.

28. Bittigau P, Sifringer M, Genz K, et al. Antiepileptic drugs and apoptotic neurodegeneration in the developing brain. Proc Natl Acad Sci U S A 2002;99:15089–94.

29. Fredriksson A, Ponten E, Gordh T, et al. Neonatal exposure to a combination of N-methyl-D-aspartate and γ-aminobutyric acid type A receptor anesthetic agents potentiates apoptotic neurodegeneration and persistent behavioral deficits. Anesthesiology 2007;107:427–36.

30. Dikranian K, Ishimaru MJ, Tenkova T, et al. Apoptosis in the in vivo mammalian forebrain. Neurobiol Dis 2001;8:359–79.

31. Dikranian K, Qin YQ, Labruyere J, et al. Ethanol-induced neuroapoptosis in the developing rodent cerebellum and related brain stem structures. Dev Brain Res 2005;155:1–13.

32. Tenkova T, Young C, Dikranian K, et al. Ethanol-induced apoptosis in the visual system during synaptogenesis. Invest Ophthalmol Vis Sci 2003;44:2809–17.

33. Young C, Klocke J, Tenkova T, et al. Ethanol-induced neuronal apoptosis in the in vivo developing mouse brain is BAX dependent. Cell Death Differ 2003;10:1148–55.

34. Shu Y, Patel SM, Pac-Soo C, et al. Xenon pretreatment attenuates anesthetic-induced apoptosis in the developing brain in comparison with nitrous oxide and hypoxia. Anesthesiology 2010;113:360–8.

35. Jiang H, Huang Y, Xu H, et al. Hypoxia inducible factor-1α is involved in the neurodegeneration induced by isoflurane in the brain of neonatal rats. J Neurochem 2012;120:453–60.

36. Young C, Straiko MM, Johnson SA, et al. Ethanol causes and lithium prevents neuroapoptosis and suppression of pERK in the infant mouse brain. Neurobiol Dis 2008;31:355–60.

37. Straiko MM, Young C, Cattano D, et al. Lithium protects against anesthesia-induced developmental neuroapoptosis. Anesthesiology 2009;110:662–8.

38. Sanders RD, Sun P, Patel S, et al. Dexmedetomidine provides cortical neuroprotection: impact on anaesthetic-induced neuroapoptosis in the rat developing brain. Acta Anaesthesiol Scand 2010;54:710–6.

39. Yon JH, Carter LB, Jevtovic-Todorovic V. Melatonin reduces the severity of anesthesia-induced apoptotic neurodegeneration in the developing rat brain. Neurobiol Dis 2006;21:522–30.

40. Ma D, Williamson P, Januszewski A, et al. Xenon mitigates isoflurane-induced neuronal apoptosis in the developing rodent brain. Anesthesiology 2007;106:746–53.

41. Sanders RD, Xu J, Shu Y, et al. Dexmedetomidine attenuates isoflurane-induced neurocognitive impairment in neonatal rats. Anesthesiology 2009;110:1077–85.

42. Olney JW, Tenkova T, Dikranian K, et al. Ethanol-induced caspase-3 activation in the in vivo developing mouse brain. Neurobiol Dis 2002;9:205–19.

43. Young C, Roth KA, Klocke BJ, et al. Role of caspase-3 in ethanol-induced developmental neurodegeneration. Neurobiol Dis 2005;20:608–14.

44. Pearn ML, Hu Y, Niesman IR, et al. Propofol neurotoxicity is mediated by p75 neurotrophin receptor activation. Anesthesiology 2012;116:352–61.
45. Yon JH, Daniel-Johnson J, Carter LB, et al. Anesthesia induces suicide in the developing rat brain via the intrinsic and extrinsic apoptotic pathways. Neuroscience 2005;135:815–27.
46. Lu LX, Yon JH, Carter LB, et al. General anesthesia activates BDNF-dependent neuroapoptosis in the developing rat brain. Apoptosis 2006;11:1603–15.
47. Zhao YL, Xiang Q, Shi QY, et al. GABAergic excitotoxicity injury of the immature hippocampal pyramidal neurons' exposure to isoflurane. Anesth Analg 2011; 113:1152–60.
48. Boscolo A, Starr JA, Sanchez V, et al. The abolishment of anesthesia-induced cognitive impairment by timely protection of mitochondria in the developing rat brain: the importance of free oxygen radicals and mitochondrial integrity. Neurobiol Dis 2012;45:1031–41.
49. Wang C, Zhang X, Liu F, et al. Anesthetic-induced oxidative stress and potential protection. ScientificWorldJournal 2010;10:1473–82.
50. Ben-Ari Y, Gaiarsa JL, Tyzio R, et al. GABA: a pioneer transmitter that excites immature neurons and generates primitive oscillations. Physiol Rev 2007;87:1215–84.
51. Yamada J, Okabe A, Toyoda H, et al. Cl- uptake promoting depolarizing GABA actions in immature rat neocortical neurones is mediated by NKCC1. J Physiol 2004;557:829–41.
52. Rivera C, Voipio J, Payne JA, et al. The K+/Cl- co-transporter KCC2 renders GABA hyperpolarizing during neuronal maturation. Nature 1999;397:251–5.
53. Zou X, Sadovova N, Patterson TA, et al. The effects of L-carnitine on the combination of, inhalation anesthetic-induced developmental, neuronal apoptosis in the rat frontal cortex. Neuroscience 2008;151:1053–65.
54. Edwards DA, Shah HP, Cao W, et al. Bumetanide alleviates epileptogenic and neurotoxic effects of sevoflurane in neonatal rat brain. Anesthesiology 2010; 112(3):567–75.
55. Head BP, Patel HH, Niesman IR, et al. Inhibition of p75 neurotrophin receptor attenuates isoflurane-mediated neuronal apoptosis in the neonatal central nervous system. Anesthesiology 2009;110:813–25.
56. Lemkuil BP, Head BP, Pearn ML, et al. Isoflurane neurotoxicity is mediated by p75NTR-RhoA activation and actin depolymerization. Anesthesiology 2011; 114:49–57.
57. Tsuchimoto T, Ueki M, Miki T, et al. Erythropoietin attenuates isoflurane-induced neurodegeneration and learning deficits in the developing mouse brain. Paediatr Anaesth 2011;21:1209–13.
58. Koo E, Oshodi T. Comparative neurotoxic effects of dexmedetomidine and ketamine in prenatal monkey brains. Abstracts of posters presented at the International Anesthesia Research Society IARS 2012 Annual Meeting, Boston, MA, May 18–21, 2012. Anesth Analg 2012;113:S-402.
59. Liu JR, Liu Q, Li J, et al. Noxious stimulation attenuates ketamine-induced neuroapoptosis in the developing rat brain. Anesthesiology 2012;117:64–71.
60. Shih J, May LD, Gonzalez HE, et al. Delayed environmental enrichment reverses sevoflurane-induced memory impairment in rats. Anesthesiology 2012;116: 586–602.
61. Mattson SN, Riley EP, Sowell ER, et al. A decrease in the size of the basal ganglia in children with fetal alcohol syndrome. Alcohol Clin Exp Res 1996;20:1088–93.
62. Riley EP, McGee CL. Fetal alcohol spectrum disorders: an overview with emphasis on changes in brain and behavior. Exp Biol Med 2005;230:357–65.

63. Ikonomidou C, Scheer I, Wilhelm T, et al. Brain morphology alterations in the basal ganglia and the hypothalamus following prenatal exposure to antiepileptic drugs. Eur J Paediatr Neurol 2007;11:297–301.
64. Zhou ZW, Shu Y, Li M, et al. The glutaminergic, GABAergic, dopaminergic but not cholinergic neurons are susceptible to anaesthesia-induced cell death in the rat developing brain. Neuroscience 2011;174:64–70.
65. Brambrink AM, Back SA, Riddle A, et al. Isoflurane-induced apoptosis of oligo-dendrocytes in the neonatal primate brain. Annals of Neurology, in press.
66. Zou X, Patterson TA, Divine RL, et al. Prolonged exposure to ketamine increases neurodegeneration in the developing monkey brain. Int J Dev Neurosci 2009;27: 727–31.
67. Olney JW, Young C, Qin YQ, et al. Ethanol-induced developmental glioapoptosis in mice and monkeys. Soc for Neurosci Annual Meeting 2005. Abstract, #916.7, published online. Available at: http://www.SFN.com. Accessed June 20, 2012.
68. De Roo M, Klauser P, Briner A, et al. Anesthetics rapidly promote synaptogen-esis during a critical period of brain development. PLoS One 2009;4:e7043.
69. Briner A, De Roo M, Dayer A, et al. Volatile anesthetics rapidly increase dendritic spine density in the rat medial prefrontal cortex during synaptogenesis. Anes-thesiology 2010;112:546–56.
70. Briner A, Nikonenko I, De Roo M, et al. Developmental stage-dependent persis-tent impact of propofol anesthesia on dendritic spines in the rat medial prefrontal cortex. Anesthesiology 2011;115:282–93.
71. Stratmann G, Sall JW, May LD, et al. Isoflurane differentially affects neurogene-sis and long-term neurocognitive function in 60-day-old and 7-day-old rats. Anesthesiology 2009;110(4):834–48.
72. Zhu C, Gao J, Karlsson N, et al. Isoflurane anesthesia induced persistent, progressive memory impairment, caused a loss of neural stem cells, and reduced neurogenesis in young, but not adult, rodents. J Cereb Blood Flow Metab 2010;30(5):1017–30.
73. Klintsova AY, Helfer JL, Calizo LH, et al. Persistent impairment of hippocampal neurogenesis in young adult rats following early postnatal alcohol exposure. Alcohol Clin Exp Res 2007;31:2073–82.
74. Stefovska VG, Uckermann O, Czuczwar M, et al. Sedative and anticonvulsant drugs suppress postnatal neurogenesis. Ann Neurol 2008;64:434–45.
75. Dobbing J, Sands J. The brain growth spurt in various mammalian species. Early Hum Dev 1979;3:79–84.
76. Rice D, Barone S Jr. Critical periods of vulnerability for the developing nervous system: evidence from human and animal models. Environ Health Perspect 2000;108:511–33.
77. Slikker W Jr, Zou X, Hotchkiss CE, et al. Ketamine-induced neuronal cell death in the perinatal rhesus monkey. Toxicol Sci 2007;98:145–58.
78. Brambrink AM, Evers AS, Avidan MS, et al. Ketamine-induced neuroapoptosis in the fetal and neonatal rhesus macaque brain. Anesthesiology 2012;116:372–84.
79. Brambrink AM, Evers AS, Avidan MS, et al. Isoflurane-induced neuroapoptosis in the neonatal rhesus macaque brain. Anesthesiology 2010;112:834–41.
80. Brambrink AM, Back SA, Avidan MS, et al. Ketamine and isoflurane anesthesia triggers neuronal and glial apoptosis in the neonatal macaque. Abstract presented at Am Soc Anesthesiol Annual Meeting. San Diego, CA, October 16–20, 2010.
81. Zou X, Liu F, Zhang X, et al. Inhalation anesthetic-induced neuronal damage in the developing rhesus monkey. Neurotoxicol Teratol 2011;33:592–7.

82. Wozniak DF, Hartman RE, Boyle MP, et al. Apoptotic neurodegeneration induced by ethanol in neonatal mice is associated with profound learning/memory deficits in juveniles followed by progressive functional recovery in adults. Neurobiol Dis 2004;17:403–14.

83. Fredriksson A, Archer T, Alm H, et al. Neurofunctional deficits and potentiated apoptosis by neonatal NMDA antagonist administration. Behav Brain Res 2004;153:367–76.

84. Paule MG, Li M, Zou X, et al. Ketamine anesthesia during the first week of life can cause long-lasting cognitive deficits in rhesus monkeys. Neurotoxicol Teratol 2011;33:220–30.

85. Anand KJS, Soriano SG. Anesthetic agents and the immature brain: are these toxic or therapeutic? Anesthesiology 2004;101:527–30.

86. Soriano SG, Loepke AW. Let's not throw the baby out with the bath water: potential neurotoxicity of anesthetic drugs in infants and children. J Neurosurg Anesthesiol 2005;17:207–9.

87. Anand KJ. Anesthetic neurotoxicity in newborns. Should we change clinical practice? Anesthesiology 2007;107:2–4.

88. DiMaggio CJ, Sun L, Kakavouli A, et al. A retrospective cohort study of the association of anesthesia and hernia repair surgery with behavioral and developmental disorders in young children. J Neurosurg Anesthesiol 2009;21:286–91.

89. DiMaggio CJ, Sun LS, Li G. Early childhood exposure to anesthesia and risk of developmental and behavioral disorders in a sibling birth cohort. Anesth Analg 2011;113:1143–51.

90. Wilder RT, Flick RP, Sprung J, et al. Early exposure to anesthesia and learning disabilities in a population-based birth cohort. Anesthesiology 2009;110:796–804.

91. Flick RP, Katusic SK, Colligan RC, et al. Cognitive and behavioral outcomes after early exposure to anesthesia and surgery. Pediatrics 2011;128:e1053–61.

92. Sprung J, Flick RP, Katusic SK, et al. Attention-deficit/hyperactivity disorder after early exposure to procedures requiring general anesthesia. Mayo Clin Proc 2012;87:120–9.

93. Thomas JJ, Choi JY, Bayman EO, et al. Does anesthesia exposure in infancy affect academic performance in childhood? IARS and SAFEKIDS International Science Symposium "Anesthetic-Induced Neonatal Neuronal Injury", International Anesthesia Research Society 2010 Annual Meeting 3/20/2010, Hawaii, Poster Session Abstract ISS – A4. Available at: http://www.IARS.org. Accessed June 20, 2012.

94. Kalkman CJ, Peelen LM, deJong TP, et al. Behavior and development in children and age at time of first anesthetic exposure. Anesthesiology 2009;110:805–12.

95. Hansen TG, Pedersen JK, Henneberg SW, et al. Academic performance in adolescence after inguinal hernia repair in infancy: a nationwide cohort study. Anesthesiology 2011;114(5):1076–85.

96. Bartels M, Althoff RR, Boomsma DI. Anesthesia and cognitive performance in children: no evidence for a causal relationship. Twin Res Hum Genet 2009;12:246–53.

97. Davidson AJ, McCann ME, Morton NS, et al. Anesthesia and outcome after neonatal surgery: the role for randomized trials. Anesthesiology 2008;109:941–4.

98. Sun LS, Li G, Dimaggio C, et al. Anesthesia and neurodevelopment in children: time for an answer? Anesthesiology 2008;109:757–61.

99. McCann M, Davidson A, Morton N, et al. An update on progress of the multi-site RCT comparing regional and general anesthesia for effects on neurodevelopmental outcome and apnea in infants – the GAS study. IARS and SAFEKIDS International Science Symposium "Anesthetic-Induced Neonatal Neuronal Injury", International Anesthesia Research Society 2010 Annual Meeting 3/20/2010, Hawaii, Poster Session Abstract ISS – A14. Available at: http://www.IARS.org. Accessed June 20, 2012.

100. Sun LS, Byrne M, Forde A, et al. Co-investigators of the PANDA Research Network. PANDA Study: status update. IARS and SAFEKIDS International Science Symposium "Anesthetic-Induced Neonatal Neuronal Injury", International Anesthesia Research Society 2010 Annual Meeting 3/20/2010, Hawaii, Poster Session Abstract ISS – A15. Available at: http://www.IARS.org. Accessed June 20, 2012.

101. Balas MC, Happ MB, Yang W, et al. Outcomes associated with delirium in older patients in surgical ICUs. Chest 2009;135:18–25.

102. Rasmussen LS. Defining postoperative cognitive dysfunction. Eur J Anaesthesiol 1998;15:761.

103. Krenk L, Rasmussen LS. Postoperative delirium and postoperative cognitive dysfunction in the elderly - what are the differences? Minerva Anestesiol 2011; 77:742–9.

104. Diegeler A, Hirsch R, Schneider F, et al. Neuromonitoring and neurocognitive outcome in off-pump versus conventional coronary bypass operation. Ann Thorac Surg 2000;69:1162–6.

105. McKhann G, Goldsborough M, Borowicz L, et al. Cognitive outcome after coronary artery bypass: a one year prospective study. Ann Thorac Surg 1997;63: 510–5.

106. Shroyer A, Grover F, Hattler B, et al. Randomized On/Off Bypass (ROOBY) study group on-pump versus off-pump coronary-artery bypass surgery. N Engl J Med 2009;361:1827–37.

107. Moller JT, Cluitmans P, Rasmussen LS, et al. Long-term postoperative cognitive dysfunction in the elderly ISPOCD1 study. ISPOCD investigators. International Study of Post-Operative Cognitive Dysfunction. Lancet 1998;351:857–61.

108. Williams-Russo P, Sharrock NE, Mattis S, et al. Cognitive effects after epidural vs general anesthesia in older adults. JAMA 1995;274:44–50.

109. Evered L, Scott DA, Silbert B, et al. Postoperative cognitive dysfunction is independent of type of surgery and anesthetic. Anesth Analg 2011;112: 1179–85.

110. Avidan MS, Evers AS. Review of clinical evidence for persistent cognitive decline or incident dementia attributable to surgery or general anesthesia. J Alzheimers Dis 2011;24:201–16.

111. Avidan MS, Searleman AC, Storandt M, et al. Long-term cognitive decline in older subjects was not attributable to noncardiac surgery or major illness. Anesthesiology 2009;111:964–70.

112. Mawhinney LJ, de Rivero Vaccari JP, Alonso OF, et al. Isoflurane/nitrous oxide anesthesia induces increases in NMDA receptor subunit NR2B protein expression in the aged rat brain. Brain Res 2012;1431:23–34.

113. Orrenius S, Zhivotovsky B, Nicotera P. Regulation of cell death: the calcium-apoptosis link. Nat Rev Mol Cell Biol 2003;4:552–65.

114. Ruiz A, Matute C, Alberdi E. Endoplasmic reticulum Ca(2+) release through ryanodine and IP(3) receptors contributes to neuronal excitotoxicity. Cell Calcium 2009;46:273–81.

115. Wei H, Liang G, Yang H. The common inhalational anesthetic isoflurane induces apoptosis via activation of inositol 1,4,5-triphosphate receptors. Anesthesiology 2008;108:251–60.

116. Zhan X, Fahlman CS, Bickler PE. Isoflurane neuroprotection in rat hippocampal slices decreases with aging: changes in intracellular Ca2+ regulation and N-methyl-D-aspartate receptor-mediated Ca2+ influx. Anesthesiology 2006; 104:995–1003.

117. Xie Z, Culley D, Dong Y. The common inhalational anesthetic isoflurane induces caspase activation and increases Aβ levels in-vivo. Ann Neurol 2008;64:618–27.

118. Perucho J, Rubio I, Casarejos MJ. Anesthesia with isoflurane increases amyloid pathology in mice models of Alzheimer's disease. J Alzheimers Dis 2010;19: 1245–57.

119. Liu W, Xu J, Wang H, et al. Isoflurane-induced spatial memory impairment by a mechanism independent of amyloid-beta levels and tau protein phosphorylation changes in aged rats. Neurol Res 2012;34:3–10.

120. Wu X, Lu Y, Dong Y, et al. The inhalational anesthetic isoflurane increases levels of proinflammatory TNF-α, IL-6, and IL-1β. Neurobiol Aging 2012;33:1364–78.

121. Rosczyk HA, Sparkman NL, Johnson RW. Neuroinflammation and cognitive function in aged mice following minor surgery. Exp Gerontol 2008;43:840–6.

122. Stratmann G, Sall JW, Bell JS, et al. Isoflurane does not affect brain cell death, hippocampal neurogenesis, or long-term neurocognitive outcome in aged rats. Anesthesiology 2010;112:305–15.

123. Makaryus R, Lee H, Yu M, et al. The metabolomic profile during isoflurane anesthesia differs from propofol anesthesia in the live rodent brain. J Cereb Blood Flow Metab 2011;31:1432–42.

124. Heyer EJ, Sharma R, Rampersad A, et al. A controlled prospective study of neuropsychological dysfunction following carotid endarterectomy. Arch Neurol 2002;59:217.

125. Monk TG, Weldon BC, Garvan CW, et al. Predictors of cognitive dysfunction after major noncardiac surgery. Anesthesiology 2008;108:18–30.

126. Mracek J, Holeckova I, Chytra I, et al. The impact of general versus local anesthesia on early subclinical cognitive function following carotid endarterectomy evaluated using P3 event-related potentials. Acta Neurochir (Wien) 2012;154: 433–8.

127. An J, Fang Q, Huang C, et al. Deeper total intravenous anesthesia reduced the incidence of early postoperative cognitive dysfunction after microvascular decompression for facial spasm. J Neurosurg Anesthesiol 2011;23:12–7.

128. Jankowski CJ, Trenerry MR, Cook DJ, et al. Cognitive and functional predictors and sequelae of postoperative delirium in elderly patients undergoing elective joint arthroplasty. Anesth Analg 2011;112:1186–93.

129. Wang H, Xu Z, Feng C, et al. Changes of learning and memory in aged rats after isoflurane inhalational anaesthesia correlated with hippocampal acetylcholine level. Ann Fr Anesth Reanim 2012;31:e61–6.

130. Lin D, Cao L, Wang Z, et al. Lidocaine attenuates cognitive impairment after isoflurane anesthesia in old rats. Behav Brain Res 2012;228:319–27.

131. Callaway JK, Jones NC, Royse CF. Isoflurane induces cognitive deficits in the Morris water maze task in rats. Eur J Anaesthesiol 2012;29:239–45.

132. Culley DJ, Baxter MG, Yukhananov R, et al. Long-term impairment of acquisition of a spatial memory task following isoflurane-nitrous oxide anesthesia in rats. Anesthesiology 2004;100:309–14.

Airway Management in Neuroanesthesiology

Michael Aziz, MD

KEYWORDS

- Airway management • Cervical spine • Video laryngoscopy • Manual inline stabilization

KEY POINTS

- Airway management for pituitary surgery. Patients with pituitary secreting tumors may present with Cushing disease or acromegaly. Those with Cushing disease are more prone to difficulties with mask ventilation and airway obstruction, although not difficult direct laryngoscopy. Those with acromegaly are at increased risk of intubation failure and should be treated conservatively.
- Airway management for functional neurosurgery. Airway emergencies may occur during awake craniotomy procedures that require immediate, but challenging airway intervention, as a patient is often fixed in a head frame. As such, some practice has moved toward the awake-asleep-awake approach to control the airway during critical portions of the procedure.
- The unstable cervical spine: rheumatoid arthritis. Arthritis of airway cartilage may increase intubation difficulty, and atlantoaxial instability may increase risk of spinal cord injury during airway interventions.
- The unstable cervical spine: traumatic injury evaluation. Patients with blunt trauma are at increased risk of unrecognized cervical spine injury, and this risk is raised in the setting of head trauma.
- The unstable cervical spine: clinical precautions and manual in line stabilization. Manual in-line stabilization effectively reduces cervical motion during airway interventions and should be applied anytime a cervical collar is removed.
- The unstable cervical spine: implications of airway interventions. All airway interventions cause some degree of cervical spine motion.
  - Mask ventilation and supraglottic airway. These interventions typically result in cervical spine flexion.
  - Direct laryngoscopy. Direct laryngoscopy is more difficult to perform when manual in-line stabilization is applied and causes cervical extension, greatest at the upper cervical levels.
  - Flexible fiberoptic intubation. Flexible fiberoptic intubation causes the least amount of cervical motion among the intubation approaches, but takes experience to master.

Continued

Disclosures: None.
Department of Anesthesiology and Perioperative Medicine, Oregon Health and Science University, Mail Code KPV 5A, 3181 SW Sam Jackson Park Road, Portland, OR 97239, USA
E-mail address: azizm@ohsu.edu

Anesthesiology Clin 30 (2012) 229–240
doi:10.1016/j.anclin.2012.04.001
1932-2275/12/$ – see front matter © 2012 Elsevier Inc. All rights reserved.

Continued

> o Rigid video laryngoscopy. Rigid video laryngoscopy improves laryngeal view and eases intubation difficulty compared with direct laryngoscopy. When manual in-line stabilization is applied, isolated segments of the cervical spine may realize less cervical motion compared with direct laryngoscopy, but the data are inconsistent.
>
> • Airway management after cervical spine surgery. Patients are at increased risk of ex-tubation failure or emergency airway management from pharyngeal edema or hema-toma. These situations occur more frequently for combined anterior–posterior approaches and for surgeries that are lengthy, have a high blood loss, or involve more than 3 cervical segments.

AIRWAY MANAGEMENT FOR PITUITARY SURGERY
Patient Preparation

The neurosurgical patient presenting for resection of a pituitary lesion may have concerns for airway management due to excess secretion of hormone from the gland. Those presenting with secretion of corticotrophs present clinically as Cushing disease. These patients can be morbidly obese and have an increased incidence of obstructive sleep apnea.[1] As such, they are prone to difficulty with bag–mask ventilation, airway obstruction, and rapid oxygen desaturation during airway management. However, difficulty with endotracheal intubation is no more frequent in this patient population than others.[2]

Contraindications for Patients

Unlike Cushing disease, patients with acromegaly from growth hormone-secreting tumors are at increased risk of difficult or failed intubation.[2,3] Historically, elective tracheostomy has been advocated for those with acromegaly involving with larynx or pharynx.[4] However, the use of awake flexible fiberoptic intubation may be used to avoid tracheostomy.[5] The mere presence of this disease state with knowledge of involvement of airway structures should raise concern for airway management, as Mallampati classification score may not independently predict difficult airway management for these patients.[6]

AIRWAY MANAGEMENT FOR FUNCTIONAL NEUROSURGERY
Patient Preparation

Intraoperative neurologic events that may necessitate airway management occur as frequently as in 16% of cases.[7] These events typically occur with a patient in a very challenging position at some distance from the anesthesia provider, possibly in a head frame with pins and fairly immobile. Furthermore, the patient may be vomiting from the neurologic event or suffering a seizure, which can make airway management more difficult. Traditional tools such as direct laryngoscopy may not be sufficient to secure the airway. Ventilation has been effectively supported with the use of a supra-glottic airway.[8]

Contraindications for Patients

Airway management is often avoided for the patient presenting for functional stereo-tactic neurosurgery. Particularly, movement disorders are masked, and the procedure is done awake with variable sedation or no sedation. However, the anesthesia provider must always be prepared for unexpected events.

Technique—Best Practices

One approach advocated for functional neurosurgery is the awake-asleep-awake technique. This technique was initially described for tumor surgery near the speech center of the brain using general endotracheal anesthesia with intraoperative extubation.[9] Today, this technique is still performed, more often with a supraglottic airway, and it may result in greater patient satisfaction.[10] However, the patient emerging from general anesthesia while surgically exposed carries inherent risks of bucking and movement in a head frame. To date, there is no reasonable comparative evidence that strongly favors 1 anesthetic technique over another for functional neurosurgery.

THE UNSTABLE CERVICAL SPINE
Avoiding Complications

The neuroanesthesiologist should be particularly concerned about the unstable cervical spine, as airway management can translate forces to compromise the spinal cord. These conditions typically arise in the setting of trauma but may also exist from arthritic disease.

Rheumatoid Arthritis

Patient preparation
The patient with rheumatoid arthritis raises particular concern. Fusion of the cricoarytenoid cartilages may progress to airway obstruction and may make tracheal intubation more difficult. Furthermore, disease involving the ligaments and odontoid can lead to antlantoaxial instability. This instability may not manifest on history and physical examination, so some authors have advocated routine screening radiographs of the neck before elective surgery for those with rheumatoid disease that may involve the cervical spine.[11] These image may already be part of the medical record on a patient who is appropriately managed for his or her cervical spine disease. There are no comparative data to suggest that screening radiographs of the cervical spine reduce complications or alter airway management techniques for the patient with rheumatoid arthritis. Patient positioning during surgery with the head resting on a flat pillow combined with a donut shaped pillow (protruding) results in the least anterior atlantodental interval compared with a flat pillow alone.[12]

Traumatic Injury Evaluation

Patient preparation
The incidence of cervical spine injury in patients suffering from blunt trauma is estimated to be 1.8%[13] The C2 vertebra is the most common level on injury, followed by the C6 and C7 levels.[14] The patient with head trauma and depressed Glasgow coma scale score is more likely to have a cervical spine injury than the patient experiencing blunt trauma without associated head injury.[15–18] Appropriately, guidelines are established within emergency medicine and trauma care to screen for cervical spine trauma and take appropriate precautions until cervical spine trauma is ruled out. The trauma patient who may be at low risk should not require further evaluation or care of the cervical spine if he or she: has no midline cervical tenderness, has no focal neurologic deficit, is alert, and has no distracting injuries. As plain radiographs may not reveal unstable ligamentous injury, computed tomography (CT) scanning is appropriate for those patients at increased risk who cannot be cleared by these standard criteria.

Clinical Precautions and Manual in-line Stabilization

Patient preparation

The patient who cannot be cleared should be maintained in cervical spine immobilization early in his or her care. Unfortunately, the cervical collar limits mouth opening[19] and can make insertion of airway devices and laryngoscopy more challenging.

Technique—best practices

Since it was first described, manual in-line stabilization (MILS) has been adopted as a practice to immobilize the spine when the cervical collar needs to be removed for situations such as airway management.[20] This practice involves a second provider fixing the head in a neutral position and applying countertraction to any suspension forces that may be applied during laryngoscopy. When MILS is effectively applied, the motion of the cervical spine is effectively limited by various airway maneuvers.[21–25]

Avoiding complications

The exclusion of MILS in patients with cervical spine injury has been associated with catastrophic neurologic events.[26–29] Therefore, MILS remains a low-cost critical intervention for airway management in the patient with potential cervical spine instability. Gerling and colleagues[23] compared cervical immobilization techniques in destabilized human cadavers and found that cervical motion is less and glottis visualization better with MILS compared with leaving the cervical collar in place alone. Soft collars alone insufficiently mobilize the cervical spine during airway management.[30]

Implications for Airway Interventions

Technique—best practices

Mask ventilation and supraglottic airways Cervical spine motion may occur during various sequences of airway management. Even preintubation maneuvers such as chin lift and jaw thrust create cervical motion in cadavers destabilized at the C1 to C2 juncture that is equal to the traction realized with intubation.[31] In a destabilized cadaver study conducted by Brimacombe and colleagues, various intubation techniques were analyzed for the effects of cervical motion[24] Mask ventilation alone produces some degree of flexion of the cervical spine that is opposite from extension forces seen with laryngoscopy devices. Supraglottic airways also produce cervical motion, but nasal fiberoptic intubation creates the least amount of cervical motion. Hauswald and colleagues[32] observed that mask ventilation produces greater cervical motion than blind intubation techniques in destabilized cadavers. Like mask ventilation, the insertion of a supraglottic airway produces flexion of the cervical spine, and posterior pressure is realized against the cervical spine.[33,34]

Direct laryngoscopy Direct laryngoscopy results in extension of the cervical spine across various segments, but most prominently at the occipitoatlantial and atlantoaxial joints.[35] Different direct laryngoscopy blade designs have been evaluated for differences in cervical motion and glottic view during laryngoscopy. The Miller blade appears to result in less cervical motion than the Macintosh or McCoy-hinged blade.[23] Furthermore, the McCoy-hinged blade does not result in any reduction in cervical spine motion compared with the conventional Macintosh blade.[36] Unfortunately, the application of MILS makes direct laryngoscopy more difficult.[37,38]

Flexible fiberoptic intubation Alternate intubation techniques have been studied to try to balance the need to limit cervical motion and the difficulty of obtaining laryngeal view when MILS is applied. Intubating supraglottic airways have been investigated; however, their failure rate may be high.[39–41] Furthermore, cervical flexion is realized across the C0 to C5 segments during intubation with these devices.[33] Flexible fiberoptic techniques may also be difficult for inexperienced providers to perform, but flexible nasal fiberoptic intubation results in less cervical motion to destabilized cadavers than use of supraglottic airway, direct laryngoscopy, intubating supraglottic airway, or even mask ventilation with chin lift and jaw thrust.[24]

Rigid video laryngoscopy Video laryngoscopy has grown in use over the past 10 years. Just recently, evidence has suggested benefit for intubation in for those patients predicted to be more difficult to intubate.[42–47] Several studies have now addressed the scenario of cervical spine pathology by artificially applying MILS in testing models. These studies are further summarized in **Table 1**. Consistently, laryngeal view is improved using video laryngoscopy compared with direct laryngoscopy in the setting of MILS.[48–52] Furthermore, a more global assessment of difficult airway management, the intubation difficulty scale score,[53] is improved with video laryngoscopy compared with direct laryngoscopy.[49–52] In one of these many studies, intubation success rate was improved with video laryngoscopy compared with direct laryngoscopy in the setting of artificially applied MILS.[48] However, video laryngoscopy may not completely overcome the intubation difficulty related to the application of MILS. In the author's study of 1 video laryngoscope, it was observed that the presence of limited cervical spine motion, either from the application of MILS or existing pathology, independently predicts video laryngoscopy failure (relative risk 1.76; 95% confidence interval [CI]: 1.01, 3.06)[42] So, while these devices provide benefit in terms of ease of intubation and may improve intubation success compared with direct laryngoscopy, they are still prone to failure in the patient with cervical spine pathology or precautions.

In terms of cervical motion, several studies have compared rigid video laryngoscopes to direct laryngoscopy by evaluating fluoroscopic images during the intubation procedure (**Table 2**). Without the application of MILS, less cervical extension may be necessary with video laryngoscopes compared with direct laryngoscopy.[54–56] When MILS is applied, the findings are inconsistent. In some studies, isolated segments of the cervical spine may realize less cervical extension compared with direct laryngoscopy;[57–59] however, another study has demonstrated no difference in cervical motion between video laryngoscopy and direct laryngoscopy when MILS is applied.[60]

The studies regarding various airway device approaches to limited cervical spine motion have yet to demonstrate any alterations in neurologic outcomes. As such, the application of techniques with the highest likelihood of success while maintaining MILS is the best approach. While flexible fiberoptic intubation may expose the cervical spine to the least amount of traction, this procedure requires significant skill and a cooperative patient if it is to be performed on an awake patient. For the anesthetized patient, this procedure still often requires jaw thrust, which may expose the patient to cervical traction. Video laryngoscopes may be easier to learn than flexible fiberoptic intubation and offer improvement in terms of intubation difficulty compared with direct laryngoscopy. As such, their use has grown for the management of the patient with cervical spine precautions. Until further evidence guides care, expert opinion continues to encourage the application of MILS with an intubation technique that is known and familiar to the laryngoscopist.

AIRWAY MANAGEMENT AFTER CERVICAL SPINE SURGERY
Extubation

Technique—best practices
A carefully planned extubation of the patient after cervical spine surgery is warranted for 2 key reasons. First, airway management may have been initially difficult because of

Table 1
Studies of video laryngoscopy on intubation performance for the patient maintained in manual in-line stabilization

Author	Device	Control	Sample	Outcome Assessed	Major Findings
Malik et al,[49] 2008	GlideScope (Verathon, Bothell, WA) AWS (Pentax, Hoya, Japan)	DL	120	Laryngeal view IDS Intubation time Success rate	Improved laryngeal view and IDS Slower intubation time No difference in success
Maharaj et al,[45] 2008	Airtraq (Prodol, Vizcaya, Spain)[a]	DL	40	IDS Intubation attempts Laryngeal view	Reduced number of intubation attempts. Improved IDS, improved laryngeal view
Smith et al,[52] 1999	WuScope (Pentax, Orangeburg, New York)	DL	87	IDS Laryngeal view, intubation attempts	Improved IDS and laryngeal view No difference in success or number of attempts
Malik et al,[50] 2009	AWS	DL	90	IDS, laryngeal view	Improved IDS and laryngeal view
Enomoto et al,[48] 2008	AWS	DL	203	Laryngeal view, intubation time, success rate	Improved laryngeal view Increased success rate Faster intubation time
Liu et al,[67] 2009	AWS	GlideScope	70	IDS, Intubation time, success rate within a defined time interval	Faster intubation time Lower IDS Improved laryngeal view and higher intubation success with AWS

Abbreviations: AWS, airway scope; DL, direct laryngoscopy; IDS, intubation difficulty scale score.
[a] Not a video laryngoscope, but often included in this category.

Table 2
Studies of cervical motion while using video laryngoscopes

Study	Device	Control	Cervical Precautions	Fluoroscopy	Major Findings
Hastings et al,[56] 1995	Bullard (Circon ACMI, Stamford, CT)	DL	None	In selected patients (C0–C4) Angle finder used in the entire sample	Reduced extension across (C0–C4)
Robitallie et al,[60] 2008	GlideScope	DL	MILS	Continuous C0–C5 during several time points	No decrease in cervical movement
Maruyama et al,[57] 2008	AWS	DL and McCoy	None	C1/C2, C3/C4	Reduced extension at adjacent vertebra
Hirabayashi et al,[55] 2007	AWS	DL	None	C0–C4	Reduced extension at all segments
Turkstra et al,[58] 2005	GlideScope Lightwand (Trachlight, Laerdal, Armonk, New York)	DL	MILS	C0–C5	Reduced C2–C5 motion with Glidescope. Reduced motion across all segments with Lightwand
Watts et al,[68] 1997	Bullard	DL	One arm with MILS One arm without	C0–C5	Reduced cervical extension in the Bullard +MILS arm
Maruyama et al,[57] 2008	AWS	DL	MILS	C0–C4	Reduced cumulative cervical motion
Turkstra et al,[59] 2009	Airtraq[a]	DL	MILS	C0–Thoracic	No difference at C1–C2 segment, less extension at C2–C5, and C5–Thoracic

Abbreviation: DL, direct laryngoscopy.
[a] Not a video laryngoscope, but often included in this category.

cervical spine immobilization or may become more difficult after a cervical spine is fused. Second, airway compromise may occur after extubation from edema or hematoma formation. Reintubation may occur as frequently as in 5% of cases after anterior cervical corpectomy, and death has been described from failed airway management.[61] In another series of 311 cervical spine surgeries, airway complications occurred in 6.1% of cases, and death occurred once.[62] Predictors of airway complications from this series included exposure of more than 3 vertebral bodies, blood loss greater than 300 mL, exposure involving upper cervical vertebra, and operative time greater than 5 hours. Furthermore, combined anterior–posterior cervical spine surgery has a higher incidence of emergent reintubation than other approaches to cervical spine surgery.[63]

In light of these feared outcomes, delayed extubation may be appropriate for those exposed to combined anterior–posterior approaches and those with operative predictors as described previously. There are no comparative data regarding extubation protocols to guide timing of the extubation. However, several useful suggestions do seem appropriate. Dexamethasone has been used as a treatment to reduce pharyngeal edema, and it may be an appropriate therapy in selected cases. Furthermore, some recovery time with the pharynx in a nondependent position should reduce the extent of pharyngeal edema. Pharyngoscopy may be performed to determine the extent of pharyngeal edema and safely predict safe extubation.[64] Similarly, a cuff leak test may reassure the clinician that an airway may remain patent after extubation.[65] Some providers further advocate extubation over an exchange catheter for ease of reintubation.[66] Certainly, the availability of specialized airway management tools with providers skilled in their use is prudent to avoid failed airway management after extubation.

SUMMARY

In summary, the neurosurgical patient has unique airway management concerns. Various associated disease states may make intubation more difficult or expose the patient to neurologic injury. The patient with potential cervical spine pathology deserves unique attention, as intubation may be more difficult from spine stabilization maneuvers. Furthermore, airway interventions expose the spine to traction, which may worsen neurologic injury. While some airway management approaches may ease intubation difficulty or expose the cervical spine to less trauma, comparative data regarding the performance of selected intubation techniques have been ineffectively compared in terms of neurologic injury. After cervical spine surgery, caution is warranted, as pharyngeal edema or hematoma formation may compromise an unsecured airway.

REFERENCES

1. Shipley JE, Schteingart DE, Tandon R, et al. Sleep architecture and sleep apnea in patients with Cushing's disease. Sleep 1992;15:514–8.
2. Nemergut EC, Zuo Z. Airway management in patients with pituitary disease: a review of 746 patients. J Neurosurg Anesthesiol 2006;18:73–7.
3. Messick JM Jr, Cucchiara RF, Faust RJ. Airway management in patients with acromegaly. Anesthesiology 1982;56:157.
4. Southwick JP, Katz J. Unusual airway difficulty in the acromegalic patient—indications for tracheostomy. Anesthesiology 1979;51:72–3.
5. Ovassapian A, Doka JC, Romsa DE. Acromegaly—use of fiberoptic laryngoscopy to avoid tracheostomy. Anesthesiology 1981;54:429–30.
6. Schmitt H, Buchfelder M, Radespiel-Troger M, et al. Difficult intubation in acromegalic patients: incidence and predictability. Anesthesiology 2000;93:110–4.

7. Venkatraghavan L, Manninen P, Mak P, et al. Anesthesia for functional neurosurgery: review of complications. J Neurosurg Anesthesiol 2006;18:64–7.
8. Skucas AP, Artru AA. Anesthetic complications of awake craniotomies for epilepsy surgery. Anesth Analg 2006;102:882–7.
9. Huncke K, Van de Wiele B, Fried I, et al. The asleep-awake-asleep anesthetic technique for intraoperative language mapping. Neurosurgery 1998;42: 1312–6.
10. Sarang A, Dinsmore J. Anaesthesia for awake craniotomy—evolution of a technique that facilitates awake neurological testing. Br J Anaesth 2003;90:161–5.
11. Kwek TK, Lew TW, Thoo FL. The role of preoperative cervical spine X-rays in rheumatoid arthritis. Anaesth Intensive Care 1998;26:636–41.
12. Tokunaga D, Hase H, Mikami Y, et al. Atlantoaxial subluxation in different intraoperative head positions in patients with rheumatoid arthritis. Anesthesiology 2006;104:675–9.
13. Crosby ET, Lui A. The adult cervical spine: implications for airway management. Can J Anaesth 1990;37:77–93.
14. Goldberg W, Mueller C, Panacek E, et al. NEXUS Group: distribution and patterns of blunt traumatic cervical spine injury. Ann Emerg Med 2001;38:17–21.
15. Blackmore CC, Emerson SS, Mann FA, et al. Cervical spine imaging in patients with trauma: determination of fracture risk to optimize use. Radiology 1999;211: 759–65.
16. Demetriades D, Charalambides K, Chahwan S, et al. Nonskeletal cervical spine injuries: epidemiology and diagnostic pitfalls. J Trauma 2000;48:724–7.
17. Hackl W, Hausberger K, Sailer R, et al. Prevalence of cervical spine injuries in patients with facial trauma. Oral Surg Oral Med Oral Pathol Oral Radiol Endod 2001;92:370–6.
18. Holly LT, Kelly DF, Counelis GJ, et al. Cervical spine trauma associated with moderate and severe head injury: incidence, risk factors, and injury characteristics. J Neurosurg 2002;96:285–91.
19. Goutcher CM, Lochhead V. Reduction in mouth opening with semi-rigid cervical collars. Br J Anaesth 2005;95:344–8.
20. Grande CM, Barton CR, Stene JK. Appropriate techniques for airway management of emergency patients with suspected spinal cord injury. Anesth Analg 1988;67:714–5.
21. Lennarson PJ, Smith D, Todd MM, et al. Segmental cervical spine motion during orotracheal intubation of the intact and injured spine with and without external stabilization. J Neurosurg 2000;92:201–6.
22. Lennarson PJ, Smith DW, Sawin PD, et al. Cervical spinal motion during intubation: efficacy of stabilization maneuvers in the setting of complete segmental instability. J Neurosurg 2001;94:265–70.
23. Gerling MC, Davis DP, Hamilton RS, et al. Effects of cervical spine immobilization technique and laryngoscope blade selection on an unstable cervical spine in a cadaver model of intubation. Ann Emerg Med 2000;36:293–300.
24. Brimacombe J, Keller C, Kunzel KH, et al. Cervical spine motion during airway management: a cinefluoroscopic study of the posteriorly destabilized third cervical vertebrae in human cadavers. Anesth Analg 2000;91:1274–8.
25. Majernick TG, Bieniek R, Houston JB, et al. Cervical spine movement during orotracheal intubation. Ann Emerg Med 1986;15:417–20.
26. Muckart DJ, Bhagwanjee S, van der Merwe R. Spinal cord injury as a result of endotracheal intubation in patients with undiagnosed cervical spine fractures. Anesthesiology 1997;87:418–20.

27. Redl G. Massive pyramidal tract signs after endotracheal intubation: a case report of spondyloepiphyseal dysplasia congenita. Anesthesiology 1998;89: 1262–4.
28. Farmer J, Vaccaro A, Albert TJ, et al. Neurologic deterioration after cervical spinal cord injury. J Spinal Disord 1998;11:192–6.
29. McLeod AD, Calder I. Spinal cord injury and direct laryngoscopy—the legend lives on. Br J Anaesth 2000;84:705–9.
30. Aprahamian C, Thompson BM, Finger WA, et al. Experimental cervical spine injury model: evaluation of airway management and splinting techniques. Ann Emerg Med 1984;13:584–7.
31. Donaldson WF 3rd, Heil BV, Donaldson VP, et al. The effect of airway maneuvers on the unstable C1-C2 segment. A cadaver study. Spine (Phila Pa 1976) 1997;22: 1215–8.
32. Hauswald M, Sklar DP, Tandberg D, et al. Cervical spine movement during airway management: cinefluoroscopic appraisal in human cadavers. Am J Emerg Med 1991;9:535–8.
33. Kihara S, Watanabe S, Brimacombe J, et al. Segmental cervical spine movement with the intubating laryngeal mask during manual in-line stabilization in patients with cervical pathology undergoing cervical spine surgery. Anesth Analg 2000; 91:195–200.
34. Keller C, Brimacombe J, Keller K. Pressures exerted against the cervical vertebrae by the standard and intubating laryngeal mask airways: a randomized, controlled, cross-over study in fresh cadavers. Anesth Analg 1999;89:1296–300.
35. Sawin PD, Todd MM, Traynelis VC, et al. Cervical spine motion with direct laryngoscopy and orotracheal intubation. An in vivo cinefluoroscopic study of subjects without cervical abnormality. Anesthesiology 1996;85:26–36.
36. MacIntyre PA, McLeod AD, Hurley R, et al. Cervical spine movements during laryngoscopy. Comparison of the Macintosh and McCoy laryngoscope blades. Anaesthesia 1999;54:413–8.
37. Heath KJ. The effect of laryngoscopy of different cervical spine immobilisation techniques. Anaesthesia 1994;49:843–5.
38. Nolan JP, Wilson ME. Orotracheal intubation in patients with potential cervical spine injuries. An indication for the gum elastic bougie. Anaesthesia 1993;48:630–3.
39. Martel M, Reardon RF, Cochrane J. Initial experience of emergency physicians using the intubating laryngeal mask airway: a case series. Acad Emerg Med 2001;8:815–22.
40. Joo HS, Kapoor S, Rose DK, et al. The intubating laryngeal mask airway after induction of general anesthesia versus awake fiberoptic intubation in patients with difficult airways. Anesth Analg 2001;92:1342–6.
41. Reardon RF, Martel M. The intubating laryngeal mask airway: suggestions for use in the emergency department. Acad Emerg Med 2001;8:833–8.
42. Aziz MF, Healy D, Kheterpal S, et al. Routine clinical practice effectiveness of the Glidescope in difficult airway management: an analysis of 2,004 Glidescope intubations, complications, and failures from two institutions. Anesthesiology 2011; 114:34–41.
43. Aziz MF, Dillman D, Fu R, et al. Comparative effectiveness of the C-MAC video laryngoscope versus direct laryngoscopy in the setting of the predicted difficult airway. Anesthesiology 2012;116:629–36.
44. Jungbauer A, Schumann M, Brunkhorst V, et al. Expected difficult tracheal intubation: a prospective comparison of direct laryngoscopy and video laryngoscopy in 200 patients. Br J Anaesth 2009;102:546–50.

45. Maharaj CH, Costello JF, Harte BH, et al. Evaluation of the Airtraq and Macintosh laryngoscopes in patients at increased risk for difficult tracheal intubation. Anaesthesia 2008;63:182–8.
46. Malik MA, Subramaniam R, Maharaj CH, et al. Randomized controlled trial of the Pentax AWS, Glidescope, and Macintosh laryngoscopes in predicted difficult intubation. Br J Anaesth 2009;103:761–8.
47. Serocki G, Bein B, Scholz J, et al. Management of the predicted difficult airway: a comparison of conventional blade laryngoscopy with video-assisted blade laryngoscopy and the GlideScope. Eur J Anaesthesiol 2010;27:24–30.
48. Enomoto Y, Asai T, Arai T, et al. Pentax-AWS, a new videolaryngoscope, is more effective than the Macintosh laryngoscope for tracheal intubation in patients with restricted neck movements: a randomized comparative study. Br J Anaesth 2008;100:544–8.
49. Malik MA, Maharaj CH, Harte BH, et al. Comparison of Macintosh, Truview EVO2, Glidescope, and Airwayscope laryngoscope use in patients with cervical spine immobilization. Br J Anaesth 2008;101:723–30.
50. Malik MA, Subramaniam R, Churasia S, et al. Tracheal intubation in patients with cervical spine immobilization: a comparison of the Airwayscope, LMA CTrach, and the Macintosh laryngoscopes. Br J Anaesth 2009;102:654–61.
51. Maharaj CH, Buckley E, Harte BH, et al. Endotracheal intubation in patients with cervical spine immobilization: a comparison of Macintosh and Airtraq laryngoscopes. Anesthesiology 2007;107:53–9.
52. Smith CE, Pinchak AB, Sidhu TS, et al. Evaluation of tracheal intubation difficulty in patients with cervical spine immobilization: fiberoptic (WuScope) versus conventional laryngoscopy. Anesthesiology 1999;91:1253–9.
53. Adnet F, Borron SW, Racine SX, et al. The intubation difficulty scale (IDS): proposal and evaluation of a new score characterizing the complexity of endotracheal intubation. Anesthesiology 1997;87:1290–7.
54. Maruyama K, Yamada T, Kawakami R, et al. Upper cervical spine movement during intubation: fluoroscopic comparison of the AirWay Scope, McCoy laryngoscope, and Macintosh laryngoscope. Br J Anaesth 2008;100:120–4.
55. Hirabayashi Y, Fujita A, Seo N, et al. Cervical spine movement during laryngoscopy using the Airway Scope compared with the Macintosh laryngoscope. Anaesthesia 2007;62:1050–5.
56. Hastings RH, Vigil AC, Hanna R, et al. Cervical spine movement during laryngoscopy with the Bullard, Macintosh, and Miller laryngoscopes. Anesthesiology 1995;82:859–69.
57. Maruyama K, Yamada T, Kawakami R, et al. Randomized cross-over comparison of cervical-spine motion with the AirWay Scope or Macintosh laryngoscope with in-line stabilization: a video–fluoroscopic study. Br J Anaesth 2008;101:563–7.
58. Turkstra TP, Craen RA, Pelz DM, et al. Cervical spine motion: a fluoroscopic comparison during intubation with lighted stylet, GlideScope, and Macintosh laryngoscope. Anesth Analg 2005;101:910–5.
59. Turkstra TP, Pelz DM, Jones PM. Cervical spine motion: a fluoroscopic comparison of the AirTraq Laryngoscope versus the Macintosh laryngoscope. Anesthesiology 2009;111:97–101.
60. Robitaille A, Williams SR, Tremblay MH, et al. Cervical spine motion during tracheal intubation with manual in-line stabilization: direct laryngoscopy versus GlideScope videolaryngoscopy. Anesth Analg 2008;106:935–41.
61. Emery SE, Smith MD, Bohlman HH. Upper airway obstruction after multilevel cervical corpectomy for myelopathy. J Bone Joint Surg Am 1991;73:544–51.

62. Sagi HC, Beutler W, Carroll E, et al. Airway complications associated with surgery on the anterior cervical spine. Spine (Phila Pa 1976) 2002;27:949–53.

63. Terao Y, Matsumoto S, Yamashita K, et al. Increased incidence of emergency airway management after combined anterior-posterior cervical spine surgery. J Neurosurg Anesthesiol 2004;16:282–6.

64. Yamashita K, Terao Y, Inadomi C, et al. Management of postoperative pharyngeal swelling after anterio-posterior cervical fusion under pharyngoscopy. Masui 2005; 54:420–2.

65. De Bast Y, De Backer D, Moraine JJ, et al. The cuff leak test to predict failure of tracheal extubation for laryngeal edema. Intensive Care Med 2002;28:1267–72.

66. Dosemeci L, Yilmaz M, Yegin A, et al. The routine use of pediatric airway exchange catheter after extubation of adult patients who have undergone maxillofacial or major neck surgery: a clinical observational study. Crit Care 2004;8: R385–90.

67. Liu EH, Goy RW, Tan BH, et al. Tracheal intubation with videolaryngoscopes in patients with cervical spine immobilization: a randomized trial of the Airway Scope and the GlideScope. Br J Anaesth 2009;103:446–51.

68. Watts AD, Gelb AW, Bach DB, et al. Comparison of the Bullard and Macintosh laryngoscopes for endotracheal intubation of patients with a potential cervical spine injury. Anesthesiology 1997;87:1335–42.

Anesthetic Considerations for Awake Craniotomy for Epilepsy and Functional Neurosurgery

Kirstin M. Erickson, MD,[a],*, Daniel J. Cole, MD[a,b]

KEYWORDS

- Awake craniotomy • Epilepsy surgery • Seizure focus resection
- Temporal lobe epilepsy • DBS implantation • Functional neurosurgery

KEY POINTS

- When an epileptic focus is immediately adjacent to eloquent cortex, such as that which controls language or motor function, the awake state optimizes the extent of resection and increases success.
- Implantation of deep brain stimulator (DBS) electrodes is performed in the awake state to facilitate microelectrode brain mapping and clinical assessment of target symptoms.
- Advances in neuromodulation techniques and growing indications for DBS make this a growth area in neuroanesthesia.
- The key to successful management of awake craniotomy patients is patient preparation.
- Dexmedetomidine or, alternatively, propofol with fentanyl or remifentanil, is a common regimen for seamless transition from the asleep or sedated state to alertness and back during craniotomy.
- Local anesthesia alone or conscious sedation with dexmedetomidine or propofol is a common choice for awake DBS implantation.

INTRODUCTION

The awake state is the anesthetic technique of choice for several neurosurgical interventions: epilepsy surgery, DBS placement, tumor or vascular lesion resection in eloquent areas, and pallidotomy. When an epileptic focus is immediately adjacent to eloquent cortex, such as that which controls language or motor function, the awake state optimizes the extent of resection and increases success.[1–4] Similarly, when targeting small groups of cells with a stimulation electrode in deep brain structures, observing the degree of symptom relief in the awake patient is essential. Although

Financial disclosures/conflicts of interest: The authors have nothing to disclose.
[a] Department of Anesthesiology, Mayo Clinic College of Medicine, 200 First Street, SE, Rochester, MN 55901, USA; [b] Department of Anesthesiology, Mayo Clinic Hospital, Mayo Clinic Arizona, 5777 East Mayo Boulevard, Phoenix, AZ 85054, USA
* Corresponding author.
E-mail address: erickson.kirstin@mayo.edu

Anesthesiology Clin 30 (2012) 241–268
doi:10.1016/j.anclin.2012.05.002
1932-2275/12/$ – see front matter © 2012 Elsevier Inc. All rights reserved.

the awake technique has other indications, including resection of tumors or vascular lesions having an impact on eloquent cortex, it was used initially to guide epileptogenic focus resection and this remains its primary role. Functional neurosurgery is currently the fastest growing indication for awake neurosurgery. An awake procedure requires good patient cooperation, anticipation of specific problems, and clinical vigilance. Neuroanesthesiologists have a wide array of anesthetic options to achieve smooth management and high patient satisfaction.

BACKGROUND
Rationale for Awake Epilepsy Surgery

Epilepsy affects approximately 0.8% to 1.7% of the population worldwide (between 2.1 and 2.7 million Americans) making it the third most common neurologic disorder in the world after stroke and Alzheimer disease.[5–7] Of those medically treated in the United States, 30% to 40% continue to have seizures.[8] Epilepsy is considered intractable when severe, frequent seizure activity cannot be adequately controlled by a reasonable trial of medications and prevents normal function or development. Many patients with intractable seizures may benefit from surgical resection. When the focus (either tumor or nonlesional focus) lies in or near eloquent brain (primary motor, sensory, memory, vision, and language cortex), an awake craniotomy, with surgical resection of the seizure focus, is often the preferred intervention.

Rationale for Awake Deep Brain Stimulator Implantation

Tremor (14.5%), Parkinson disease (7%), and dystonia (1.8%) represent 3 of the most common movement disorders.[9] Each of these disorders may become refractory to medication and cause significant disability in otherwise healthy individuals. Such disability may be significantly ameliorated by electrical stimulation of specific deep brain structures unique to each disorder. Effectiveness of DBS for idiopathic essential tremor, idiopathic Parkinson disease, and dystonia has been well documented in the literature.[10–34]

The mechanism by which DBS modifies neuronal activity to intercede in movement disorders is not known.[35] Target sites differ according to the specific disorder (**Table 1**). Neuronal effects of stimulation at each site vary as well. Both inhibition and activation of γ-aminobutyric acid (GABA) cells are reported depending on the location of stimulation.[36,37] Real-time voltammetry, measuring local brain chemicals at the lead tip, has recorded an evoked release of dopamine with electrical stimulation and may provide greater insight into mechanisms of efficacy.[38]

INDICATIONS
Indications for Resection of Seizure Focus

Patients with epilepsy are considered candidates for resection when a sufficient trial of antiepileptic drugs (AEDs) has failed to attain adequate control and when there is reasonable likelihood that an operation will benefit the patients. Judging the adequacy of AED trials for a given patient must be done in context of the prognosis and severity of the specific epileptic type.[39] In most centers, an interdisciplinary team, including neurologists, neurophysiologists, social workers, radiologists, and neurosurgeons, decides whether a patient meets these criteria.

Surgical treatment is most beneficial for patients with partial epilepsy due to discrete structural lesions (benign or neoplastic) and specific surgically remediable syndromes, including mesial temporal lobe epilepsy, which is described as the most common type of epilepsy and the most refractory to pharmacotherapy.[40–42]

Table 1
Indications and target areas for deep brain stimulation

	Target Cells
Established Indications	
Idiopathic essential tremor	VIM thalamus, PSA[a]
Idiopathic Parkinson disease—tremor, dyskinesia, rigidity, bradykinesia, and motor fluctuations	STN, GPi
Dystonia	GPi
Emerging Indications (Investigational)	
Obsessive compulsive disorder	Right nucleus accumbens, STN, VC/VS
Refractory epilepsy	Various (anterior nucleus of the thalamus to cerebellum)
Tremor caused by multiple sclerosis	VIM thalamus
Tourette syndrome	Centromedian-parafascicular complex, anterior thalamus, GPi
Chronic pain	PAG/PVG, thalamus
Major depression	Cg25, nucleus accumbens, VC/VS
Indications Under Early Investigation	
Other tremor (kinetic, poststroke, posthead trauma, PSP)	VIM thalamus, STN, PPTg
Alzheimer disease	Hypothalamus
Minimally conscious and vegetative states	Mesencephalic reticular formation, central thalamus

Abbreviations: Cg25, subgenual cingulate cortex; PAG, periaquaductal gray; PPTg, nucleus tegmenti pedunculopontine; PSA, posterior subthalamic area; PSP, progressive supranuclear palsy; PVG, periventricular gray; VC/VS, ventral capsule/ventral striatum; VIM thalamus, ventral intermediate nucleus of the thalamus.
[a] PSA is nontraditional for idiopathic essential tremor.

Lesions or foci are commonly located in the temporal lobe and may be in or near the functional cortex, depending on the hemisphere. A variety of tests may be performed to locate the seizure focus (**Box 1**). Eloquent cortex includes Wernicke speech area in the dominant temporal lobe, Broca speech area in the dominant frontal lobe, and the motor strip. Areas associated with memory, both verbal and visuospatial, have also been mapped to the temporal lobes, although intraoperative testing of these functions has proved complex and time consuming.[43,44] When intraoperative brain mapping requires neurologic assessment of speech or other function, an awake procedure is indicated to achieve maximal resection of epileptic cortex and maximal preservation of function.

Benefits of an awake craniotomy include greater extent of resection[2–4]; better preservation of language function[1,45]; shorter hospitalization[46,47] and thereby reduced costs[48]; decreased use of invasive monitors[46,49,50]; decreased postoperative anesthetic complications, including nausea and vomiting[51]; and decreased risk of permanent deficit.[45,52–55] One retrospective comparison found no difference in seizure-free outcomes after awake resections versus those done under general anesthesia.[56]

Indications for DBS Implantation

DBS implantation is an elective intervention offered to significantly improve quality of life in movement disorders. DBS is indicated for the treatment of idiopathic essential

---

Box 1
Diagnostic tests used in evaluation for resection of epileptogenic foci

Tests of epileptic excitability

Noninvasive electroencephalogram (EEG)

Video EEG, long-term monitoring

Outpatient long-term EEG monitoring

Invasive EEG

    Intraoperative electrocorticography

    Stereotactic depth-electrode, long-term recording

    Subdural grid or strip, long-term recording

Ictal single-photon emission CT (SPECT)

Subtraction ictal SPECT coregistered to MRI (SISCOM)

Functional MRI (fMRI)[a]

Interictal and ictal magnetoencephalography (MEG)[a]

Tests for structural abnormalities

X-ray films, CT, and other radiographic studies

MRI

Magnetic resonance spectroscopy (MR SPECT)

Tests for functional deficit

Interictal positron emission tomography (PET)

Interictal SPECT

Neuropsychological batteries

Intracarotid amobarbital (Wada test)

Interictal EEG

MR SPECT

Interictal MEG[a]

Tests of normal cortical function (cortical mapping)

Intraoperative electrocorticography (ECoG)

Extraoperative subdural grid recording

Intracarotid amobarbital (Wada test)

PET

fMRI

MEG[a]

Magnetic source imaging or MEG coregistered to MRI (MSI)[a]

[a] Considered experimental for this indication.
  Adapted from Engel Jr J. Surgery for seizures. N Engl J Med 1996;334:647–52; with permission.

---

tremor (FDA approval, 1997), idiopathic Parkinson disease (FDA approval, 2002), and dystonia (FDA approval, 2003).[57] DBS is an emerging/experimental treatment for obsessive-compulsive disorder (FDA humanitarian device exemption, 2009),[57–64] refractory epilepsy (FDA approval, 2010),[65–71] tremor caused by multiple sclerosis,[72–76]

Tourette syndrome,[77–80] chronic pain,[81–87] major depression,[88–91] other tremors (kinetic, poststroke, posttraumatic, progressive supranuclear palsy, and so forth),[92–97] Alzheimer disease,[98,99] and minimally conscious and vegetative states.[100–102]

In general, patients are offered DBS only after medical management of the specific condition is no longer effective and disease progression reaches the point of causing disability. Earlier, milder disease symptoms do not outweigh the risks of the procedure, whereas later stage problems, for example permanent skeletal changes in dystonia, may not respond to DBS.

Contraindications to DBS Implantation

Contraindications to DBS include coagulopathy, recent use of antiplatelet medication, and uncontrolled hypertension, because these are associated with an increased risk of intracranial hemorrhage.[103,104] The need for ongoing electroconvulsive shock therapy or diathermy treatments (deep tissue heat treatments) is also a contraindication to DBS insertion. The need for MRI seems not to preclude DBS implantation, because it has been demonstrated to be safe by several investigators (including a review of more than 4000 cases).[105–107] Procedures requiring electrocautery are not absolutely contraindicated after DBS placement but should be avoided when possible.[108–110] If electrocautery must be used, recommendations include preoerative and postoperative program alterations to the DBS generator, use of bipolar rather than monopolar cautery, and use of the lowest energy and shortest amount of time possible.[111]

SURGICAL PROCEDURE
Resection of Epileptic Focus

Although craniotomy, ECoG, and resection may be done in 1 procedure, these are often separated into 2 operations. In this approach, a craniotomy for placement of subdural grid electrodes is done under general anesthesia, although awake craniotomy for grid placement guided by cortical stimulation (to identify the sensorimotor cortex and to reproduce the patient's aura) has been described.[112] Postoperatively, a period of ictal electrocorticographic recordings and cortical stimulation further delineates the site of seizure onset and functional anatomy. Return to the operating room occurs days to weeks later for grid removal and definitive resection of the epileptogenic center. This is when the awake technique is most often required. A limited resection of epileptogenic brain is performed after using bipolar stimulation to identify motor or language sites (**Fig. 1**). Continuous ECoG is performed to rule out confounding subclinical seizure activity as a cause of speech or motor errors. Guidance from cortical stimulation is correlated to 3-D MRI. Function is continuously monitored during resection (**Fig. 2**). When ECoG is used to reproduce a seizure aura, iced saline may be subsequently administered directly on the cortex to stop the epileptic activity. Closure of the dura, bone flap, and scalp is routine.

Surgical Technique for DBS Implantation

DBS implantation, likewise, may be performed in a single operation or as a 2-stage procedure. The initial stage, consisting of microelectrode implantation, is when the awake state is required. Subsequent implantation of the pulse generator (battery unit) may be done immediately or days later and is performed under general anesthetic.

In contrast to epilepsy surgery, a bur hole is sufficient to pass the microelectrode to its target. A rigid head frame holds the patient's head and an immediate, preoperative MRI is obtained to reference internal anatomy to external coordinates (**Fig. 3**). Imaging

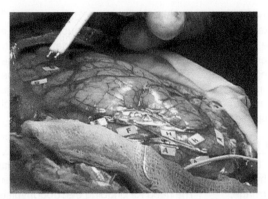

Fig. 1. Open craniotomy showing the cortical surface of a patient with bipolar stimulation using an Ojemann bipolar stimulator while testing appropriate neurologic function in an awake patient. Cortical labels shown include A (arm), F (face), and H (hand). (*Courtesy of* Fredric B. Meyer, MD.)

aids are use to plan a linear trajectory from parietal surface to thalamus or structures near-thalamus, which avoids vasculature and ventricles. Once the styleted electrode lead is in place, microelectrode recordings (MERs) demonstrate changes in spontaneous neuronal firing as the electrode enters different nuclear or thalamic brain tissue. Recordings of both spontaneous neuronal discharge and changes in discharges with patient movement guide lead placement. Macrostimulation then begins and patients are observed for specific symptom amelioration and for adverse effects or unpleasant sensations resulting from stimulation. High-frequency stimulation (above 100 Hz) seems to improve symptoms whereas low frequencies have no effect.[113] The stylet is removed when satisfactory feedback is observed, and the lead is ready for tunneled connection to the pulse generator.

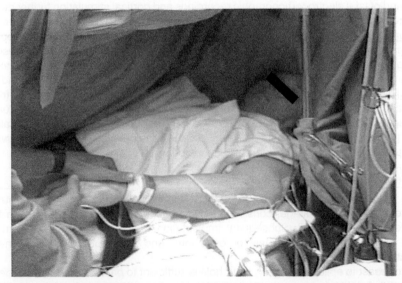

Fig. 2. An awake patient is positioned supine in pinion and under surgical drapes awake and is undergoing motor testing of the left upper extremity. (*Courtesy of* Fredric B. Meyer, MD.)

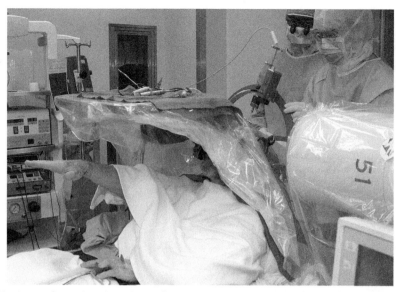

Fig. 3. An awake patient is positioned in a semisitting position with head in a Leksell head frame and under widely spread surgical drapes. A left-sided DBS electrode has been placed via a bur hole, and symptom relief (lack of tremor) is demonstrated in the outstretched right upper extremity during macrostimulation.

PATIENT SELECTION AND PREOPERATIVE EVALUATION

For either procedure, attention should focus on issues critical for the awake patient, in particular, mental maturity and the airway. Good rapport between patient and anesthesiologist as well as among all members of the operating room team cannot be overemphasized in making the procedure as safe and smooth as possible (**Box 2**).

The importance of selecting motivated, mature patients who are able to cope in a strange and stressful environment for an extended period of time is crucial.[114] Anxiety disorder, low tolerance for pain, or psychiatric disorders, such as schizophrenia, may preclude candidacy because there is little pharmacologic rescue that can be offered to awake patients, with their head fixed with penetrating pins within a stereotactic head holder, who has a psychological crisis, without sacrificing the entire awake technique. Screening may include tests of concentration or personality inventory aimed at discovering traits incompatible with cooperative performance in the operating room. Claustrophobia, if severe, may complicate positioning because usually surgical drapes must hang near the immobilized face and can cause a sense of smothering. Careful draping with a more open access to a patient's face, or perhaps the intermittent use of cool air blown over the face, may minimize this fearful sensation.[115] Movement disorders may also compromise a motionless surgical field, although one case report describes the use of regional blocks to eliminate involuntary extremity movements in a patient with unilateral spontaneous movements.[116]

The airway must also be carefully considered. Ease of mask airway, Mallampati score, intubation history, and other predictors of difficulty with laryngoscopy should be assessed with an eye to potential for obstruction, wheezing, or other compromise. Obesity, gastroesophageal reflux, and chronic cough or wheezing may be contraindications of an awake procedure, depending on severity. Airway factors affect planning

---

Box 2
Considerations for preoperative anesthetic evaluation of the patient for awake craniotomy for epilepsy or for awake DBS implantation

Patient cooperation

    Age/maturity

    Anxiety/claustrophobia/emotional stability

    Psychiatric disorders

Airway

    Intubation history

    Airway patency (obesity, obstructive sleep apnea, asthma or other pulmonary disease)

    Airway examination (ease of ability to mask ventilate, to insert laryngeal mask airway [LMA], to intubate)

    Gastroesophageal reflux

Disease state

    Epilepsy

        Form

        Frequency

        Treatment (medications taken)

    Movement disorder

        Type of symptoms

        Severity in off-medication state

        Treatment (medications taken)

Intracranial pressure

Nausea and vomiting

Hemodynamic stability

Adapted from Bonhomme V, Born JD, Hans P. Prise en charge anesthesique des craniotomies en état vigile. Ann Fr Anesth Reanim 2004;23:391; with permission.

---

for intracranial pressure control because brain relaxation by hyperventilation is not attainable in sedated, spontaneously breathing patients.

As with any type of anesthetic, anticipation of specific difficulties is a mainstay of care in the awake craniotomy. Type and frequency of seizures, medication regimen, and serum levels, if applicable, may limit candidacy. Other factors, including size of tumor (if present), hemorrhagic risk, and hemodynamic stability, are considered in conjunction with the surgeon.

PATIENT PREPARATION
Epilepsy Surgery

The procedure is discussed between the patient and the neurosurgeon; although awake brain surgery initially sounds frightening to a patient, once its purpose is carefully explained and reassurance given, the response is usually one of acceptance.[48,114,117,118] After initial preparation, the surgeon, neurologists, neurophysiologists, and speech pathologists review specific language testing (naming, reading, repeating, and responding) or motor testing (facial and extremity movement) that is done in the operating room. In some centers, a test run of patient positioning and language testing in the operating room is done the day before surgery.[119]

Deep Brain Stimulator Implantation

As for awake craniotomy for epilepsy, detailed descriptions of the rationale and of the procedure reassure and motivate patients. A multidisciplinary team reviews and optimizes current treatment and ensures that patients are well informed and have appropriate expectations. Some patients must be in an off-medication state. Similar to awake craniotomy, pediatric patients have also tolerated DBS well with good preparation.[120–123]

POSITIONING

Positioning of awake patients is paramount. The anatomy of interest to all involved—anesthesiologist, surgeon, neurologist, and neurophysiologist—is the patient's head. Access to the surgical field, airway, speech, sight, and facial expression must all be made possible without causing the patient to feel smothered. The patient must remain in rigid pinion fixation or, at minimum, lie motionless on an operating table for several hours. If pinion or epidural skull clamp fixation is not used (necessary for stereotactic techniques), the patient's head may rest in a donut-shaped gel pad or other conformed pillow but must nonetheless remain immobile for several hours.[124] Both the supine and lateral positions are described for epilepsy surgery without report of difficulty. When the supine position is used for seizure focus resection, the head is turned to expose the temporal lobe and to allow gravity to aid frontal lobe retraction (**Fig. 4**). A supine or semisitting position is used for DBS implantation (see **Fig. 3**). A soft mattress, padding of the extremities, and avoidance of extreme head rotation allow the patient to remain still and provide protection from injuries of stretch and pressure. A wide-open geometry of surgical drapes helps to minimize claustrophobia, whereas sufficient blanket coverage and a forced air-warming blanket maintain modesty and body temperature (see **Figs. 2** and **3**). This arrangement also allows eye contact with the patient and provides a clear view for the patient to name objects or pictures. If motor testing is done, a view of the patient's arm and hand as well as face is important (see **Figs. 2** and **3**). In some centers, a microphone is placed near the patient's head or a video camera records the patient's face for viewing by the surgical team.[125,126]

ANESTHETIC MONITORING

Little more than routine monitoring is necessary for either epilepsy surgery or DBS implantation. At the authors' institution, invasive measures are usually not used because neither laboratory assessment nor beat-to-beat blood pressure monitoring is usually indicated intraoperatively, although at some centers these are reportedly used routinely. Type and size of venous access can be directed by the expectations of blood loss and need for administration of hypertonic solutions (eg, hypertonic saline or mannitol). Medical comorbidities should guide this determination. Exhaled carbon dioxide monitoring is essential to both airway vigilance and prevention of cerebral edema/increased brain volume. Precordial Doppler is placed to monitor for venous air embolism in sitting or semisitting patients. A urinary catheter, if used, may be placed under sedation and prevents discomfort due to bladder distention (although the urinary catheter may cause a sense of urgency in some patients).

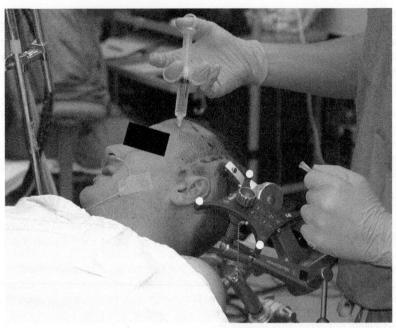

Fig. 4. A patient is positioned supine in pinion and Mayfield head holder, with his head turned, for seizure focus resection. The skin incision is marked and local infiltration of the scalp is in progress while patient is sedated. Nasal cannula for oxygen is taped to the face. The ECoG technician is in the background. (*Courtesy of* Fredric B. Meyer, MD.)

EXPANDED ROLE OF THE ANESTHESIOLOGIST

With any awake patient, and perhaps especially during an awake craniotomy, the role of the anesthesiologist broadens from clinician and physiologist to encompass the roles of coach, confidant, and interpreter. Beyond making frequent inquiries of a patient, the anesthesiologist must remain vigilant of the patient's rate and depth of breathing, skin color, and facial expression. An anesthesiologist may need to facilitate patient communication with the surgeon and give encouragement and reassurance to the patient.

ANESTHETIC MANAGEMENT

A variety of anesthetic techniques have been described to safeguard the airway and to provide good operative conditions in an awake state during the critical portion of eloquent brain mapping. Currently, the 2 general techniques in the literature are asleep-awake-asleep (AAA) and monitored anesthetic care (MAC), with sedation.

Although no generally accepted guidelines for managing awake epilepsy procedures exist at this time, it has been suggested that monitored anesthetic care should be the standard approach.[127] For DBS implantation, sedation or simply local anesthesia is strongly favored in the literature, although long-term success after placement under general anesthesia is reported.[111,128–131] Neuroleptanalgesia is also described for awake craniotomy but is no longer widely used, because the technique is associated with excessive sedation and a higher incidence of pain and seizures.[49]

Newer medications, such as dexmedetomidine, propofol and remifentanil, are shorter acting, provide better pain control, result in fewer adverse effects, and affect neurocognitive testing less than drugs, such as droperidol.[49,132–134] The degree of proconvulsant or anticonvulsant activity of various anesthetic medications is an important consideration during seizure focus resection (**Table 2**). For DBS implantation, light sedation for bur hole and closure or a solely local anesthetic technique is used at many institutions.[128] Propofol attenuates MERs during DBS insertion (to a varying degree depending on deep brain site) whereas dexmedetomidine has little effect on MERs and dissipates quickly to facilitate macrostimulation and motor testing.[135–137] Remifentanil also seems to have little influence on MERs.[136]

Premedication

The goal of premedication is to achieve anxiolysis without oversedation. Other goals may include prevention of nausea, seizure, reflux, pain, hemodynamic instability, or other adverse effects. Oral clonidine, midazolam, alprazolam, and droperidol have all been used to provide anxiolysis, and some amnesia of initial events, although

Table 2
Common anesthetic medications and adjuvants and their associated epileptogenicity (anticonvulsant or proconvulsant activity)

Medication	Epileptogenicity
Propofol	Anticonvulsant at sedative doses
Dexmedetomidine	Possible anticonvulsant activity/possible proconvulsant
Thiopental	Anticonvulsant/proconvulsant in low doses
Midazolam	Anticonvulsant
Diazepam	Anticonvulsant
Methohexital	Anticonvulsant/proconvulsant at low doses
Ketamine	Proconvulsant/anticonvulsant in doses used to treat status epilepticus
Etomidate	Proconvulsant/anticonvulsant in doses used to treat status epilepticus
Nitrous oxide	Likely no effect on EEG/possibly mildly proconvulsant
Isoflurane	Anticonvulsant/possibly mildly proconvulsant
Sevoflurane	Anticonvulsant/possibly mildly proconvulsant
Desflurane	Not proconvulsant
Local anesthetics	Anticonvulsant in low doses/proconvulsant in toxic doses
Opioids (fentanyl, remifentanil, alfentanil, sufentanil)	Proconvulsant in patients with epilepsy
Meperidine	Metabolite normeperidine is proconvulsant
Droperidol	No effect on EEG although may lower seizure threshold
Metoclopramide	No effect on EEG
Ondansetron/granisetron	No effect on EEG
Succinylcholine	EEG activation due to muscle afferent input and increased cerebral blood flow
Vecuronium/rocuronium	No effect on EEG
Atracurium/cisatracurium	Metabolite laudanosine is theoretically proconvulsant

oversedation may be a risk with even small doses of any of these. Droperidol should be avoided in patients with Parkinson disease and dystonia.[138] Clonidine, an α_2-agonist, provides blood pressure control as well and is less likely to induce cognitive impairment. Midazolam may help prevent nausea.[139,140] Benzodiazepines may occasionally produce paradoxic agitation. For this reason, and in order not to risk oversedation and compromise of the neurologic examination, some anesthesia providers do not routinely give any sedative premedication.[141,142] Metoclopramide (metoclopramide blocks dopamine receptors and can cause extrapyramidal side effects), ondansetron, ranitidine, and sodium bicitrate, or similar medications in these classes may be given for prevention of nausea, reflux, or aspiration pneumonia. Depending on the frequency of seizures, patients may receive an oral loading dose of phenytoin or other AED. Dexamethasone may be given for elevated intracranial pressure or prevention of nausea.[143] Acetaminophen was given routinely in one trial for mild analgesia.[117]

Local Anesthetics

With any anesthetic technique for awake craniotomy, adequate local anesthesia is critical to minimizing opioid and sedative requirements and avoiding airway compromise. A neurosurgeon will often depend on consultation with an anesthesiologist to determine maximal dose limits for the local anesthetic. Bupivacaine, levobupivacaine, and ropivacaine are chosen for their long duration of action.[144] Levobupivacaine and ropivacaine are reported to have less cardiac and neurotoxicity in animals.[145] Local anesthetic is used at the pinion sites (if 3-point rigid pinion fixation is used), scalp, and dura (see **Fig. 4**). Plasma levels of local anesthetics have been shown to increase rapidly after scalp infiltration, reaching a peak in 12 to 15 minutes, but without producing signs of toxicity.[146,147] Reinfiltration at closure, although several hours later, is usually not necessary due to the duration of local anesthetic and institution of moderate sedation and analgesia or general anesthesia. An alternative to local field block by a surgeon is the use of regional nerve block of the scalp.[148]

Asleep-Awake-Asleep Technique

The AAA technique calls for general anesthesia, with or without the use of an airway, during the opening and closing portions and emergence of patients in the interim. This technique has also been described as a prolonged wake-up test with removal and replacement of an airway device and is used more often for epilepsy surgery than for DBS insertion. Most often patients are induced with propofol and a short-acting opioid or pulses of fentanyl or a remifentanil infusion, and in some centers target-controlled infusions are used. Propofol infusion rates range from 75 μg/kg/min to 250 μg/kg/min in reports. Sufentanil and alfentanil are cited less frequently but are also easily managed opioids due to their short duration of action. Nitrous oxide may be added. A volatile anesthetic has been used by some anesthesiologists for the initial craniotomy opening, although a residual dose of a volatile anesthetic interferes with ECoG testing. The rates of anesthetic infusion are adjusted to provide deep general anesthesia at the beginning and end of the case and to provide a responsive patient during testing. Propofol is turned off 15 minutes before ECoG recordings, because propofol has a predominantly suppressive effect at sedative doses and interferes with ECoG interpretation.[133] Rates as low as 10 μg/kg/min, however, are reported not to interfere with ECoG.[149] More often, only a low infusion of opioid, such as remifentanil (0.01 μg/kg/min to 0.05 μg/kg/min), is continued during the awake portion.[119,149] The rate of opioid infusion can be adjusted independently of propofol to improve patient comfort or alter the rate of a patient's breathing during spontaneous ventilation. Dexmedetomidine can be used and has been shown to not suppress epileptiform activity on EEG and not interfere with ECoG or MERs at low doses.[137,150–154] One study showed that an infusion rate of dexmedetomidine, 0.2 μg/kg/h, did not affect ECoG recordings.[151]

An LMA is the airway device most often used for the sleep portions due to its ease of insertion, removal, and reinsertion without changing the position of a patient's head (and disruption of the surgical field). Controversy as to whether the LMA represents a secure airway is by no means settled, but in this arena, case reports and chart reviews report low complication rates for using the LMA as an airway device in the spontaneously breathing patient as well as a rescue airway.[114,155] Although this provides good patient comfort and satisfaction, significant sedation can interfere with intraoperative testing.[137] Successful AAA technique without airway manipulation is reported in a retrospective series of pediatric DBS insertion procedures.[123]

In earlier AAA reports, placement of a cuffed endotracheal tube is described as well, including the technique of extubation and reintubation over a tube exchanger,[156] although this may interfere with language testing or, at a minimum, with patient comfort. Fiberoptic intubation is an option for replacement of a cuffed endotracheal tube in pinion fixation.

Monitored Anesthesia Care

The more commonly advocated technique is MAC, also called conscious sedation, for the opening and closing portions of the procedure. Pulses or infusions of many of the same medications—propofol and fentanyl and its analogs—are used as for the AAA technique but at lower doses. Low-dose dexmedetomidine infusion has become a useful choice for MAC during awake craniotomy.

MAC perhaps better achieves the goal of providing a smooth transition to alertness and obviates the difficulties of airway intervention. Oxygen by nasal cannula or face-mask is used. The airway is not manipulated, although a nasal trumpet or oral airway can be helpful for patients with obstructive breathing.[50] Care must be taken to prevent an enriched oxygen environment to develop near the surgical site, because use of electrocautery in this situation may precipitate a surgical site fire. Target-controlled infusions or patient-controlled administration methods have been used.[134,157] Midazolam is a frequently reported adjunct for epilepsy procedures but is avoided for DBS implantation. Suggested doses of remifentanil range from 0.03 to 0.09 μg/kg/min.[118,149,158] Propofol doses are often between 30 μg/kg/min and 180 μg/kg/min.[118,149,158–160] When the dura is opened, it is possible to continue a low-dose infusion of remifentanil or dexmedetomidine throughout the awake portion to achieve a state in which the patient is relaxed but fully arousable to perform testing and respond to questions. Doses in the range of 0.005 μg/kg/min to 0.01 μg/kg/min for remifentanil or 0.02 μg/kg/h to 0.5 μg/kg/h for dexmedetomidine are described for use in this manner.[114,141,149,161–166] These do not interfere with cognitive testing or cortical mapping. For DBS implantation, dexmedetomidine, from 0.2 μg/kg/h to 0.8 μg/kg/h, seems to preserve movement disorder symptoms as well as MERs, although there are currently no prospective data in this area.[137,154]

If propofol and remifentanil are used for seizure focus resection, propofol is turned off 10 to 15 minutes before testing or cortical mapping, and the remifentanil infusion is stopped (or decreased) approximately 2 minutes before testing. Sedation is deepened at the conclusion of all testing and is maintained until skin closure. Just before emergence, a dose of longer-acting opioid is sometimes administered, such as 5 mg to 10 mg of morphine,[114,149] for postoperative analgesia. Johnson and Egan[149] used pharmacokinetic simulations to show that rapid decreases in effect site concentration are achieved by such infusion management during awake craniotomy.

Medications

Several specific medication effects have been studied with regard to awake craniotomy for epilepsy and functional neurosurgery.

Propofol, although providing good patient satisfaction and antiemetic and antiepileptic effects, may cause oversedation and poor operating conditions. Propofol is associated with hypoventilation, although this is less of a problem when a target-controlled infusion is used or when opioids are not added.[114,134] During DBS insertion, less propofol may be required in patients with Parkinson disease than is predicted by target-controlled infusion models.[167]

Opioid-based techniques are associated with increased reports of seizures and nausea.[142] Among opioids, none of the short-acting fentanyl congeners, including the ultra–short-acting remifentanil and alfentanil, used for awake craniotomy has been shown to be superior to its peers. Comparisons of fentanyl with sufentanil and alfentanil, and remifentanil with fentanyl, do not show any differences in complications and all provided good clinical conditions although a case report described severe remifentanil-induced opioid tolerance in a 16 year old.[118,142,168] The desirable brevity of action common to these opioids may require the use of a longer-acting opioid for postoperative pain control.[168] The problems of respiratory depression and increased brain volume (discussed previously) as well as airway obstruction and desaturation are common to all opioids.

Dexmedetomidine, the selective α_2-agonist, has been used for both MAC and AAA management of awake craniotomy and DBS implantation since the first case report by Bekker and colleagues in 2001.[141,150,151,154,161–166,169] The successful use of dexmedetomidine has even been reported in children as young as 12 years.[163,166] Dexmedetomidine provides analgesia with minimal respiratory depression (little risk of hypercapnea), cooperative sedation, anxiolysis without agitation or hangover effect, and hemodynamic stability. Lower doses are suggested for awake craniotomy, because higher doses can impair patient responsiveness.[170] It may be used alone for sedation and analgesia, or with volatile, nitrous oxide, or total intravenous anesthesia as an adjunct to smooth induction, and emergence. Dexmedetomidine alone may be ideal for DBS implantation because it does not depend on GABAergic pharmacology and also does not suppress target symptoms, such as tremor or dyskinesia.[137,153,154] High-dose dexmedetomidine, however, has been shown to interfere with MERs.[137] Likewise, Oda and colleagues[152] reported changes in ECoG recordings during epilepsy surgery with dexmedetomidine use at higher doses (discussed previously). The main disadvantages of dexmedetomidine include hypotension and bradycardia, which are reported to be dose related and treatable, if not preventable.[171]

Anesthetics and Microelectrode Recordings

One of the main purposes of the awake state for DBS placement is to avoid interference of general anesthesia with MERs from deep brain structures.

Benzodiazepines seem to abolish MERs and may induce dyskinesias.[103,128,172] Although there are no prospective data, it seems that anesthetics do not uniformly depress MERs but rather differ by disease as well as by deep brain site/nuclei. For example, desflurane seems to depress MERs from the globus pallidus internus (GPi) in Parkinson disease but not in dystonia.[173] Reports of GPi recordings, both unaffected and depressed by propofol, have been published.[135–137,154,174–176]

In contrast, MERs from the subthalamic nucleus (STN) seem relatively more robust under anesthesia, which has been attributed to its lower GABA input compared with the GPi.[177] Benzodiazepines seem to abolish MERs and may induce dyskinesias.[172]

Dexmedetomidine infusion without loading dose, titrated to an arousable level of consciousness, has been shown to produce MERs from the STN no different from those in the awake state.[136,137] Likewise, propofol and remifentanil seem to have little influence on STN MERs.[136] Adequate STN MERs have been described even under general anesthesia.[178]

COMPLICATIONS

Fortunately, complications are infrequent during and after awake neurosurgery, due in part to the great amount of care taken with patient selection and preparation. For DBS surgery, overall complication rates are so disparate (8.6% up to 54%) that one meta-analysis concluded no meaningful range could be cited.[17,153,169,179–184] The inconsistency is attributed to differences in practice, surgeon experience, basic definition of complications, duration of postoperative recording, and the paucity of systematic prospective recording.[183] Nevertheless, in one prospective study with a high rate of reported complications (54%), adverse events led to no significant difference in quality of life outcomes after DBS insertion ($P = .22$).[183] Regardless, adverse events associated with DBS insertion deserve extra consideration due to the elective nature of the procedure.

Nausea and Vomiting

Nausea and vomiting are infrequent during awake craniotomy for tumors as well as for epileptic foci, likely related to use of propofol, lack of reversal medications, and lack of opioid use.[50,51]

Airway Complications

Airway complications and desaturation, not surprisingly, occur more frequently during awake craniotomy, because sedation is used in conjunction with an unprotected airway. In a large retrospective review, 0.6% of patients under AAA technique had airway complications (requiring intubation, LMA, or nasal airway), two-thirds of whom were obese.[50] None had any adverse sequelae. Incidence of many of these complications has been shown to decrease in recent years with increased experience.[50,114,185] Although some reports describe up to 16% of cases requiring intubation,[119] in the authors' and other investigators' experience, the need for intubation during awake craniotomy is rare.[186,187] Two retrospective studies report the incidence of respiratory complications from 1.6% to 2.2% during DBS implantation.[169,179]

Cerebral Edema

Likewise, hypoventilation and increased brain volume are reported complications of awake craniotomy. Brain swelling may interfere with resection and dural and cranial closure. The large review of complications by Skucas and Artru[50] reported 2 of 332 propofol-based AAA cases involved brain swelling due to hypoventilation. It was thought that only 1 of the 2 (in which a significant hemorrhage with dural opening was sustained) suffered an adverse event as a result of increased brain volume. A prospective trial included 1 of 25 patients who required emergent intubation for brain swelling with no further sequelae after conversion to general anesthesia.[119] Other investigators report hypoventilation but no detrimental increase in brain volume.[114,134,185] During DBS surgery, cerebral edema is also rare. One prospective study reported 0.7% of patients suffered hydrocephalus, although no explicit association with hypoventilation was given.[183]

Seizure

Intraoperative seizure is a risk in this population. Although reports suggest seizures occur infrequently,[50] an unchecked seizure in awake patients in pinion with an unsecured airway is a potential crisis. During DBS implantation, one prospective study of complications reported a seizure rate of 0.06% (as a percentage of procedures),[183] whereas other reports range from 0.8% to 4.5% of patients.[169,179,188,189] Although confounded by duplication in published data, the largest literature review of seizures reports a range of 0% to 10% but without a clear explanation for the variation.[190] The majority (74%) of seizures occurred near the time of lead implantation and many of these patients also sustained intracranial hemorrhage.[190]

Suggested risk factors for seizure include abnormality on postoperative imaging (hemorrhage, edema, and ischemia),[189] hemorrhage,[189,190] age greater than 60 years,[189] transventricular electrode trajectories,[189] and multiple sclerosis.[191] Fortunately, seizures stimulated by cortical mapping during craniotomy for epilepsy are usually aborted by the surgeon stopping the stimulation or delivering ice-cold saline directly onto the cortical surface. Seizures that are spontaneous or do not stop with these measures are treated with small doses of benzodiazepine, propofol, or barbiturate. Rarely do these require intubation. A postictal period may interfere with neurocognitive testing.

Hemorrhage

Bleeding is one of the most feared surgical complications during DBS implantation because it is less easily controlled through a bur hole than via an open craniotomy and because of the functional structures at stake in the area of bleeding. Fortunately, it is rare. Reported frequency of bleeding ranges from 0.9% per procedure[192] to 2.2%[179] to 10%[183] and up to 34.4%.[106] In Zrinzo and coworkers' review of consecutive cases (214 patients, 417 electrodes), 0.5% of hemorrhage was asymptomatic, 0.5% was symptomatic, and 0% resulted in permanent deficit.[192] The investigators identified hypertension and age as risk factors and excluded diagnosis, gender, and previous use of anticoagulants.[192] Surgical risk factors associated with hemorrhage included the use of MERs (in contrast to "image-guided and image-verified" or macrostimulation-guided lead placement), number of microelectrode passes, and transventricular lead trajectories.[192]

Hemodynamic Instability

Hemodynamic changes, including hypertension, hypotension, and tachycardia, were found more frequent, albeit not harmful, to patients when promptly treated with awake craniotomy by the AAA technique than under general anesthesia.[50] During DBS insertion in awake patients, hypertension has been associated with intracranial hemorrhage.[104,193] In one report of 172 DBS procedures plus 6 ablative procedures, 3.9% of patients had systemic arterial blood pressure greater than 160/90 mm Hg for 2 consecutive readings 5 minutes apart (3.9%).[179] Five of 6 patients had a history of hypertension, and all were treated without sequelae.[179] Nevertheless, hypertension requires prompt treatment. Two investigators suggest goals for systolic blood pressure of less than 140 mm Hg or no more than a 20% to 30% decrease from a patient's usual level.[154,193] Rozet and colleagues[154] found improved blood pressure management and less use of antihypertensive medications in patients who were given dexmedetomidine compared with unsedated patients.

Venous Air Embolism

Venous air embolism in awake craniotomy patients is apparently no more frequent than in craniotomy under general anesthesia.[194] In the sitting or semisitting position for DBS insertion, however, venous air embolism occurs with an incidence of 4.5%, as recorded by precordial Doppler, and is often signaled by coughing.[123,195–198] Maintaining hemodynamic stability and communicating with the neurosurgeon while bone wax and/or cautery are applied are priorities when air embolism is encountered.

Agitation and Other Complications

Patient agitation and movement can be managed by altering sedative medications and making other small changes in a patient's immediate surroundings, such as temperature, amount of light, and padding, although rarely more drastic measures, including conversion to general anesthesia are necessary. Care must be taken to observe for and quickly address emergence delirium in patients having AAA care. In the setting of emergence delirium, patients may cause severe injury to themselves (eg, scalp injury or brain herniation) or members of the operating room team. Other reported intraoperative complications in awake craniotomy patients are apparently no more frequent than in craniotomy in the same position under general anesthesia.[194] Excessive sedation during DBS placement may occur as a result of low central dopamine in the off-medication state in unsedated patients with Parkinson disease.[199] Stroke, other neurologic deficit, and death are all rare events in prospective data of DBS surgery (0.007% each).[183] Tension pneumocephalus associated with cerebrospinal fluid drainage from the bur hole has also been described.[195] Complications are managed best if anticipated and prevented through patient selection, preparation, and appropriate use of medication.

SUMMARY

A variety of anesthetic methods, with and without airway manipulation, are available to facilitate awake intraoperative examinations and cortical stimulation, which allow more aggressive resection of epileptogenic foci in functionally important brain regions. Currently, dexmedetomidine or, alternatively, propofol with fentanyl or remifentanil, is the most commonly chosen regimen for seamless transition from the asleep or sedated state to alertness and back during craniotomy. Careful patient selection and preparation combined with attentive cooperation of the medical team are the foundation for a smooth awake procedure. With improved pharmacologic agents and variety of techniques at the neuroanesthesiologist's disposal, awake craniotomy has become an elegant approach to epileptic focus resection in functional cortex and treatment of movement disorders by DBS.

REFERENCES

1. Sahjpaul RL. Awake craniotomy: controversies, indications and techniques in the surgical treatment of temporal lobe epilepsy. Can J Neurol Sci 2000; 27(Suppl 1):S55–63 [discussion: S92–6].
2. De Benedictis A, Moritz-Gasser S, Duffau H. Awake mapping optimizes the extent of resection for low-grade gliomas in eloquent areas. Neurosurgery 2010;66(6):1074–84 [discussion: 1084].
3. Duffau H, Lopes M, Arthuis F, et al. Contribution of intraoperative electrical stimulations in surgery of low grade gliomas: a comparative study between two series without (1985-96) and with (1996-2003) functional mapping in the same institution. J Neurol Neurosurg Psychiatry 2005;76(6):845–51.
4. Reithmeier T, Krammer M, Gumprecht H, et al. Neuronavigation combined with electrophysiological monitoring for surgery of lesions in eloquent brain areas in 42 cases: a retrospective comparison of the neurological outcome and the

quality of resection with a control group with similar lesions. Minim Invasive Neurosurg 2003;46(2):65–71.

5. Organization WH. Neurological disorders: public health challenges. Available at: http://www.who.int/mental_health/neurology/neurodiso/en/index.html. Accessed March 8, 2012.

6. Hirtz D, Thurman DJ, Gwinn-Hardy K, et al. How common are the "common" neurologic disorders? Neurology 2007;68(5):326–37.

7. Foundation E. Epilepsy and seizure statistics. Available at: http://www.epilepsyfoundation.org/aboutepilepsy/index.cfm/statistics. Accessed March 8, 2012.

8. Kwan P, Brodie MJ. Early identification of refractory epilepsy. N Engl J Med 2000;342(5):314–9.

9. Wenning GK, Kiechl S, Seppi K, et al. Prevalence of movement disorders in men and women aged 50-89 years (Bruneck Study cohort): a population-based study. Lancet Neurol 2005;4(12):815–20.

10. Benabid AL, Pollak P, Gervason C, et al. Long-term suppression of tremor by chronic stimulation of the ventral intermediate thalamic nucleus. Lancet 1991; 337(8738):403–6.

11. Schuurman PR, Bosch DA, Bossuyt PM, et al. A comparison of continuous thalamic stimulation and thalamotomy for suppression of severe tremor. N Engl J Med 2000;342(7):461–8.

12. Tasker RR. Deep brain stimulation is preferable to thalamotomy for tremor suppression. Surg Neurol 1998;49(2):145–53 [discussion: 153–4].

13. Pahwa R, Lyons KE, Wilkinson SB, et al. Comparison of thalamotomy to deep brain stimulation of the thalamus in essential tremor. Mov Disord 2001;16(1):140–3.

14. Blond S, Caparros-Lefebvre D, Parker F, et al. Control of tremor and involuntary movement disorders by chronic stereotactic stimulation of the ventral intermediate thalamic nucleus. J Neurosurg 1992;77(1):62–8.

15. Koller W, Pahwa R, Busenbark K, et al. High-frequency unilateral thalamic stimulation in the treatment of essential and parkinsonian tremor. Ann Neurol 1997; 42(3):292–9.

16. Limousin P, Speelman JD, Gielen F, et al. Multicentre European study of thalamic stimulation in parkinsonian and essential tremor. J Neurol Neurosurg Psychiatry 1999;66(3):289–96.

17. Hariz MI, Shamsgovara P, Johansson F, et al. Tolerance and tremor rebound following long-term chronic thalamic stimulation for Parkinsonian and essential tremor. Stereotact Funct Neurosurg 1999;72(2–4):208–18.

18. Blomstedt P, Hariz GM, Hariz MI, et al. Thalamic deep brain stimulation in the treatment of essential tremor: a long-term follow-up. Br J Neurosurg 2007; 21(5):504–9.

19. DiLorenzo DJ, Jankovic J, Simpson RK, et al. Long-term deep brain stimulation for essential tremor: 12-year clinicopathologic follow-up. Mov Disord 2010;25(2): 232–8.

20. Benabid AL, Chabardes S, Mitrofanis J, et al. Deep brain stimulation of the subthalamic nucleus for the treatment of Parkinson's disease. Lancet Neurol 2009; 8(1):67–81.

21. Deuschl G, Schade-Brittinger C, Krack P, et al. A randomized trial of deep-brain stimulation for Parkinson's disease. N Engl J Med 2006;355(9):896–908.

22. Krack P, Batir A, Van Blercom N, et al. Five-year follow-up of bilateral stimulation of the subthalamic nucleus in advanced Parkinson's disease. N Engl J Med 2003;349(20):1925–34.

23. Limousin P, Krack P, Pollak P, et al. Electrical stimulation of the subthalamic nucleus in advanced Parkinson's disease. N Engl J Med 1998;339(16):1105–11.
24. Lanotte MM, Rizzone M, Bergamasco B, et al. Deep brain stimulation of the subthalamic nucleus: anatomical, neurophysiological, and outcome correlations with the effects of stimulation. J Neurol Neurosurg Psychiatry 2002;72(1):53–8.
25. Weaver FM, Follett K, Stern M, et al. Bilateral deep brain stimulation vs best medical therapy for patients with advanced Parkinson disease: a randomized controlled trial. JAMA 2009;301(1):63–73.
26. Moro E, Lozano AM, Pollak P, et al. Long-term results of a multicenter study on subthalamic and pallidal stimulation in Parkinson's disease. Mov Disord 2010; 25(5):578–86.
27. Bronte-Stewart H, Louie S, Batya S, et al. Clinical motor outcome of bilateral subthalamic nucleus deep-brain stimulation for Parkinson's disease using image-guided frameless stereotaxy. Neurosurgery 2010;67(4):1088–93 [discussion: 1093].
28. Coubes P, Roubertie A, Vayssiere N, et al. Treatment of DYT1-generalised dystonia by stimulation of the internal globus pallidus. Lancet 2000;355(9222): 2220–1.
29. Coubes P, Cif L, El Fertit H, et al. Electrical stimulation of the globus pallidus internus in patients with primary generalized dystonia: long-term results. J Neurosurg 2004;101(2):189–94.
30. Holloway KL, Baron MS, Brown R, et al. Deep brain stimulation for dystonia: a meta-analysis. Neuromodulation 2006;9(4):253–61.
31. Kiss ZH, Doig-Beyaert K, Eliasziw M, et al. The Canadian multicentre study of deep brain stimulation for cervical dystonia. Brain 2007;130(Pt 11):2879–86.
32. Kupsch A, Benecke R, Muller J, et al. Pallidal deep-brain stimulation in primary generalized or segmental dystonia. N Engl J Med 2006;355(19):1978–90.
33. Vidailhet M, Vercueil L, Houeto JL, et al. Bilateral deep-brain stimulation of the globus pallidus in primary generalized dystonia. N Engl J Med 2005;352(5): 459–67.
34. Hung SW, Hamani C, Lozano AM, et al. Long-term outcome of bilateral pallidal deep brain stimulation for primary cervical dystonia. Neurology 2007;68(6): 457–9.
35. Dostrovsky JO, Lozano AM. Mechanisms of deep brain stimulation. Mov Disord 2002;17(Suppl 3):S63–8.
36. Ashby P, Rothwell JC. Neurophysiologic aspects of deep brain stimulation. Neurology 2000;55(12 Suppl 6):S17–20.
37. Benazzouz A, Hallett M. Mechanism of action of deep brain stimulation. Neurology 2000;55(12 Suppl 6):S13–6.
38. Van Gompel JJ, Chang SY, Goerss SJ, et al. Development of intraoperative electrochemical detection: wireless instantaneous neurochemical concentration sensor for deep brain stimulation feedback. Neurosurg Focus 2010;29(2):E6.
39. Engel J Jr. Surgery for seizures. N Engl J Med 1996;334(10):647–52.
40. Engel J Jr, Wiebe S, French J, et al. Practice parameter: temporal lobe and localized neocortical resections for epilepsy. Epilepsia 2003;44(6):741–51.
41. Engel J Jr. Etiology as a risk factor for medically refractory epilepsy: a case for early surgical intervention. Neurology 1998;51(5):1243–4.
42. Langfitt JT. Cost-effectiveness of anterotemporal lobectomy in medically intractable complex partial epilepsy. Epilepsia 1997;38(2):154–63.
43. Ojemann GA, Schoenfield-McNeill J. Activity of neurons in human temporal cortex during identification and memory for names and words. J Neurosci 1999;19(13):5674–82.

44. Ojemann GA. The neurobiology of language and verbal memory: observations from awake neurosurgery. Int J Psychophysiol 2003;48(2):141–6.
45. Sanai N, Mirzadeh Z, Berger MS. Functional outcome after language mapping for glioma resection. N Engl J Med 2008;358(1):18–27.
46. Taylor MD, Bernstein M. Awake craniotomy with brain mapping as the routine surgical approach to treating patients with supratentorial intraaxial tumors: a prospective trial of 200 cases. J Neurosurg 1999;90(1):35–41.
47. Blanshard HJ, Chung F, Manninen PH, et al. Awake craniotomy for removal of intracranial tumor: considerations for early discharge. Anesth Analg 2001; 92(1):89–94.
48. Jaaskelainen J, Randell T. Awake craniotomy in glioma surgery. Acta Neurochir Suppl 2003;88:31–5.
49. Danks RA, Rogers M, Aglio LS, et al. Patient tolerance of craniotomy performed with the patient under local anesthesia and monitored conscious sedation. Neurosurgery 1998;42(1):28–34 [discussion: 34–6].
50. Skucas AP, Artru AA. Anesthetic complications of awake craniotomies for epilepsy surgery. Anesth Analg 2006;102(3):882–7.
51. Manninen PH, Tan TK. Postoperative nausea and vomiting after craniotomy for tumor surgery: a comparison between awake craniotomy and general anesthesia. J Clin Anesth 2002;14(4):279–83.
52. Chang EF, Potts MB, Keles GE, et al. Seizure characteristics and control following resection in 332 patients with low-grade gliomas. J Neurosurg 2008; 108(2):227–35.
53. Duffau H, Peggy Gatignol ST, Mandonnet E, et al. Intraoperative subcortical stimulation mapping of language pathways in a consecutive series of 115 patients with Grade II glioma in the left dominant hemisphere. J Neurosurg 2008;109(3):461–71.
54. Sanai N, Berger MS. Glioma extent of resection and its impact on patient outcome. Neurosurgery 2008;62(4):753–64 [discussion: 264–6].
55. Serletis D, Bernstein M. Prospective study of awake craniotomy used routinely and nonselectively for supratentorial tumors. J Neurosurg 2007;107(1):1–6.
56. Kim CH, Chung CK, Lee SK. Longitudinal change in outcome of frontal lobe epilepsy surgery. Neurosurgery 2010;67(5):1222–9 [discussion: 1229].
57. Administration USFaD. Recently-approved devices. Available at: http://www.fda.gov/MedicalDevices/ProductsandMedicalProcedures/DeviceApprovalsand Clearances/Recently-ApprovedDevices/default.htm. Accessed February 8, 2012.
58. Greenberg BD, Malone DA, Friehs GM, et al. Three-year outcomes in deep brain stimulation for highly resistant obsessive-compulsive disorder. Neuropsychopharmacology 2006;31(11):2384–93.
59. Jimenez-Ponce F, Velasco-Campos F, Castro-Farfan G, et al. Preliminary study in patients with obsessive-compulsive disorder treated with electrical stimulation in the inferior thalamic peduncle. Neurosurgery 2009;65(Suppl 6):203–9 [discussion: 209].
60. Mian MK, Campos M, Sheth SA, et al. Deep brain stimulation for obsessive-compulsive disorder: past, present, and future. Neurosurg Focus 2010;29(2): E10.
61. de Koning PP, Figee M, van den Munckhof P, et al. Current status of deep brain stimulation for obsessive-compulsive disorder: a clinical review of different targets. Curr Psychiatry Rep 2011;13(4):274–82.
62. Mallet L, Polosan M, Jaafari N, et al. Subthalamic nucleus stimulation in severe obsessive-compulsive disorder. N Engl J Med 2008;359(20):2121–34.

63. Nuttin B, Cosyns P, Demeulemeester H, et al. Electrical stimulation in anterior limbs of internal capsules in patients with obsessive-compulsive disorder. Lancet 1999;354(9189):1526.
64. Huff W, Lenartz D, Schormann M, et al. Unilateral deep brain stimulation of the nucleus accumbens in patients with treatment-resistant obsessive-compulsive disorder: Outcomes after one year. Clin Neurol Neurosurg 2010;112(2):137–43.
65. Fisher RS, Uematsu S, Krauss GL, et al. Placebo-controlled pilot study of centromedian thalamic stimulation in treatment of intractable seizures. Epilepsia 1992;33(5):841–51.
66. Fisher R. Initial Results of SANTE Trial. American Epilepsy Society 62nd Annual Meeting. Seattle, December 7, 2008.
67. Fisher R, Salanova V, Witt T, et al. Electrical stimulation of the anterior nucleus of thalamus for treatment of refractory epilepsy. Epilepsia 2010;51(5):899–908.
68. Lega BC, Halpern CH, Jaggi JL, et al. Deep brain stimulation in the treatment of refractory epilepsy: update on current data and future directions. Neurobiol Dis 2010;38(3):354–60.
69. Lockman J, Fisher RS. Therapeutic brain stimulation for epilepsy. Neurol Clin 2009;27(4):1031–40.
70. Davis R, Emmonds SE. Cerebellar stimulation for seizure control: 17-year study. Stereotact Funct Neurosurg 1992;58(1–4):200–8.
71. Velasco F, Carrillo-Ruiz JD, Brito F, et al. Double-blind, randomized controlled pilot study of bilateral cerebellar stimulation for treatment of intractable motor seizures. Epilepsia 2005;46(7):1071–81.
72. Hooper J, Taylor R, Pentland B, et al. A prospective study of thalamic deep brain stimulation for the treatment of movement disorders in multiple sclerosis. Br J Neurosurg 2002;16(2):102–9.
73. Herzog J, Hamel W, Wenzelburger R, et al. Kinematic analysis of thalamic versus subthalamic neurostimulation in postural and intention tremor. Brain 2007;130(Pt 6):1608–25.
74. Mandat T, Koziara H, Tutaj M, et al. Thalamic deep brain stimulation for tremor among multiple sclerosis patients. Neurol Neurochir Pol 2010;44(6):542–5.
75. Thevathasan W, Schweder P, Joint C, et al. Permanent tremor reduction during thalamic stimulation in multiple sclerosis. J Neurol Neurosurg Psychiatry 2011; 82(4):419–22.
76. Torres CV, Moro E, Lopez-Rios AL, et al. Deep brain stimulation of the ventral intermediate nucleus of the thalamus for tremor in patients with multiple sclerosis. Neurosurgery 2010;67(3):646–51 [discussion: 651].
77. Vandewalle V, van der Linden C, Groenewegen HJ, et al. Stereotactic treatment of Gilles de la Tourette syndrome by high frequency stimulation of thalamus. Lancet 1999;353(9154):724.
78. Maciunas RJ, Maddux BN, Riley DE, et al. Prospective randomized double-blind trial of bilateral thalamic deep brain stimulation in adults with Tourette syndrome. J Neurosurg 2007;107(5):1004–14.
79. Servello D, Porta M, Sassi M, et al. Deep brain stimulation in 18 patients with severe Gilles de la Tourette syndrome refractory to treatment: the surgery and stimulation. J Neurol Neurosurg Psychiatry 2008;79(2):136–42.
80. Porta M, Brambilla A, Cavanna AE, et al. Thalamic deep brain stimulation for treatment-refractory Tourette syndrome: two-year outcome. Neurology 2009; 73(17):1375–80.

81. Katayama Y, Yamamoto T, Kobayashi K, et al. Deep brain and motor cortex stimulation for post-stroke movement disorders and post-stroke pain. Acta Neurochir Suppl 2003;87:121–3.

82. Bittar RG, Kar-Purkayastha I, Owen SL, et al. Deep brain stimulation for pain relief: a meta-analysis. J Clin Neurosci 2005;12(5):515–9.

83. Hamani C, Schwalb JM, Rezai AR, et al. Deep brain stimulation for chronic neuropathic pain: long-term outcome and the incidence of insertional effect. Pain 2006;125(1-2):188–96.

84. Schoenen J, Di Clemente L, Vandenheede M, et al. Hypothalamic stimulation in chronic cluster headache: a pilot study of efficacy and mode of action. Brain 2005;128(Pt 4):940–7.

85. Green AL, Owen SL, Davies P, et al. Deep brain stimulation for neuropathic cephalalgia. Cephalalgia 2006;26(5):561–7.

86. Fontaine D, Lanteri-Minet M, Ouchchane L, et al. Anatomical location of effective deep brain stimulation electrodes in chronic cluster headache. Brain 2010; 133(Pt 4):1214–23.

87. Franzini A, Messina G, Cordella R, et al. Deep brain stimulation of the posteromedial hypothalamus: indications, long-term results, and neurophysiological considerations. Neurosurg Focus 2010;29(2):E13.

88. Schlaepfer TE, Cohen MX, Frick C, et al. Deep brain stimulation to reward circuitry alleviates anhedonia in refractory major depression. Neuropsychopharmacology 2008;33(2):368–77.

89. Mayberg HS, Lozano AM, Voon V, et al. Deep brain stimulation for treatment-resistant depression. Neuron 2005;45(5):651–60.

90. Lozano AM, Mayberg HS, Giacobbe P, et al. Subcallosal cingulate gyrus deep brain stimulation for treatment-resistant depression. Biol Psychiatry 2008;64(6):461–7.

91. Malone DA Jr, Dougherty DD, Rezai AR, et al. Deep brain stimulation of the ventral capsule/ventral striatum for treatment-resistant depression. Biol Psychiatry 2009;65(4):267–75.

92. Vesper J, Funk T, Kern B, et al. Thalamic deep brain stimulation: present state of the art. Neurosurg Q 2000;10(4):252–60.

93. Nguyen JP, Degos JD. Thalamic stimulation and proximal tremor. A specific target in the nucleus ventrointermedius thalami. Arch Neurol 1993;50(5): 498–500.

94. Broggi G, Brock S, Franzini A, et al. A case of posttraumatic tremor treated by chronic stimulation of the thalamus. Mov Disord 1993;8(2):206–8.

95. Benabid AL, Pollak P, Gao D, et al. Chronic electrical stimulation of the ventralis intermedius nucleus of the thalamus as a treatment of movement disorders. J Neurosurg 1996;84(2):203–14.

96. Bergmann KJ, Salak VL. Subthalamic stimulation improves levodopa responsive symptoms in a case of progressive supranuclear palsy. Parkinsonism Relat Disord 2008;14(4):348–52.

97. Brusa L, Iani C, Ceravolo R, et al. Implantation of the nucleus tegmenti pedunculopontini in a PSP-P patient: safe procedure, modest benefits. Mov Disord 2009;24(13):2020–2.

98. Laxton AW, Tang-Wai DF, McAndrews MP, et al. A phase I trial of deep brain stimulation of memory circuits in Alzheimer's disease. Ann Neurol 2010;68(4): 521–34.

99. Mannu P, Rinaldi S, Fontani V, et al. Radio electric asymmetric brain stimulation in the treatment of behavioral and psychiatric symptoms in Alzheimer disease. Clin Interv Aging 2011;6:207–11.

100. Tsubokawa T, Yamamoto T, Katayama Y, et al. Deep-brain stimulation in a persistent vegetative state: follow-up results and criteria for selection of candidates. Brain Inj 1990;4(4):315–27.

101. Schiff ND, Giacino JT, Kalmar K, et al. Behavioural improvements with thalamic stimulation after severe traumatic brain injury. Nature 2007;448(7153):600–3.

102. Sen AN, Campbell PG, Yadla S, et al. Deep brain stimulation in the management of disorders of consciousness: a review of physiology, previous reports, and ethical considerations. Neurosurg Focus 2010;29(2):E14.

103. Hutchinson WL, Lozano A. Microelectrode recording in movement disorder surgery. In: Lozano A, editor. Movement disorder surgery, vol. 15. Basel (Switzerland): Karger; 2000. p. 103–17.

104. Binder DK, Rau GM, Starr PA. Risk factors for hemorrhage during microelectrode-guided deep brain stimulator implantation for movement disorders. Neurosurgery 2005;56(4):722–32 [discussion: 722–32].

105. Zrinzo L, Yoshida F, Hariz MI, et al. Clinical safety of brain magnetic resonance imaging with implanted deep brain stimulation hardware: large case series and review of the literature. World Neurosurg 2011;76(1-2):164–72 [discussion: 169–73].

106. Chhabra V, Sung E, Mewes K, et al. Safety of magnetic resonance imaging of deep brain stimulator systems: a serial imaging and clinical retrospective study. J Neurosurg 2010;112(3):497–502.

107. Huston OO, Watson RE, Bernstein MA, et al. Intraoperative magnetic resonance imaging findings during deep brain stimulation surgery. J Neurosurg 2011;115(4):852–7.

108. Martinelli PT, Schulze KE, Nelson BR. Mohs micrographic surgery in a patient with a deep brain stimulator: a review of the literature on implantable electrical devices. Dermatol Surg 2004;30(7):1021–30.

109. Milligan DJ, Milligan KR. Deep brain neuro-stimulators and anaesthesia. Anaesthesia 2007;62(8):852–3.

110. Weaver J, Kim SJ, Lee MH, et al. Cutaneous electrosurgery in a patient with a deep brain stimulator. Dermatol Surg 1999;25(5):415–7.

111. Poon CC, Irwin MG. Anaesthesia for deep brain stimulation and in patients with implanted neurostimulator devices. Br J Anaesth 2009;103(2):152–65.

112. Cohen-Gadol AA, Britton JW, Collignon FP, et al. Nonlesional central lobule seizures: use of awake cortical mapping and subdural grid monitoring for resection of seizure focus. J Neurosurg 2003;98(6):1255–62.

113. Johnson MD, Miocinovic S, McIntyre CC, et al. Mechanisms and targets of deep brain stimulation in movement disorders. Neurotherapeutics 2008;5(2):294–308.

114. Sarang A, Dinsmore J. Anaesthesia for awake craniotomy–evolution of a technique that facilitates awake neurological testing. Br J Anaesth 2003;90(2):161–5.

115. Brock-Utne JG. Awake craniotomy. Anaesth Intensive Care 2001;29(6):669.

116. Gebhard RE, Berry J, Maggio WW, et al. The successful use of regional anesthesia to prevent involuntary movements in a patient undergoing awake craniotomy. Anesth Analg 2000;91(5):1230–1.

117. Whittle IR, Midgley S, Georges H, et al. Patient perceptions of "awake" brain tumour surgery. Acta Neurochir (Wien) 2005;147(3):275–7 [discussion: 277].

118. Manninen PH, Balki M, Lukitto K, et al. Patient satisfaction with awake craniotomy for tumor surgery: a comparison of remifentanil and fentanyl in conjunction with propofol. Anesth Analg 2006;102(1):237–42.

119. Picht T, Kombos T, Gramm HJ, et al. Multimodal protocol for awake craniotomy in language cortex tumour surgery. Acta Neurochir (Wien) 2006;148(2):127–37 [discussion: 137–8].

120. Lipsman N, Ellis M, Lozano AM. Current and future indications for deep brain stimulation in pediatric populations. Neurosurg Focus 2010;29(2):E2.

121. Air EL, Ostrem JL, Sanger TD, et al. Deep brain stimulation in children: experience and technical pearls. J Neurosurg Pediatr 2011;8(6):566–74.

122. Walcott BP, Nahed BV, Kahle KT, et al. Deep brain stimulation for medically refractory life-threatening status dystonicus in children. J Neurosurg Pediatr 2012;9(1):99–102.

123. Sebeo J, Deiner SG, Alterman RL, et al. Anesthesia for pediatric deep brain stimulation. Anesthesiol Res Pract 2010;2010:1–4.

124. Leuthardt EC, Fox D, Ojemann GA, et al. Frameless stereotaxy without rigid pin fixation during awake craniotomies. Stereotact Funct Neurosurg 2002;79(3-4):256–61.

125. Bernstein M. Outpatient craniotomy for brain tumor: a pilot feasibility study in 46 patients. Can J Neurol Sci 2001;28(2):120–4.

126. Costello TG, Cormack JR. Anaesthesia for awake craniotomy: a modern approach. J Clin Neurosci 2004;11(1):16–9.

127. Meyer FB, Bates LM, Goerss SJ, et al. Awake craniotomy for aggressive resection of primary gliomas located in eloquent brain. Mayo Clin Proc 2001;76(7):677–87.

128. Venkatraghavan L, Luciano M, Manninen P. Review article: anesthetic management of patients undergoing deep brain stimulator insertion. Anesth Analg 2010;110(4):1138–45.

129. Venkatraghavan L, Manninen P. Anesthesia for deep brain stimulation. Curr Opin Anaesthesiol 2011;24(5):495–9.

130. Bilotta F, Rosa G. 'Anesthesia' for awake neurosurgery. Curr Opin Anaesthesiol 2009;22(5):560–5.

131. Harries AM, Kausar J, Roberts SA, et al. Deep brain stimulation of the subthalamic nucleus for advanced Parkinson disease using general anesthesia: long-term results. J Neurosurg 2012;116(1):107–13.

132. Archer DP, McKenna JM, Morin L, et al. Conscious-sedation analgesia during craniotomy for intractable epilepsy: a review of 354 consecutive cases. Can J Anaesth 1988;35(4):338–44.

133. Herrick IA, Craen RA, Gelb AW, et al. Propofol sedation during awake craniotomy for seizures: electrocorticographic and epileptogenic effects. Anesth Analg 1997;84(6):1280–4.

134. Herrick IA, Craen RA, Gelb AW, et al. Propofol sedation during awake craniotomy for seizures: patient-controlled administration versus neurolept analgesia. Anesth Analg 1997;84(6):1285–91.

135. Steigerwald F, Hinz L, Pinsker MO, et al. Effect of propofol anesthesia on pallidal neuronal discharges in generalized dystonia. Neurosci Lett 2005;386(3):156–9.

136. Maciver MB, Bronte-Stewart HM, Henderson JM, et al. Human subthalamic neuron spiking exhibits subtle responses to sedatives. Anesthesiology 2011;115(2):254–64.

137. Elias WJ, Durieux ME, Huss D, et al. Dexmedetomidine and arousal affect subthalamic neurons. Mov Disord 2008;23(9):1317–20.

138. Mason LJ, Cojocaru TT, Cole DJ. Surgical intervention and anesthetic management of the patient with Parkinson's disease. Int Anesthesiol Clin 1996;34(4):133–50.

139. Bauer KP, Dom PM, Ramirez AM, et al. Preoperative intravenous midazolam: benefits beyond anxiolysis. J Clin Anesth 2004;16(3):177–83.
140. Heidari SM, Saryazdi H, Saghaei M. Effect of intravenous midazolam premedication on postoperative nausea and vomiting after cholecystectomy. Acta Anaesthesiol Taiwan 2004;42(2):77–80.
141. Almeida AN, Tavares C, Tibano A, et al. Dexmedetomidine for awake craniotomy without laryngeal mask. Arq Neuropsiquiatr 2005;63(3B):748–50.
142. Gignac E, Manninen PH, Gelb AW. Comparison of fentanyl, sufentanil and alfentanil during awake craniotomy for epilepsy. Can J Anaesth 1993;40(5 Pt 1): 421–4.
143. Chen MS, Hong CL, Chung HS, et al. Dexamethasone effectively reduces postoperative nausea and vomiting in a general surgical adult patient population. Chang Gung Med J 2006;29(2):175–81.
144. Kerscher C, Zimmermann M, Graf BM, et al. [Scalp blocks. A useful technique for neurosurgery, dermatology, plastic surgery and pain therapy]. Anaesthesist 2009;58(9):949–58 [quiz: 959–60] [in German].
145. Ohmura S, Kawada M, Ohta T, et al. Systemic toxicity and resuscitation in bupivacaine-, levobupivacaine-, or ropivacaine-infused rats. Anesth Analg 2001; 93(3):743–8.
146. Costello TG, Cormack JR, Hoy C, et al. Plasma ropivacaine levels following scalp block for awake craniotomy. J Neurosurg Anesthesiol 2004;16(2):147–50.
147. Costello TG, Cormack JR, Mather LE, et al. Plasma levobupivacaine concentrations following scalp block in patients undergoing awake craniotomy. Br J Anaesth 2005;94(6):848–51.
148. Girvin JP. Resection of intracranial lesions under local anesthesia. Int Anesthesiol Clin 1986;24(3):133–55.
149. Johnson KB, Egan TD. Remifentanil and propofol combination for awake craniotomy: case report with pharmacokinetic simulations. J Neurosurg Anesthesiol 1998;10(1):25–9.
150. Talke P, Stapelfeldt C, Garcia P. Dexmedetomidine does not reduce epileptiform discharges in adults with epilepsy. J Neurosurg Anesthesiol 2007;19(3):195–9.
151. Souter MJ, Rozet I, Ojemann JG, et al. Dexmedetomidine sedation during awake craniotomy for seizure resection: effects on electrocorticography. J Neurosurg Anesthesiol 2007;19(1):38–44.
152. Oda Y, Toriyama S, Tanaka K, et al. The effect of dexmedetomidine on electrocorticography in patients with temporal lobe epilepsy under sevoflurane anesthesia. Anesth Analg 2007;105(5):1272–7.
153. Rozet I. Anesthesia for functional neurosurgery: the role of dexmedetomidine. Curr Opin Anaesthesiol 2008;21(5):537–43.
154. Rozet I, Muangman S, Vavilala MS, et al. Clinical experience with dexmedetomidine for implantation of deep brain stimulators in Parkinson's disease. Anesth Analg 2006;103(5):1224–8.
155. Gadhinglajkar S, Sreedhar R, Abraham M. Anesthesia management of awake craniotomy performed under asleep-awake-asleep technique using laryngeal mask airway: report of two cases. Neurol India 2008;56(1):65–7.
156. Shuer LM. Epilepsy surgery: surgical considerations. In: Jaffe RA, Samuels SI, editors. Anesthesiologist's manual of surgical procedures. 2nd edition. Philadelphia: Lippincott Williams & Wilkins; 1999. p. 54–5.
157. Hans P, Bonhomme V, Born JD, et al. Target-controlled infusion of propofol and remifentanil combined with bispectral index monitoring for awake craniotomy. Anaesthesia 2000;55(3):255–9.

158. Keifer JC, Dentchev D, Little K, et al. A retrospective analysis of a remifentanil/ propofol general anesthetic for craniotomy before awake functional brain mapping. Anesth Analg 2005;101(2):502–8.
159. Hagberg CA, Gollas A, Berry JM. The laryngeal mask airway for awake craniotomy in the pediatric patient: report of three cases. J Clin Anesth 2004;16(1): 43–7.
160. Klimek M, Verbrugge SJ, Roubos S, et al. Awake craniotomy for glioblastoma in a 9-year-old child. Anaesthesia 2004;59(6):607–9.
161. Bekker AY, Kaufman B, Samir H, et al. The use of dexmedetomidine infusion for awake craniotomy. Anesth Analg 2001;92(5):1251–3.
162. Mack PF, Perrine K, Kobylarz E, et al. Dexmedetomidine and neurocognitive testing in awake craniotomy. J Neurosurg Anesthesiol 2004;16(1):20–5.
163. Ard J, Doyle W, Bekker A. Awake craniotomy with dexmedetomidine in pediatric patients. J Neurosurg Anesthesiol 2003;15(3):263–6.
164. Ard JL Jr, Bekker AY, Doyle WK. Dexmedetomidine in awake craniotomy: a technical note. Surg Neurol 2005;63(2):114–6 [discussion 116–7].
165. Moore TA 2nd, Markert JM, Knowlton RC. Dexmedetomidine as rescue drug during awake craniotomy for cortical motor mapping and tumor resection. Anesth Analg 2006;102(5):1556–8.
166. Everett LL, van Rooyen IF, Warner MH, et al. Use of dexmedetomidine in awake craniotomy in adolescents: report of two cases. Paediatr Anaesth 2006;16(3): 338–42.
167. Fabregas N, Rapado J, Gambus PL, et al. Modeling of the sedative and airway obstruction effects of propofol in patients with Parkinson disease undergoing stereotactic surgery. Anesthesiology 2002;97(6):1378–86.
168. Stricker PA, Kraemer FW, Ganesh A. Severe remifentanil-induced acute opioid tolerance following awake craniotomy in an adolescent. J Clin Anesth 2009; 21(2):124–6.
169. Khatib R, Ebrahim Z, Rezai A, et al. Perioperative events during deep brain stimulation: the experience at cleveland clinic. J Neurosurg Anesthesiol 2008;20(1): 36–40.
170. Bustillo MA, Lazar RM, Finck AD, et al. Dexmedetomidine may impair cognitive testing during endovascular embolization of cerebral arteriovenous malformations: a retrospective case report series. J Neurosurg Anesthesiol 2002;14(3): 209–12.
171. Cormack JR, Orme RM, Costello TG. The role of alpha2-agonists in neurosurgery. J Clin Neurosci 2005;12(4):375–8.
172. Davies A. Midazolam-induced dyskinesia. Palliat Med 2000;14(5):435–6.
173. Sanghera MK, Grossman RG, Kalhorn CG, et al. Basal ganglia neuronal discharge in primary and secondary dystonia in patients undergoing pallidotomy. Neurosurgery 2003;52(6):1358–70 [discussion: 1370–3].
174. Yamada K, Goto S, Kuratsu J, et al. Stereotactic surgery for subthalamic nucleus stimulation under general anesthesia: a retrospective evaluation of Japanese patients with Parkinson's disease. Parkinsonism Relat Disord 2007; 13(2):101–7.
175. Maltete D, Navarro S, Welter ML, et al. Subthalamic stimulation in Parkinson disease: with or without anesthesia? Arch Neurol 2004;61(3):390–2.
176. Hertel F, Zuchner M, Weimar I, et al. Implantation of electrodes for deep brain stimulation of the subthalamic nucleus in advanced Parkinson's disease with the aid of intraoperative microrecording under general anesthesia. Neurosurgery 2006;59(5):E1138 [discussion: E1138].

177. Benarroch EE. Subthalamic nucleus and its connections: anatomic substrate for the network effects of deep brain stimulation. Neurology 2008;70(21): 1991–5.
178. Sutcliffe AJ, Mitchell RD, Gan YC, et al. General anaesthesia for deep brain stimulator electrode insertion in Parkinson's disease. Acta Neurochir 2011;153(3):621–7.
179. Venkatraghavan L, Manninen P, Mak P, et al. Anesthesia for functional neurosurgery: review of complications. J Neurosurg Anesthesiol 2006;18(1):64–7.
180. Goodman RR, Kim B, McClelland S 3rd, et al. Operative techniques and morbidity with subthalamic nucleus deep brain stimulation in 100 consecutive patients with advanced Parkinson's disease. J Neurol Neurosurg Psychiatry 2006;77(1):12–7.
181. Lyons KE, Pahwa R. Deep brain stimulation and essential tremor. J Clin Neurophysiol 2004;21(1):2–5.
182. Lyons KE, Koller W, Wilkinson S, et al. Long term safety and efficacy of unilateral deep brain stimulation of the thalamus for parkinsonian tremor. J Neurol Neurosurg Psychiatry 2001;71(5):682–4.
183. Burdick AP, Fernandez HH, Okun MS, et al. Relationship between higher rates of adverse events in deep brain stimulation using standardized prospective recording and patient outcomes. Neurosurg Focus 2010;29(2):E4.
184. Videnovic A, Metman LV. Deep brain stimulation for Parkinson's disease: prevalence of adverse events and need for standardized reporting. Mov Disord 2008; 23(3):343–9.
185. Berkenstadt H, Perel A, Hadani M, et al. Monitored anesthesia care using remifentanil and propofol for awake craniotomy. J Neurosurg Anesthesiol 2001;13(3): 246–9.
186. Duffau H, Capelle L, Denvil D, et al. Usefulness of intraoperative electrical subcortical mapping during surgery for low-grade gliomas located within eloquent brain regions: functional results in a consecutive series of 103 patients. J Neurosurg 2003;98(4):764–78.
187. Sinha PK, Koshy T, Gayatri P, et al. Anesthesia for awake craniotomy: a retrospective study. Neurol India 2007;55(4):376–81.
188. Kenney C, Simpson R, Hunter C, et al. Short-term and long-term safety of deep brain stimulation in the treatment of movement disorders. J Neurosurg 2007; 106(4):621–5.
189. Pouratian N, Reames DL, Frysinger R, et al. Comprehensive analysis of risk factors for seizures after deep brain stimulation surgery. Clinical article. J Neurosurg 2011;115(2):310–5.
190. Coley E, Farhadi R, Lewis S, et al. The incidence of seizures following Deep Brain Stimulating electrode implantation for movement disorders, pain and psychiatric conditions. Br J Neurosurg 2009;23(2):179–83.
191. Johnson RD, Qadri SR, Joint C, et al. Perioperative seizures following deep brain stimulation in patients with multiple sclerosis. Br J Neurosurg 2010; 24(3):289–90.
192. Zrinzo L, Foltynie T, Limousin P, et al. Reducing hemorrhagic complications in functional neurosurgery: a large case series and systematic literature review. J Neurosurg 2012;116(1):84–94.
193. Gorgulho A, De Salles AA, Frighetto L, et al. Incidence of hemorrhage associated with electrophysiological studies performed using macroelectrodes and microelectrodes in functional neurosurgery. J Neurosurg 2005;102(5):888–96.
194. Bonhomme V, Born JD, Hans P. [Anaesthetic management of awake craniotomy]. Ann Fr Anesth Reanim 2004;23(4):389–94 [in French].

195. Hooper AK, Okun MS, Foote KD, et al. Venous air embolism in deep brain stimulation. Stereotact Funct Neurosurg 2009;87(1):25–30.
196. Deogaonkar A, Avitsian R, Henderson JM, et al. Venous air embolism during deep brain stimulation surgery in an awake supine patient. Stereotact Funct Neurosurg 2005;83(1):32–5.
197. Moitra V, Permut TA, Penn RM, et al. Venous air embolism in an awake patient undergoing placement of deep brain stimulators. J Neurosurg Anesthesiol 2004;16(4):321–2.
198. Suarez S, Ornaque I, Fabregas N, et al. Venous air embolism during Parkinson surgery in patients with spontaneous ventilation. Anesth Analg 1999;88(4): 793–4.
199. Stacy M. Sleep disorders in Parkinson's disease: epidemiology and management. Drugs Aging 2002;19(10):733–9.

Multimodal Intracranial Monitoring: Implications for Clinical Practice

Matthew A. Kirkman, MBBS, BSc,[a,b],
Martin Smith, MBBS, FRCA, FFICM[a],*

KEYWORDS

- Intracranial monitoring • Brain hypoxia/ischemia • Intracranial pressure
- Brain oxygenation • Brain metabolism

KEY POINTS

- The aims of intracranial monitoring are to provide early warning of secondary brain hypoxia/ischemia and cellular energy crisis and guide individualized therapy.
- Several techniques are available for global and regional monitoring of cerebral hemodynamics, oxygenation, and metabolism.
- Cerebral oxygenation monitoring assesses the balance between cerebral oxygen delivery and utilization, and thereby the adequacy of cerebral perfusion, and is increasingly used whenever intracranial pressure (ICP) monitoring is indicated.
- Each monitoring technique has specific advantages and inherent shortcomings and several modalities combined (multimodal monitoring) more reliably inform treatment decisions.
- Developments in multimodality monitoring have allowed a move away from rigid physiologic target setting to an individually tailored, patient-specific approach.
- The ideal technique would deliver noninvasive monitoring of cerebral oxygenation, hemodynamics, and metabolism over multiple regions of interest simultaneously.

The monitoring of perioperative and critically ill neurologic patients has become increasingly complex. Besides the close monitoring and assessment of cardiac and respiratory functions, several neurologic monitoring techniques are available to identify or predict the occurrence of secondary brain insults and guide therapeutic interventions. The indications for intracranial monitoring are summarized in **Box 1**.

Disclosures: MS is part funded by the Department of Health National Institute for Health Research Centres funding scheme via the University College London Hospitals/University College London Biomedical Research Centre.
Conflicts of interest: None.
[a] The National Hospital for Neurology and Neurosurgery, University College London Hospitals, Queen Square, London WC1N 3BG, UK; [b] Imperial College London, London SW7 2AZ, UK
* Corresponding author.
E-mail address: martin.smith@uclh.nhs.uk

Anesthesiology Clin 30 (2012) 269–287
doi:10.1016/j.anclin.2012.05.007
1932-2275/12/$ – see front matter © 2012 Elsevier Inc. All rights reserved.

anesthesiology.theclinics.com

Box 1
Indications for neuromonitoring

1. Monitoring the healthy but at-risk brain
2. Monitoring temporal changes in the pathophysiology of the injured brain and its response to treatment
3. Early detection of secondary adverse events
4. Guiding individualized, patient-specific therapy

Several techniques are available for global and regional brain monitoring and these provide early warning of impending brain hypoxia/ischemia and allow optimization of cerebral hemodynamics, oxygenation, and metabolism. In the neurocritical care unit (NCCU), developments in multimodality monitoring have enabled a move away from rigid physiologic target settings to an individually tailored, patient-specific approach. Each neuromonitoring modality has its own advantages and specific shortcomings (**Table 1**), and multimodal monitoring allows comparisons across variables and provides greater confidence for making treatment decisions.[1,2] This review describes current perioperative and NCCU neuromonitoring techniques and discusses their clinical relevance.

INTRACRANIAL PRESSURE MONITORING

ICP is usually monitored via an intraventricular catheter or intraparenchymal microsensor; other techniques have a substantially lower accuracy and are now rarely used.[3] ICP monitoring via an intraventricular catheter is the gold standard and measures global ICP. In vivo calibration and therapeutic drainage of cerebrospinal fluid (CSF) are possible but catheter placement can be difficult and there is a significant risk of catheter-related ventriculitis during prolonged monitoring.[4] Antibiotic-impregnated or silver-coated catheters may reduce infection rates.[5] Modern microtransducer-tipped and fiberoptic catheter systems are sited directly into brain parenchyma through a cranial access device or in the subdural space via a burr hole or craniotomy. The complication rates, including infection risk, are minimal[3] but measured ICP may not be representative of global pressure because of the presence of intraparenchymal pressure gradients in the injured brain.[6] Although microtransducer systems are reliable, they may drift during long-term monitoring, and in vivo recalibration is not possible.[4]

ICP monitoring allows for calculation of cerebral perfusion pressure (CPP), the difference between mean arterial pressure and ICP, and identification and analysis of pathologic ICP waveforms. Indices of cerebrovascular pressure reactivity and pressure-volume compensatory reserve may also be derived.[7] Indications for perioperative ICP monitoring include traumatic brain injury (TBI), hydrocephalus, intracranial hemorrhage (ICH), and surgery for large brain tumors with mass effect. Postoperative ICP monitoring is indicated if there is a risk of intracranial hypertension, particularly if a patient remains sedated. ICP monitoring is recommended by expert consensus guidelines to facilitate ICP- and CPP-directed therapy after severe TBI in all salvageable patients with an abnormal cranial CT scan and in patients with a normal scan if 2 or more of the following features are present: age greater than 40 years, unilateral or bilateral motor posturing, and systolic blood pressure less than 90 mm Hg.[8] It is also increasingly used after subarachnoid hemorrhage (SAH) and ICH.[9] Although evidence from randomized controlled trials confirming the benefit of monitoring and managing ICP is lacking, ICP monitoring is widely accepted as a low-risk, high-yield, and cost-effective intervention after TBI. Several studies using multi-modal brain monitoring indicate that brain hypoxia and ischemia can occur even in the presence of optimal ICP and CPP control, and there is a shift toward monitoring cerebral oxygenation in many patients in whom ICP monitoring is indicated.[10]

CEREBRAL BLOOD FLOW

Modern cerebral imaging techniques deliver sophisticated hemodynamic and meta-bolic information over multiple regions of interest. They, however, provide only snap-shot images, have limited availability, and require transfer of patients to specialized imaging facilities. Positron emission tomography (PET) is widely used as a diagnostic and clinical research tool and is increasing understanding of the pathophysiology of brain injury as well as allowing data from bedside monitors of perfusion and oxygen-ation to be compared with actual measures of cerebral blood flow (CBF) and oxygen consumption.[11]

Kety-Schmidt and Radioactive Tracer Methods

The first practical method of measuring CBF was described by Kety and Schmidt in 1945 (see Ref.[12] for the methodology). This forms the basis of many CBF measure-ment techniques in use today and remains the gold standard against which new methods of measurement are validated. A modification of the technique using inhala-tion or injection of xenon Xe 133 (^{133}Xe) can be used to measure absolute CBF, by calculation of the exponential clearance of ^{133}Xe from the brain using scalp scintillation counters and the creation of 2-D maps of cortical blood flow.[13] The methodologic accuracy and specificity depends on the number of detectors, but high spatial reso-lution is possible. ^{133}Xe is rapidly cleared so repeat studies within 30 minutes are possible. Although this method can be applied at the bedside and is a useful research tool, perioperative clinical applications are limited.

Continuous Quantitative CBF Monitoring

Laser Doppler flowmetry (LDF) and thermal diffusion flowmetry (TDF) are invasive continuous monitors of regional CBF (rCBF). Through access to exposed cortex (eg, via a burr hole), LDF provides reliable local cortical blood flow measurements based on assessment of the Doppler shift of laser light by moving red blood cells.[14] It is limited by arbitrary units and extremely localized measurements but has been used to reliably detect postoperative ischemia in SAH.[15] TDF, alternatively, offers quantita-tive assessment of rCBF in absolute flow units. The TDF catheter consists of a therm-istor heated to a few degrees above tissue temperature and a proximally located temperature probe. Temperature differences between the two reflect heat transfer and this can be translated into rCBF measurements. Although TDF provides a sensi-tive, real-time assessment of rCBF,[16] clinical data are limited and there have been some concerns about its accuracy and reliability.[17]

Transcranial Doppler Ultrasonography

Introduced in 1982, transcranial Doppler ultrasonography (TCD) is an established, noninvasive technique for assessing cerebral hemodynamics in real time[18] and trans-lates with relative ease into the operating room.[19] TCD uses ultrasound waves to measure blood flow velocity (FV) through large cerebral vessels from the Doppler shift caused by red blood cells moving through the field of view. It measures relative changes rather than actual CBF. The TCD FV waveform resembles an arterial pulse

Table 1
Applications of bedside neuromonitoring techniques and their relative advantages and disadvantages

Technique	Established Neurocritical Care Applications	Established Perioperative Applications	Advantages	Disadvantages
ICP (ventricular catheter)	Yes	Yes	Gold standard Measures global pressure Therapeutic drainage of CSF In vivo calibration	Placement can be difficult Risk of hemorrhage Risk of infection
ICP (microsensor)	Yes	Yes	Robust technology Intraparenchymal/subdural placement Easy to place with low procedural complication rate Low infection risk	Small drift over time In vivo calibration not possible Measures localized pressure
TCD	Yes	Yes	Noninvasive Assesses regional blood FV Real time with good temporal resolution	Only assesses relative flow Operator dependent Failure rate of 5%–10% (absent acoustic window) Measures FV only in large vessels
Sjvo$_2$	Yes	Yes	Represents balance between flow and metabolism	Invasive Global and insensitive to regional changes Risk of vein thrombosis, hematoma, carotid puncture

			Advantages	Limitations
Ptio₂	Yes	Yes	Bedside gold standard for oxygenation monitoring Represents balance between flow and metabolism Real time	Invasive Measures regional oxygen tension Utility dependent on probe location Subject to drift
NIRS	Research	Yes	Noninvasive Real time Assessment of several regions of interest NIRS-guided brain protection strategies during cardiac surgery	Dependent on derived algorithms Lack of standardization between commercial oximeters Signals affected by extracranial blood
MD	Yes	Research	Measurement of local brain tissue biochemistry Early detection of hypoxic/ischemic injury Monitor of cellular bioenergetic distress Measurement of novel biomarkers	Focal measure Thresholds for abnormality uncertain Small risk of catheter-related hemorrhage
cEEG	Yes	Yes	Noninvasive Real time Correlates with ischemic and metabolic changes	Skilled interpretation required Affected by anesthetic/sedative agents Sensitivity and specificity issues
ECoG	Research	Research	As for cEEG	As for cEEG Invasive Limited availability

Abbreviations: CBF, cerebral blood flow; cEEG, continuous electroencephalography; CVR, cerebrovascular reactivity; ECoG, electrocorticography; ICP, intracranial pressure; MD, microdialysis; NIRS, near-infrared spectroscopy; PtiO₂, brain tissue oxygen tension monitoring; SjvO₂ , jugular venous oximetry; TCD, transcranial Doppler.

wave and may be quantified into peak systolic, end diastolic, and mean FVs and pulsatility index. Pulsatility index provides an assessment of distal cerebrovascular resistance.

TCD is widely used during carotid endarterectomy and can quantify the risk of cerebral ischemia during carotid cross-clamping.[20] TCD variables correlate well with subsequent electroencephalographic (EEG) changes suggestive of ischemia and have been used as an indication for shunt placement.[21] Emboli can be detected as characteristic short-duration, high-intensity chirps, and waveform analysis allows differentiation between air and particulate emboli.[22]

TCD is routinely used in the perioperative and intensive care management of patients during surgical or neuroradiologic treatment of intracranial aneurysms and has a key role in the diagnosis and management of delayed cerebral ischemia (DCI).[23] Consecutive TCD examinations should be performed after SAH, and FV greater than 120 cm/s to 140 cm/s or FV increases greater than 50 cm/s/d from baseline are generally accepted as indicative of developing or established cerebral vasospasm–related DCI. The accuracy of TCD has been assessed using receiver operator characteristic analysis, and mean middle cerebral artery FV thresholds of 100 cm/s and 160 cm/s were most accurate for the detection of angiographic and clinical vasospasm, respectively.[24] There is considerable interindividual variation, however, and a recent study analyzing 1877 TCD examinations found that almost 40% of patients with clinical evidence of DCI never had FVs that exceeded 120 cm/s.[25] Treatment decisions should, therefore, not be based on TCD findings alone. Because changes in CBF itself affect FV, the Lindegaard ratio, which compares FV in the ipsilateral middle cerebral artery and internal carotid artery and is unaffected by changes in CBF, is often used.[26] A ratio greater than 3.0 is indicative of vasospasm and values greater than 6 suggest severe spasm.

TCD may also be used to monitor the integrity of pressure autoregulation and CO_2 reactivity and as a noninvasive estimate of ICP,[27] although the absolute accuracy of the latter is only ±10 mm Hg to 15 mm Hg, making it unsuitable for routine clinical use.[28] Contralateral hemispheric pulsatility index is a predictor of outcome after ICH,[29] and transcranial ultrasound duplex sonography–measured hematoma volume correlates well with CT-derived volume, providing a bedside monitor of hematoma expansion after ICH.[30]

MEASUREMENT OF CEREBROVASCULAR REACTIVITY

Cerebrovascular reactivity (CVR) is a key component of cerebral autoregulation and its absence renders the brain more susceptible to secondary ischemic insults. Because CVR may be disturbed or abolished by intracranial pathology and some anesthetic agents, the ability to monitor CVR in the perioperative period and on the NCCU is an attractive proposition.[31]

Pressure Reactivity Index

Methods of testing static and dynamic autoregulation are well established but most are interventional and intermittent.[32] The ICP response to arterial blood pressure (ABP) changes depends on the pressure reactivity of cerebral vessels, and disturbed pressure reactivity implies disturbed pressure autoregulation. A pressure reactivity index (PRx) can be derived from the continuous monitoring and analysis of slow waves in ABP and ICP as a surrogate and continuous marker of global cerebral autoregulation.[7,33] Under normal circumstances, increased ABP leads to cerebral vasoconstriction within 5 to 15 seconds and a secondary reduction of cerebral blood volume (CBV) and ICP. When CVR is impaired, CBV and ICP increase passively with ABP with opposite effects occurring during reduced ABP. PRx is determined by calculating the moving correlation coefficient of consecutive time averaged data points of ICP and ABP recorded over a 4-minute period.[7,33] A negative value for PRx, when ABP is inversely correlated with ICP, indicates a normal CVR, and a positive value a nonreactive cerebrovascular circulation. PRx correlates with standard measures of cerebral autoregulation and allows determination of optimal CPP after TBI.[34] Abnormal PRx is predictive of poor outcome after brain injury.[35,36]

Oxygen Pressure Reactivity Index

The oxygen reactivity index (ORx) is the correlation between brain tissue oxygen partial pressure (Ptio$_2$) and CPP and, as with PRx, positive and negative values for ORx indicate disturbed and intact autoregulation, respectively.[37] Disturbed ORx is predictive of poor outcome after TBI and SAH.[37,38] Because Ptio$_2$ is a focal measure, ORx may better represent regional autoregulation than PRx. In a small prospective pilot study, 5 patients with ICH had deranged perihematomal ORx but only 1 had abnormal PRx, suggesting the presence of focal but not global autoregulatory failure.[39]

Noninvasive Measures of Cerebral Autoregulation

CVR can be assessed continuously and noninvasively using the moving correlation between ABP and TCD-derived mean and systolic FVs.[40] Near-infrared spectroscopy (NIRS)-derived hemoglobin and tissue oxygenation indices have also been used as noninvasive measures of cerebral autoregulation (discussed later).[41]

MEASUREMENT OF CEREBRAL OXYGENATION

Cerebral oxygenation monitoring assesses the balance between cerebral oxygen delivery and utilization and, therefore, the adequacy of cerebral perfusion. Several bedside methods of monitoring global and regional cerebral oxygenation are available.

Jugular Venous Oximetry

Jugular venous oxygen saturation (Sjvo$_2$) assesses the balance between global cerebral oxygen delivery and metabolic demand and provides a nonquantitative estimate of the adequacy of cerebral perfusion.[42] Normal Sjvo$_2$ is 55% to 75% and interpretation of changes is straightforward (**Fig. 1**). Jugular venous desaturation may indicate cerebral hypoperfusion secondary to decreased CPP or hypocapnea, whereas Sjvo$_2$ greater than 85% indicates relative hyperemia or ateriovenous shunting and is

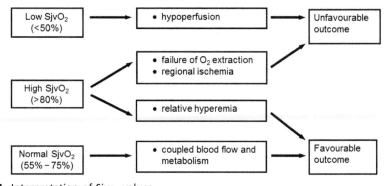

Fig. 1. Interpretation of Sjvo$_2$ values.

frequently associated with poor outcome.[43] Derived variables, such as the arterial-to-jugular venous oxygen concentration difference (AjvDo$_2$), have also been extensively studied as an assessment of CBF.[44] Sjvo$_2$ has been used to detect impaired cerebral perfusion after TBI and SAH, with prolonged or multiple desaturation less than 50% associated with poor neurologic outcome.[45] Various intraoperative uses have also been described.[46]

Disadvantages of Sjvo$_2$ monitoring include its invasive nature, the procedural risks (carotid puncture, vein thrombosis, and hematoma), and, because it is a global measure, its inability to detect regional ischemia.[47] Sjvo$_2$ reflects global cerebral oxygenation only if the dominant jugular bulb is cannulated but, in practice, the right side is often chosen.[48] Although widely used for decades, Sjvo$_2$ monitoring is being superseded by newer modalities.

Brain Tissue Oxygen Tension

Intraparenchymal brain tissue oxygen tension (Ptio$_2$) is increasingly measured whenever ICP monitoring is indicated and has become the gold standard bedside monitor of cerebral oxygenation.[49,50] The Ptio$_2$ monitor most frequently used in clinical practice (Licox, Integra, Plainsboro, New Jersey) incorporates a closed polarographic (Clark-type) cell with reversible electrochemical electrodes. A run-in period is required because Ptio$_2$ readings in the first hour postinsertion are unreliable and this limits intraoperative applications. Ptio$_2$ provides a highly focal measurement of cerebral oxygenation and, although offering the potential for selective monitoring of critically perfused tissue, accurate probe placement is crucial and global changes may be missed.[47]

Brain Ptio$_2$ is a complex and highly dynamic variable that represents the interaction between cerebral oxygen delivery and demand (oxygen metabolism)[50] as well as tissue oxygen diffusion gradients.[51] PET studies have confirmed correlations between Ptio$_2$ and rCBF[52] and regional venous oxygen saturation[11] and, therefore, Ptio$_2$ most likely represents a balance between CBF, oxygen extraction fraction, and Pao$_2$. It is affected by many physiologic variables, including Fio$_2$ (and therefore Pao$_2$), mean arterial pressure, and CPP.[53,54] Normal brain Ptio$_2$ values are in the region of 35 mm Hg to 50 mm Hg[55] and PET studies suggest that the ischemic threshold lies below 14 mm Hg.[53] Critical values should be considered, however, within a range rather than as a precise threshold, and ischemia is best defined by both duration and depth of hypoxia.[56]

Ptio$_2$ monitoring allows rapid detection of cerebral ischemia and the possibility of initiating therapy before irreversible neuronal damage occurs. It has been used during aneurism surgery[57] and is more effective than other methods at detecting ischemia.[58] Brain oxygenation improves as ICP reduces and CPP increases after decompressive craniectomy, and Ptio$_2$ monitoring may, therefore, assist in the selection of those who might benefit from surgical decompression.[59] Reduced Ptio$_2$ (usually defined as <15 mm Hg) correlates with poor outcome after TBI and SAH,[60,61] with evidence of a dose-response relationship.[56] Perihematomal reduction in Ptio$_2$ correlates with poor outcome after ICH.[62] Preliminary evidence suggests that Ptio$_2$-guided therapy in combination with ICP-guided and CPP-guided therapy reduces mortality and improves outcome in survivors after severe TBI compared with ICP-guided and CPP-guided therapy alone.[63] Although various maneuvers, such as increasing CPP, manipulation of sedation, and increasing Fio$_2$, may all improve Ptio$_2$, which intervention or combination of interventions is most effective at modulating outcome is unclear. The responsiveness of brain hypoxia to an intervention seems, however, to be a prognostic factor, with reversal of hypoxia associated with reduced mortality.[64] Although evidence from randomized controlled trials on the utility of Ptio$_2$-directed therapy on outcome in acute brain injury (ABI) is awaited, many NCCUs already incorporate $Ptio_2$-directed therapy into treatment algorithms.

Near-Infrared Spectroscopy

NIRS is a noninvasive technique based on the transmission and absorption of near-infrared light (700–1000 nm) as it passes through tissue. Oxygenated and deoxygenated hemoglobin have characteristic and different absorption spectra in the near infrared and their relative concentrations in tissue can be determined by the relative absorption of light at these wavelengths.

Earlier NIRS monitors were limited to measuring changes in the concentrations of oxyhemoglobin and deoxyhemoglobin but more modern devices incorporating spatially resolved spectroscopy provide an absolute measure of regional cerebral tissue oxygen saturation ($rSco_2$).[65] This is a reliable and continuous measure of the balance between cerebral oxygen delivery and utilization and, because NIRS interrogates arterial, venous, and capillary blood within the field of view, the derived saturation represents a tissue oxygen saturation measured from these 3 compartments. Recent advances, including frequency (or domain)-resolved spectroscopy and time-resolved spectroscopy, allow measurement of absolute concentrations of oxyhemoglobin and deoxyhemoglobin.[66] NIRS has also been used to measure rCBF and CBV but these indications have not been validated.[67] Cytochrome-c oxidase (CCO) is the terminal complex of the electron transfer chain and NIRS-derived measurement of CCO has been validated in animal studies as a measure of changes in cellular energy status.[68] It has recently become possible to measure changes in the concentration of CCO in human adults using NIRS.[69]

There is a plethora of commercial NIRS-based cerebral oximeters but a lack of standardization. Different manufacturers use different nomenclature, although most provide an absolute measure of $rSco_2$ and display this as a simple percentage value. The algorithms and even the variables measured vary, however, making comparisons between studies and devices difficult.[66,70] In the past decade, there has been a rapid expansion of the clinical experience of cerebral oximetry and there is some evidence that NIRS-guided brain protection protocols might lead to a reduction in perioperative neurologic complications, in particular, postoperative cognitive dysfunction, after cardiac surgery.[71] NIRS-based cerebral oximetry is also widely used to monitor the adequacy of cerebral oxygenation during carotid surgery and has similar accuracy and reproducibility in the detection of cerebral ischemia compared with other monitoring modalities and some advantages in terms of simplicity and temporal resolution.[21] It is currently impossible, however, to specify an $rSco_2$ threshold that can be widely applied to guide shunt placement or detect cerebral hypoxia/ischemia during carotid endarterectomy; reductions in $rSco_2$ between 5% and 25% from baseline have been reported as potential ischemic thresholds.[65]

There are no data to support the routine application of NIRS during surgery under general anesthesia and its application in neurosurgical anesthesia and after brain injury, where it might be expected to have a key monitoring role, is undefined. There are limited high-quality data in this area. A small observational study of 18 TBI patients identified an association between increasing length of time with $rSco_2$ values less than or equal to 60% and mortality, intracranial hypertension, and compromised CPP.[72] The utility of NIRS after ABI is confounded by the optical complexity of the injured brain. Intracranial hematoma, cerebral edema, and subarachnoid blood may invalidate some of the assumptions on which NIRS algorithms are based and the importance of this is not always appreciated. Newer technology will play an important role in overcoming these issues and a recently introduced time-resolved spectroscopy system was able to predict vasospasm with high sensitivity in poor-grade SAH patients.[73] A broadband NIRS system optimized for the measurement of CCO in adults has been used to demonstrate oxidation in cerebral mitochondrial redox state during normobaric hyperoxia after TBI.[74] Recent work has also focused on the noninvasive and continuous measurement of CVR using NIRS-derived hemoglobin and oxygenation variables.[75,76]

There are several concerns about the clinical application of NIRS and the one most often highlighted is the potential for contamination of the signal by extracranial tissue. Some commercial systems use 2 detectors and a subtraction-based algorithm to address this issue, assuming that the detecting optode closest to the emitter receives light that has passed mainly through the scalp whereas that arriving at the farthest detector has mainly passed through brain tissue. Although the proprietary algorithms on which this assumption is based are not published, there is weighting in favor of intracerebral tissue with an interoptode spacing greater than 4 cm. Spatially resolved spectroscopy has high sensitivity and specificity for intracranial changes, so its wider application effectively resolves this problem.[77] Claims for absolute rSco$_2$ thresholds for the determination of cerebral ischemia/hypoxia should be treated with caution and the wide intraindividual and interindividual baseline variability in Sco$_2$ means that NIRS is best used as a trend monitor.

NIRS has potential advantages compared with other neuromonitoring techniques; it is noninvasive, has high temporal and spatial resolution, and offers simultaneous measurement over multiple regions of interest. Although a single NIRS-based device could provide regional monitoring of cerebral oxygenation, hemodynamics, and cerebral cellular energy status, technologic advances are necessary before these techniques can be introduced more widely into clinical practice.[78]

CEREBRAL MICRODIALYSIS

Cerebral microdialysis (MD) is a well-established laboratory tool increasingly used as a bedside monitor for the online analysis of brain tissue biochemistry to provide unique information regarding the cellular metabolic environment. A miniature MD catheter is placed into brain tissue and diffusion of molecules across the semipermeable dialysis membrane at its tip allows collection of substances from the brain extracellular fluid (ECF) in the microdialysate (**Figs. 2** and **3**). Commercial assays for glucose, lactate, pyruvate, glycerol, and glutamate are available for use with a semiautomated analyser

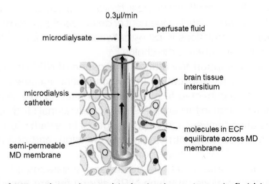

Fig. 2. Schematic of MD catheter located in brain tissue. Isotonic fluid is pumped through the MD catheter at a rate of 0.3 µL min^{-1}. Molecules at high concentration in the brain ECF equilibrate across the semipermeable MD membrane and can be analyzed in the microdialysate.

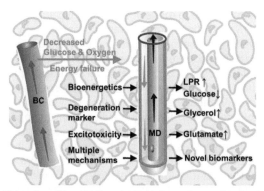

Fig. 3. Schematic of blood capillary (BC) and MD catheter located in brain tissue. The effects of decreased brain glucose and oxygen supply and cellular energy failure can be monitored by the bedside measurement of biomarkers of bioenergetics, cellular degeneration, and excitotoxicty. Additional, novel biomarkers can also be measured in the research setting.

(M-dialysis AB, Solna, Sweden), delivering bedside data usually at hourly intervals (**Table 2**). Subsequent offline analysis of the dialysate allows a myriad other biomarkers to be measured. It is recommended that the MD catheter be placed in at-risk tissue (ie, adjacent to a mass lesion or, in the case of an aneurism, in the territory of the parent vessel), allowing biochemical changes to be measured in the area of brain most vulnerable to secondary insult.[79]

The majority of clinical experience with cerebral MD relates to monitoring in patients with TBI and SAH.[80,81] Severe cerebral hypoxia/ischemia is typically associated with marked increases in the lactate:pyruvate ratio (LPR) and LPR greater than 20 to 25 is associated with poor outcome after TBI.[82] Anerobic glycolysis may occur not only because of hypoxia/ischemia but also because of mitochondrial failure and ineffective utilization of delivered oxygen, and cerebral MD offers a unique opportunity to monitor such cellular dysfunction and ensuing metabolic crisis.[83,84] Glycerol is a marker of ischemic cell damage and increased MD glycerol concentrations are associated with poor outcome after TBI.[85] Increased levels of excitatory amino acids and reduced brain ECF glucose levels may also predict, or be associated with, metabolic catastrophes after ABI.[57,86] Catheters with a higher membrane molecular weight cutoff (100 kDa) offer the potential to measure a host of novel biomarkers in the research setting.[87,88]

Table 2
Bedside cerebral microdialysis-derived biomarkers of secondary brain injury

Variable	Interpretation	Comments
Glucose <1.5–2.0 mmol/L	Hypoxia/ischemia Reduced cerebral glucose supply Cerebral hyperglycolysis	Affected by serum glucose concentration
LPR >20–25	Hypoxia/ischemia Cellular redox state Bioenergetic crisis	Reliable biomarker of ischemia Tissue hypoxic threshold for raised LPR not established
Glycerol >100 μmol/L	Hypoxia/ischemia Cell membrane degradation	Overspill of glycerol from systemic circulation may confound results
Glutamate >15–20 μmol/L	Hypoxia/ischemia Excitotoxicty	Large interpatient and intrapatient variability

MD is an attractive technique to monitor impending ischemia during neurovascular procedures when early detection might prevent or minimize damage by prompting a change in operative or anesthetic management. In one study, increases in lactate, LPR, and glutamate were associated with reductions in brain $Ptio_2$ during aneurysm surgery.[57] The clinical applications of cerebral MD are currently limited by technology and, although the standard hourly sampling rate is sufficient for most NCCU applications, it is unlikely to offer adequate time resolution for intraoperative use. A continuous rapid-sampling cerebral MD technique suitable for intraoperative applications has been described but is not currently available for clinical use.[89]

Because cerebral MD measures changes at the cellular level, it has the potential to detect abnormalities before changes can be detected by more conventional monitoring techniques or clinical status. In recent studies, LPR greater than 25 and glycerol concentration greater than 100 μmol/L were associated with a significantly higher risk of imminent intracranial hypertension after ABI,[90] and a rise in LPR and glycerol predicted the occurrence of DCI after SAH 11 to 23 hours before its clinical appearance.[91] A large cohort study demonstrated that early MD markers are correlated with long-term outcome, suggesting that therapeutic modulation of the cellular energy crisis that accompanies ABI might improve outcome.[92]

There are several caveats to the interpretation of MD values. There is no established value above which the LPR is considered indicative of tissue hypoxia,[93] although thresholds of greater than 25 and greater than 40 are often applied.[81] Glycerol can leak from the plasma through the blood-brain barrier, and high brain ECF glycerol levels may occur because of systemic factors, such as triglyceride breakdown.[80] Lactate may be an energy substrate for the brain and is not solely an indicator of anaerobic metabolism,[94] highlighting the importance of using the LPR rather than lactate alone. For these reasons, MD variables should not be interpreted in isolation. The future success of cerebral MD depends on the choice of biomarker; their sensitivity, specificity, and predictive value for secondary neurochemical events, and the availability of practical methods for analysis of biomarkers.

CONTINUOUS ELECTROENCEPHALOGRAPHY

Nonconvulsive seizures and nonconvulsive status epilepticus occur more frequently after ABI than previously recognized (possibly in up to one-third of patients) and continuous EEG (cEEG) has a key role in their detection.[95] Nonconvulsive seizures and nonconvulsive status epilepticus may also occur in patients without neurologic disease, for example, in severe sepsis.[96] In patients with ABI, integrating cEEG into multimodal neuromonitoring strategies has identified associations between seizures, intracranial hypertension, and metabolic derangements.[97] cEEG is limited by its attenuation by anesthetic and sedative agents and is a resource-intense technology, requiring skilled personnel for interpretation. Telemedicine may increase the adoption of cEEG by allowing interpretation away from the bedside[98] and there is also a drive toward the development of automated seizure detection software. Randomized clinical trials investigating the effects of cEEG-guided treatment are urgently required.

Cortical spreading depolarizations (SDs) are pathologic events detected by electrocorticography.[99,100] SDs are characterized by near-complete sustained depolarization of neurons and astrocytes, resulting in secondary injury related to mitochondrial damage, accumulation of intracellular calcium, and excitotoxicity. It has been suggested that more than half of TBI patients and approximately 70% of SAH patients experience SDs at some stage.[101,102] SDs are independently associated with unfavorable outcome after TBI[103] and may represent a potential target for therapy.[99] A definite cause-effect relationship, however, is not proved. Furthermore, it is still not entirely clear what SDs actually represent and it has been suggested that they might in part play a protective role after ABI.[104] Detection of SDs currently requires placement of an electrode strip directly onto the brain surface, limiting its routine use in the NCCU. Developments in scalp EEG and NIRS technology are likely to lead to noninvasive measurement methods. Until then, management should focus on controlling variables, such as pyrexia, hypoxia, hypoglycemia, and systemic hypotension, which are known to increase the incidence and duration of SDs.[105]

FUTURE TECHNOLOGY

There have been several recent technologic developments that may have an impact on future neuromonitoring practices. A multiparameter probe that measures ICP, Ptio2, and temperature is already available (Raumedic AG, Münchberg, Germany) and other companies are likely to follow suit and possibly incorporate CBF measurement. Stereotactic placement of invasive probes will target regions of interest with greater accuracy and may find a place in selected patients. Fiberoptic pulse oximetry has been used to estimate cerebral arterial oxygen saturation[106] and a prototype invasive probe combining NIRS and indocyanine green dye dilution has been used to simultaneously monitor ICP, CBF, and CBV.[107] The feasibility of noninvasive continuous bedside monitoring of cerebral oxygenation and CBF has also been assessed using a hybrid optical device comprising diffuse correlation spectroscopy and NIRS.[108] Finally, multimodal cerebral monitoring generates large and complex data sets, and systems that analyze and present information in a user-friendly format at the bedside are essential to maximize its clinical relevance.[1,109]

SUMMARY

Given the physiologic complexity of the human brain, it is not surprising that a single variable or device is unable to adequately monitor all aspects of cerebral physiology and pathophysiology. It is for this reason that multimodality monitoring, including combined measures of cerebral perfusion, oxygenation, and metabolic status, is often recommended. Such monitoring may provide an extended window for the prevention, early detection, and treatment of ongoing hypoxic/ischemic neuronal injury and, thereby, improve outcome. Technical advances are likely to lead to the development of noninvasive monitors that deliver continuous, multisite measurement of cerebral hemodynamics, oxygenation, and metabolism over multiple regions of interest simultaneously.

REFERENCES

1. Oddo M, Villa F, Citerio G. Brain multimodality monitoring: an update. Curr Opin Crit Care 2012;18:111–8.
2. Tisdall MM, Smith M. Multimodal monitoring in traumatic brain injury: current status and future directions. Br J Anaesth 2007;99:61–7.
3. Smith M. Monitoring intracranial pressure in traumatic brain injury. Anesth Analg 2008;106:240–8.
4. Zhong J, Dujovny M, Park HK, et al. Advances in ICP monitoring techniques. Neurol Res 2003;25:339–50.
5. Babu MA, Patel R, Marsh WR, et al. Strategies to decrease the risk of ventricular catheter infections: a review of the evidence. Neurocrit Care 2012;16:194–202.

6. Sahuquillo J, Poca MA, Arribas M, et al. Interhemispheric supratentorial intracranial pressure gradients in head-injured patients: are they clinically important? J Neurosurg 1999;90:16–26.
7. Czosnyka M, Pickard JD. Monitoring and interpretation of intracranial pressure. J Neurol Neurosurg Psychiatry 2004;75:813–21.
8. The Brain Trauma Foundation. The American Association of Neurological Surgeons. The Joint Section on Neurotrauma and Critical Care. Indications for intracranial pressure monitoring. J Neurotrauma 2007;24:S37–44.
9. Spiotta AM, Provencio JJ, Rasmussen PA, et al. Brain monitoring after subarachnoid hemorrhage: lessons learned. Neurosurgery 2011;69:755–66.
10. Chen HI, Stiefel MF, Oddo M, et al. Detection of cerebral compromise with multimodality monitoring in patients with subarachnoid hemorrhage. Neurosurgery 2011;69:53–63.
11. Gupta AK, Hutchinson PJ, Fryer T, et al. Measurement of brain tissue oxygenation performed using positron emission tomography scanning to validate a novel monitoring method. J Neurosurg 2002;96:263–8.
12. Kety SS, Schmidt CF. The determination of cerebral blood flow in man by the use of nitrous oxide in low concentrations. Am J Physiol 1945;143:53–5.
13. Anderson RE. Cerebral blood flow xenon-133. Neurosurg Clin N Am 1996;7: 703–8.
14. Bolognese P, Miller JI, Heger IM, et al. Laser-Doppler flowmetry in neurosurgery. J Neurosurg Anesthesiol 1993;5:151–8.
15. Johnson WD, Bolognese P, Miller JI, et al. Continuous postoperative ICBF monitoring in aneurysmal SAH patients using a combined ICP-laser Doppler fiberoptic probe. J Neurosurg Anesthesiol 1996;8:199–207.
16. Jaeger M, Soehle M, Schuhmann MU, et al. Correlation of continuously monitored regional cerebral blood flow and brain tissue oxygen. Acta Neurochir (Wien) 2005;147:51–6.
17. Vajkoczy P, Horn P, Thome C, et al. Regional cerebral blood flow monitoring in the diagnosis of delayed ischemia following aneurysmal subarachnoid hemorrhage. J Neurosurg 2003;98:1227–34.
18. Aaslid R, Markwalder TM, Nornes H. Noninvasive transcranial Doppler ultrasound recording of flow velocity in basal cerebral arteries. J Neurosurg 1982; 57:769–74.
19. Kincaid MS, Douville CM, Lam AM. Perioperative use of transcranial Doppler. Anesth Analg 2005;100:291–2.
20. Dunne VG, Besser M, Ma WJ. Transcranial Doppler in carotid endarterectomy. J Clin Neurosci 2001;8:140–5.
21. Moritz S, Kasprzak P, Arlt M, et al. Accuracy of cerebral monitoring in detecting cerebral ischemia during carotid endarterectomy: a comparison of transcranial Doppler sonography, near-infrared spectroscopy, stump pressure, and somatosensory evoked potentials. Anesthesiology 2007;107:563–9.
22. Ringelstein EB, Droste DW, Babikian VL, et al. Consensus on microembolus detection by TCD. International Consensus Group on Microembolus Detection. Stroke 1998;29:725–9.
23. Springborg JB, Frederiksen HJ, Eskesen V, et al. Trends in monitoring patients with aneurysmal subarachnoid haemorrhage. Br J Anaesth 2005; 94:259–70.
24. Mascia L, Fedorko L, terBrugge K, et al. The accuracy of transcranial Doppler to detect vasospasm in patients with aneurysmal subarachnoid hemorrhage. Intensive Care Med 2003;29:1088–94.

25. Carrera E, Schmidt JM, Oddo M, et al. Transcranial Doppler for predicting delayed cerebral ischemia after subarachnoid hemorrhage. Neurosurgery 2009;65:316–23.
26. Lindegaard KF, Nornes H, Bakke SJ, et al. Cerebral vasospasm diagnosis by means of angiography and blood velocity measurements. Acta Neurochir (Wien) 1989;100:12–24.
27. Kincaid MS. Transcranial Doppler ultrasonography: a diagnostic tool of increasing utility. Curr Opin Anaesthesiol 2008;21:552–9.
28. Czosnyka M, Matta BF, Smielewski P, et al. Cerebral perfusion pressure in head-injured patients: a noninvasive assessment using transcranial Doppler ultrasonography. J Neurosurg 1998;88:802–8.
29. Wang W, Yang Z, Liu L, et al. Relationship between transcranial Doppler variables in acute stage and outcome of intracerebral hemorrhage. Neurol Res 2011;33:487–93.
30. Perez ES, Delgado-Mederos R, Rubiera M, et al. Transcranial duplex sonography for monitoring hyperacute intracerebral hemorrhage. Stroke 2009;40:987–90.
31. Dagal A, Lam AM. Cerebral autoregulation and anesthesia. Curr Opin Anaesthesiol 2009;22:547–52.
32. Rasulo FA, Balestreri M, Matta B. Assessment of cerebral pressure autoregulation. Curr Opin Anaesthesiol 2002;15:483–8.
33. Czosnyka M, Hutchinson PJ, Balestreri M, et al. Monitoring and interpretation of intracranial pressure after head injury. Acta Neurochir Suppl 2006;96:114–8.
34. Steiner LA, Czosnyka M, Piechnik SK, et al. Continuous monitoring of cerebrovascular pressure reactivity allows determination of optimal cerebral perfusion pressure in patients with traumatic brain injury. Crit Care Med 2002;30:733–8.
35. Diedler J, Sykora M, Rupp A, et al. Impaired cerebral vasomotor activity in spontaneous intracerebral hemorrhage. Stroke 2009;40:815–9.
36. Rasulo FA, Girardini A, Lavinio A, et al. Are optimal cerebral perfusion pressure and cerebrovascular autoregulation related to long-term outcome in patients with aneurysmal subarachnoid hemorrhage? J Neurosurg Anesthesiol 2012;24:3–8.
37. Jaeger M, Schuhmann MU, Soehle M, et al. Continuous assessment of cerebrovascular autoregulation after traumatic brain injury using brain tissue oxygen pressure reactivity. Crit Care Med 2006;34:1783–8.
38. Jaeger M, Schuhmann MU, Soehle M, et al. Continuous monitoring of cerebrovascular autoregulation after subarachnoid hemorrhage by brain tissue oxygen pressure reactivity and its relation to delayed cerebral infarction. Stroke 2007;38:981–6.
39. Diedler J, Karpel-Massler G, Sykora M, et al. Autoregulation and brain metabolism in the perihematomal region of spontaneous intracerebral hemorrhage: an observational pilot study. J Neurol Sci 2010;295:16–22.
40. Sorrentino E, Budohoski KP, Kasprowicz M, et al. Critical thresholds for transcranial Doppler indices of cerebral autoregulation in traumatic brain injury. Neurocrit Care 2011;14:188–93.
41. Lee JK, Kibler KK, Benni PB, et al. Cerebrovascular reactivity measured by near-infrared spectroscopy. Stroke 2009;40:1820–6.
42. Schell RM, Cole DJ. Cerebral monitoring: jugular venous oximetry. Anesth Analg 2000;90:559–66.
43. Dagal A, Lam AM. Cerebral blood flow and the injured brain: how should we monitor and manipulate it? Curr Opin Anaesthesiol 2011;24:131–7.

44. Macmillan CS, Andrews PJ. Cerebrovenous oxygen saturation monitoring: practical considerations and clinical relevance. Intensive Care Med 2000;26:1028–36.

45. Robertson CS, Gopinath SP, Goodman JC, et al. SjvO2 monitoring in head-injured patients. J Neurotrauma 1995;12:891–6.

46. Matta BF, Lam AM, Mayberg TS, et al. A critique of the intraoperative use of jugular venous bulb catheters during neurosurgical procedures. Anesth Analg 1994;79:745–50.

47. Gupta AK, Hutchinson PJ, al-Rawi P, et al. Measuring brain tissue oxygenation compared with jugular venous oxygen saturation for monitoring cerebral oxygenation after traumatic brain injury. Anesth Analg 1999;88:549–53.

48. Lam JM, Chan MS, Poon WS. Cerebral venous oxygen saturation monitoring: is dominant jugular bulb cannulation good enough? Br J Neurosurg 1996;10:357–64.

49. Nortje J, Gupta AK. The role of tissue oxygen monitoring in patients with acute brain injury. Br J Anaesth 2006;97:95–106.

50. Rose JC, Neill TA, Hemphill JC III. Continuous monitoring of the microcirculation in neurocritical care: an update on brain tissue oxygenation. Curr Opin Crit Care 2006;12:97–102.

51. Rosenthal G, Hemphill JC III, Sorani M, et al. Brain tissue oxygen tension is more indicative of oxygen diffusion than oxygen delivery and metabolism in patients with traumatic brain injury. Crit Care Med 2008;36:1917–24.

52. Scheufler KM, Rohrborn HJ, Zentner J. Does tissue oxygen-tension reliably reflect cerebral oxygen delivery and consumption? Anesth Analg 2002;95:1042–8.

53. Johnston AJ, Steiner LA, Coles JP, et al. Effect of cerebral perfusion pressure augmentation on regional oxygenation and metabolism after head injury. Crit Care Med 2005;33:189–95.

54. McLeod AD, Igielman F, Elwell C, et al. Measuring cerebral oxygenation during normobaric hyperoxia: a comparison of tissue microprobes, near-infrared spectroscopy, and jugular venous oximetry in head injury. Anesth Analg 2003;97:851–6.

55. Hoffman WE, Charbel FT, Edelman G. Brain tissue oxygen, carbon dioxide, and pH in neurosurgical patients at risk for ischemia. Anesth Analg 1996;82:582–6.

56. van den Brink WA, van Santbrink H, Steyerberg EW, et al. Brain oxygen tension in severe head injury. Neurosurgery 2000;46:868–76.

57. Kett-White R, Hutchinson PJ, Czosnyka M, et al. Effects of variation in cerebral haemodynamics during aneurysm surgery on brain tissue oxygen and metabolism. Acta Neurochir Suppl 2002;81:327–9.

58. Jodicke A, Hubner F, Boker DK. Monitoring of brain tissue oxygenation during aneurysm surgery: prediction of procedure-related ischemic events. J Neurosurg 2003;98:515–23.

59. Stiefel MF, Heuer GG, Smith MJ, et al. Cerebral oxygenation following decompressive hemicraniectomy for the treatment of refractory intracranial hypertension. J Neurosurg 2004;101:241–7.

60. Meixensberger J, Jaeger M, Vath A, et al. Brain tissue oxygen guided treatment supplementing ICP/CPP therapy after traumatic brain injury. J Neurol Neurosurg Psychiatry 2003;74:760–4.

61. van Santbrink H, van den Brink WA, Steyerberg EW, et al. Brain tissue oxygen response in severe traumatic brain injury. Acta Neurochir (Wien) 2003;145:429–38.

62. Ko SB, Choi HA, Parikh G, et al. Multimodality monitoring for cerebral perfusion pressure optimization in comatose patients with intracerebral hemorrhage. Stroke 2011;42:3087–92.

63. Spiotta AM, Stiefel MF, Gracias VH, et al. Brain tissue oxygen-directed management and outcome in patients with severe traumatic brain injury. J Neurosurg 2010;113:571–80.
64. Bohman LE, Heuer GG, Macyszyn L, et al. Medical management of compromised brain oxygen in patients with severe traumatic brain injury. Neurocrit Care 2011;14:361–9.
65. Smith M. Shedding light on the adult brain: a review of the clinical applications of near-infrared spectroscopy. Phil Trans R Soc 2011;369:4452–69.
66. Ferrari M, Quaresima V. Near infrared brain and muscle oximetry: from discovery to current applications. J Near Infrared Spectrosc 2012;20:1–14.
67. Ferrari M, Mottola L, Quaresima V. Principles, techniques, and limitations of near infrared spectroscopy. Can J Appl Physiol 2004;29:463–87.
68. Springett R, Wylezinska M, Cady EB, et al. Oxygen dependency of cerebral oxidative phosphorylation in newborn piglets. J Cereb Blood Flow Metab 2000;20:280–9.
69. Tisdall MM, Tachtsidis I, Leung TS, et al. Near-infrared spectroscopic quantification of changes in the concentration of oxidized cytochrome c oxidase in the healthy human brain during hypoxemia. J Biomed Opt 2007;12: 024002.
70. Highton D, Elwell C, Smith M. Noninvasive cerebral oximetry: is there light at the end of the tunnel? Curr Opin Anaesthesiol 2010;23:576–81.
71. Vohra HA, Modi A, Ohri SK. Does use of intra-operative cerebral regional oxygen saturation monitoring during cardiac surgery lead to improved clinical outcomes? Interact Cardiovasc Thorac Surg 2009;9:318–22.
72. Dunham CM, Ransom KJ, Flowers LL, et al. Cerebral hypoxia in severely brain-injured patients is associated with admission Glasgow Coma Scale score, computed tomographic severity, cerebral perfusion pressure, and survival. J Trauma 2004;56:482–9.
73. Yokose N, Sakatani K, Murata Y, et al. Bedside monitoring of cerebral blood oxygenation and hemodynamics after aneurysmal subarachnoid hemorrhage by quantitative time-resolved near-infrared spectroscopy. World Neurosurg 2010;73:508–13.
74. Tisdall MM, Tachtsidis I, Leung TS, et al. Increase in cerebral aerobic metabolism by normobaric hyperoxia after traumatic brain injury. J Neurosurg 2008;109: 424–32.
75. Zweifel C, Castellani G, Czosnyka M, et al. Noninvasive monitoring of cerebrovascular reactivity with near infrared spectroscopy in head-injured patients. J Neurotrauma 2010;27:1951–8.
76. Zweifel C, Castellani G, Czosnyka M, et al. Continuous assessment of cerebral autoregulation with near-infrared spectroscopy in adults after subarachnoid hemorrhage. Stroke 2010;41:1963–8.
77. Al-Rawi PG, Smielewski P, Kirkpatrick PJ. Evaluation of a near-infrared spectrometer (NIRO 300) for the detection of intracranial oxygenation changes in the adult head. Stroke 2001;32:2492–500.
78. Smith M, Elwell C. Near-infrared spectroscopy: shedding light on the injured brain. Anesth Analg 2009;108:1055–7.
79. Bellander BM, Cantais E, Enblad P, et al. Consensus meeting on microdialysis in neurointensive care. Intensive Care Med 2004;30:2166–9.
80. Hillered L, Vespa PM, Hovda DA. Translational neurochemical research in acute human brain injury: the current status and potential future for cerebral microdialysis. J Neurotrauma 2005;22:3–41.

81. Tisdall MM, Smith M. Cerebral microdialysis: research technique or clinical tool. Br J Anaesth 2006;97:18–25.

82. Zauner A, Doppenberg EM, Woodward JJ, et al. Continuous monitoring of cerebral substrate delivery and clearance: initial experience in 24 patients with severe acute brain injuries. Neurosurgery 1997;41:1082–91.

83. Kim-Han JS, Kopp SJ, Dugan LL, et al. Perihematomal mitochondrial dysfunction after intracerebral hemorrhage. Stroke 2006;37:2457–62.

84. Vespa P, Bergsneider M, Hattori N, et al. Metabolic crisis without brain ischemia is common after traumatic brain injury: a combined microdialysis and positron emission tomography study. J Cereb Blood Flow Metab 2005;25:763–74.

85. Clausen T, Alves OL, Reinert M, et al. Association between elevated brain tissue glycerol levels and poor outcome following severe traumatic brain injury. J Neurosurg 2005;103:233–8.

86. Vespa PM, McArthur D, O'Phelan K, et al. Persistently low extracellular glucose correlates with poor outcome 6 months after human traumatic brain injury despite a lack of increased lactate: a microdialysis study. J Cereb Blood Flow Metab 2003;23:865–77.

87. Goodman JC, Robertson CS. Microdialysis: is it ready for prime time? Curr Opin Crit Care 2009;15:110–7.

88. Petzold A, Tisdall MM, Girbes AR, et al. In vivo monitoring of neuronal loss in traumatic brain injury: a microdialysis study. Brain 2011;134:464–83.

89. Bhatia R, Hashemi P, Razzaq A, et al. Application of rapid-sampling, online microdialysis to the monitoring of brain metabolism during aneurysm surgery. Neurosurgery 2006;58(Suppl 2):313–20.

90. Belli A, Sen J, Petzold A, et al. Metabolic failure precedes intracranial pressure rises in traumatic brain injury: a microdialysis study. Acta Neurochir (Wien) 2008; 150:461–9.

91. Skjoth-Rasmussen J, Schulz M, Kristensen SR, et al. Delayed neurological deficits detected by an ischemic pattern in the extracellular cerebral metabolites in patients with aneurysmal subarachnoid hemorrhage. J Neurosurg 2004;100:8–15.

92. Timofeev I, Carpenter KL, Nortje J, et al. Cerebral extracellular chemistry and outcome following traumatic brain injury: a microdialysis study of 223 patients. Brain 2011;134:484–94.

93. Hutchinson PJ, Gupta AK, Fryer TF, et al. Correlation between cerebral blood flow, substrate delivery, and metabolism in head injury: a combined microdialysis and triple oxygen positron emission tomography study. J Cereb Blood Flow Metab 2002;22:735–45.

94. Gallagher CN, Carpenter KL, Grice P, et al. The human brain utilizes lactate via the tricarboxylic acid cycle: a 13C-labelled microdialysis and high-resolution nuclear magnetic resonance study. Brain 2009;132:2839–49.

95. Claassen J, Mayer SA, Kowalski RG. Detection of electrographic seizures with continuous EEG monitoring in critically ill patients. Neurology 2004;62:1743–8.

96. Oddo M, Carrera E, Claassen J, et al. Continuous electroencephalography in the medical intensive care unit. Crit Care Med 2009;37:2051–6.

97. Friedman D, Claassen J, Hirsch LJ. Continuous electroencephalogram monitoring in the intensive care unit. Anesth Analg 2009;109:506–23.

98. Vespa PM. Multimodality monitoring and telemonitoring in neurocritical care: from microdialysis to robotic telepresence. Curr Opin Crit Care 2005;11:133–8.

99. Dreier JP. The role of spreading depression, spreading depolarization and spreading ischemia in neurological disease. Nat Med 2011;17:439–47.

100. Fabricius M, Fuhr S, Bhatia R, et al. Cortical spreading depression and peri-infarct depolarization in acutely injured human cerebral cortex. Brain 2006; 129:778–90.
101. Dreier JP, Woitzik J, Fabricius M, et al. Delayed ischaemic neurological deficits after subarachnoid haemorrhage are associated with clusters of spreading depolarizations. Brain 2006;129:3224–37.
102. Strong AJ, Fabricius M, Boutelle MG, et al. Spreading and synchronous depressions of cortical activity in acutely injured human brain. Stroke 2002;33:2738–43.
103. Hartings JA, Bullock MR, Okonkwo DO, et al. Spreading depolarisations and outcome after traumatic brain injury: a prospective observational study. Lancet Neurol 2011;10:1058–64.
104. Yanamoto H, Miyamoto S, Tohnai N, et al. Induced spreading depression activates persistent neurogenesis in the subventricular zone, generating cells with markers for divided and early committed neurons in the caudate putamen and cortex. Stroke 2005;36:1544–50.
105. Lauritzen M, Dreier JP, Fabricius M, et al. Clinical relevance of cortical spreading depression in neurological disorders: migraine, malignant stroke, subarachnoid and intracranial hemorrhage, and traumatic brain injury. J Cereb Blood Flow Metab 2011;31:17–35.
106. Phillips JP, Langford RM, Chang SH, et al. Cerebral arterial oxygen saturation measurements using a fiber-optic pulse oximeter. Neurocrit Care 2010;13: 278–85.
107. Keller E, Froehlich J, Muroi C, et al. Neuromonitoring in intensive care: a new brain tissue probe for combined monitoring of intracranial pressure (ICP) cerebral blood flow (CBF) and oxygenation. Acta Neurochir Suppl 2011;110:217–20.
108. Kim MN, Durduran T, Frangos S, et al. Noninvasive measurement of cerebral blood flow and blood oxygenation using near-infrared and diffuse correlation spectroscopies in critically brain-injured adults. Neurocrit Care 2010;12:173–80.
109. Hemphill JC, Andrews P, De Georgia M. Multimodal monitoring and neurocritical care bioinformatics. Nat Rev Neurol 2011;7:451–60.

Monitoring and Intraoperative Management of Elevated Intracranial Pressure and Decompressive Craniectomy

Shih-Shan Lang, MD[a],*, W. Andrew Kofke, MD, MBA, FCCM[a,b],
Michael F. Stiefel, MD, PhD[c]

KEYWORDS

- Elevated intracranial pressure • Decompressive craniectomy
- Intraoperative management • Intracranial hypertension

KEY POINTS

- Elevated intracranial pressure can be caused by a variety of underlying conditions.
- Several physiologic and pharmacologic factors have a significant impact on intracranial hypertension, mostly caused by changes on cerebral blood volume, flow, and oxygenation.
- There are many therapies that can be used to decrease intracranial pressure ranging from pharmacologic to surgical decompressive removal of the calvarium.
- Special consideration is made for the anesthetic management of these patients perioperatively.

There are numerous clinical scenarios wherein critically ill patients may present with neurologic dysfunction as a result of ischemia, trauma, or neuroexcitation. Neurons and its supporting elements may be damaged in a virtually unnoticeable manner or there may be widespread neuronal loss and tissue infarction. Any of these scenarios may include a period of decreased cerebral perfusion pressure (CPP), which is usually caused by intracranial hypertension from elevated intracranial pressure (ICP). Prolonged, elevated ICP leads to compromised cerebral blood flow (CBF), which

Disclosures: None.
[a] Department of Neurosurgery, University of Pennsylvania, 3400 Spruce Street 3rd Floor Silverstein, Philadelphia, PA 19104, USA; [b] Department of Anesthesiology and Critical Care, University of Pennsylvania, 3400 Spruce Street 3rd Floor Silverstein, Philadelphia, PA 19104, USA; [c] Department of Neurosurgery, Westchester Medical Center, New York Medical College, Munger Pavilion, Valhalla, NY 10595, USA
* Corresponding author.
E-mail address: shihshan.lang@uphs.upenn.edu

Anesthesiology Clin 30 (2012) 289–310
doi:10.1016/j.anclin.2012.05.008   anesthesiology.theclinics.com
1932-2275/12/$ – see front matter © 2012 Elsevier Inc. All rights reserved.

transitions to permanent neuronal loss, infarction, and possibly even brain death. Even though elevated ICP arises from a variety of causes, it often ends in a distinct neurosurgical procedure intended to ameliorate the impact or cause of intracranial hypertension. This neurosurgical procedure of decompressive craniectomy has been widely used in the management of patients with refractory elevated ICP.

INTRACRANIAL HYPERTENSION

The brain, spinal cord, cerebrospinal fluid (CSF), and blood are encased in the skull and vertebral canal, thus constituting a nearly incompressible system. In a totally incompressible system, pressure would vary linearly with increased volume. However, there is capacitance in the system, which is thought to be provided by the intervertebral spaces and the vasculature. Once this capacitance is exhausted, the ICP increases dramatically with increased intracranial volume (**Fig. 1**). This increase is based on the following relation: CBF = (MAP-ICP)/CVR, where *MAP* is mean arterial pressure and *CVR* is cerebrovascular resistance. The relationship between increasing ICP and the associated decrements in CBF is not a straightforward linear curve. MAP may increase with ICP elevations,[1] and CVR decreases with decreasing CPP to maintain CBF until maximal vasodilatation occurs (**Fig. 2**).[2–5] This maximal vasodilatation, with increased cerebral blood volume (CBV), is thought to occur when CPP is less than or equal to 50 mm Hg, although there is considerable heterogeneity in this value among individuals.[6] A convincing argument, put forth by Drummond,[7] is that the lower limit of autoregulation is probably closer to 70 mm Hg. Therefore, increasing ICP is often associated with cerebral vasodilatation or increasing MAP to maintain CBF, which makes the assessment and therapeutic decision making a complex process.

Normal ICP is less than 10 mm Hg. Sustained ICP greater than 20 mm Hg is generally associated with the need for escalation of ICP-reducing interventions.[8,9] However, this number, 20 mm Hg, is an epidemiologically derived number found in traumatic brain injury (TBI) studies that indicate patients do worse with ICP greater than 20 mm Hg.[9] Physiologically, simply elevating ICP to greater than 20 mm Hg does not necessarily correlate with decrements in CBF, provided the previously noted compensatory mechanisms occur.[10] Nonetheless, mass lesions or CSF outflow obstructions

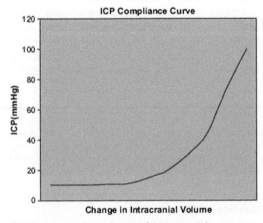

Fig. 1. The relationship between the volume of intracranial contents and pressure. Initial increases in volume have little effect on ICP until a threshold of capacitive exhaustion is reached after which pressure increases abruptly.

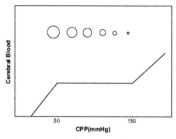

Fig. 2. Relationship between CBF and perfusion pressure. CBF stays constant between CPP perfusion pressures of approximately 50 to 150 mm Hg. The changing vascular caliber required to accomplish this (with associated change in cerebral blood volume) is depicted across the top.

that increase ICP can exhaust compensatory mechanisms. Eventually, compromise of CBF occurs, which initially manifests as an abnormality in the distal runoff of the cerebral circulation. As the process continues, compromise of diastolic perfusion arises. This compromise makes the normally continuous (through systole and diastole) CPP become discontinuous (**Fig. 3**).[11] Further compromise of CBF results in anaerobic metabolism, exacerbation of edema, and ultimately intracranial circulatory arrest.[11,12] Therefore, early detection of elevated ICP is critical to intervene and treat before this lethal sequence of events.

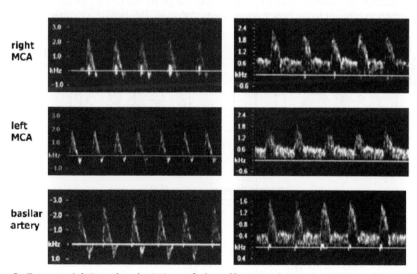

Fig. 3. Transcranial Doppler depiction of the effects in decreasing CPP on blood flow velocity. Initially, at normal perfusion pressure, a normal waveform is evident with blood flow present during systole and diastole. Increasing ICP with associated decreased CPP encroaches on diastolic flow until ICP exceeds diastolic blood pressure, at which point diastolic flow stops. Continued increase in ICP to exceed systolic blood pressure produces total intracranial circulatory arrest throughout systole and diastole, producing the to-and-fro waveform on the right, indicating blood pumping against the swollen brain and bouncing backward within the basal arteries of the brain. MCA, middle cerebral artery. (*From* Reinhard M, Petrick M, Steinfurth G, et al. Acute increase in intracranial pressure revealed by transcranial Doppler sonography. J Clin Ultrasound 2003;31:326; with permission.)

There are generally 2 types of intracranial hypertension categorized according to CBF: hyperemic or oligemic (**Fig. 4**). Although conceptualized as a dichotomous process, the real physiology is undoubtedly more of a continuum. In the normal state, increases in CBF are not typically associated with increased ICP because the normal capacitive mechanisms absorb the excess intracranial blood volume. However, in the situation of disordered intracranial compliance, small increases in intracranial volume caused by increased CBF produce increases in ICP.[3,13]

Elevated ICP has traditionally been considered to be a concern because it indicates that cerebral perfusion might be jeopardized. However, it is unclear whether it is appropriate to be concerned about high ICP inducing intracranial oligemia when the cause of the high ICP is intracranial hyperemia. There have been no specific answers to this targeted question, although there have been some studies that allow reasonable inferences about the significance of hyperemic intracranial hypertension. For many years, it has been known that brief noxious stimuli momentarily increase ICP in the setting of decreased intracranial compliance. Recent studies have reported that such situations are associated with hyperemia,[14] suggesting that hyperemic intracranial hypertension may not be a dangerous situation.[15] However, there are a few reasons to be concerned about this hyperemia. First, elevated ICP caused by hyperemia in one area of the brain may increase ICP, which leads to the compromise of CBF in other areas of the brain in which regional CBF (rCBF) is already marginal. Second, increased ICP in one area of the brain may produce gradients that could potentially escalate to a herniation syndrome. Third, inappropriate hyperemia may predispose the brain to worsened edema or hemorrhage, as seen in other hyperperfusion syndromes.[13,16,17] Thus, hyperemic intracranial hypertension has the theoretical potential to be deleterious but this phenomenon has yet to be conclusively demonstrated. Intubation, or other temporary

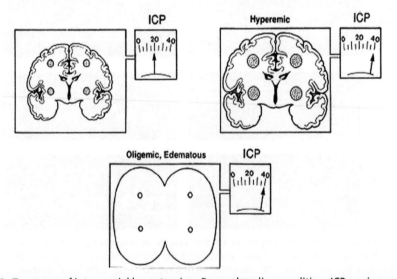

Fig. 4. Two types of intracranial hypertension. From a baseline condition, ICP can increase in 2 ways. One is via an increase in cerebral blood volume associated with reflex vasodilation caused by moderate blood pressure decreases or by hyperemia. The second mechanism of intracranial hypertension is via malignant brain edema or other expanding masses encroaching on the vascular bed to produce intracranial ischemia. (*From* Kofke WA, Wechsler L. Neurointensive care. In: Albin M, editor. Textbook of neurosanesthesia. New York: McGraw-Hill; 1997. p. 1247–348; with permission.)

noxious stimuli that momentarily increase ICP, have not been proven to have long-term consequences.[18]

In contrast, oligemic intracranial hypertension is associated with compromised cerebral perfusion.[19] This finding is supported by the high mortality observed in patients with head trauma in whom ICP increases and CBF decreases because of brain edema after a TBI.[9,20] Transcranial Doppler and CBF studies on these patients have demonstrated that CBF is low and perfusion is discontinuous during the cardiac cycle (see **Fig. 3**).[11,20] In addition, jugular venous bulb oxygenation data indicate that O2 extraction is markedly increased,[21] suggesting anaerobic metabolism is occurring.[20] In this setting, noxious stimuli can further increase the ICP, which produces the situation of hyperemic on oligemic intracranial hypertension. Presumably, in this setting, the hyperemic increase in ICP acts to further compromise rCBF in areas of edema.

PLATEAU WAVES

In a seminal article, Lundberg[22] monitored ICP in hundreds of patients and identified characteristic pressure waves. One category of these waves was described as plateau waves, which are known to be associated with increased CBV.[2] These waves occur when the ICP abruptly increases in response to systemic blood pressure levels, which are occasionally accompanied by neurologic deterioration. Rosner and Becker[3] analyzed the data and provided evidence that suggests that CBV dysautoregulation is responsible for plateau waves. They intensively monitored cats after inducing mild head trauma and observed that mild blood pressure decrements to a mean of approximately 70 to 80 mm Hg preceded the development of plateau waves (**Fig. 5**). Normally, CBV in autoregulating brain tissue increases with decreasing blood pressure. However, this increase in CBV is nonlinear because there is an exponential increase in CBV as the perfusion pressure reaches less than 80 mm Hg (**Fig. 6**).[3,23] A small decrease in blood pressure, even within the normotensive range, produces exponential increases in CBV in a setting of abnormal intracranial compliance, with the ICP at the elbow of the ICP-intracranial volume curve. Therefore, a small decrease in blood pressure introduces an exponential CBV change on an exponential ICP relation, which results in an abrupt and significant ICP increase. Plateau waves spontaneously resolve with a hypertensive response or with hyperventilation, which both act to oppose the increase in CBV. To develop a plateau wave, there must be an area of the brain with normally reactive vasculature in contrast to a dysautoregulating area with a mass effect and overall elevated ICP; this becomes a situation of heterogeneous autoregulation (**Fig. 7**). Typically, within the normal autoregulatory range, changes in

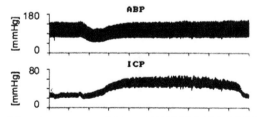

Fig. 5. In an animal head trauma model, a trivial-appearing and transient decrease in systemic arterial blood pressure in the setting of borderline, precipitates sufficient cerebral vasodilatation to markedly increase the intracranial pressure. Restoration of CPP is associated with abolition of the plateau wave. (*Adapted from* Schmidt B, Czosnyka M, Schwarze JJ, et al. Cerebral vasodilatation causing acute intracranial hypertension: a method for noninvasive assessment. J Cereb Blood Flow Metab 1999;19:990–6; with permission.)

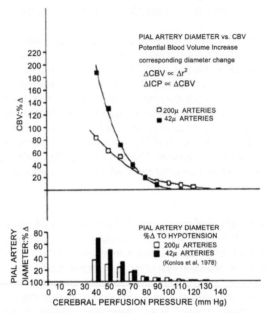

Fig. 6. Vasodilatation occurs at a logarithmic rate as CPP is reduced. ICP will increase at a proportional rate within each pressure range, with the most rapid increase occurring less than a CPP of 80 mmHg. (*From* Rosner M, Becker D. The etiology of plateau waves: a theoretical model and experimental observations. In: Ishii S, Nagai H, Brock M, editors. Intracranial pressure. New York: Springer-Verlag; 1983. p. 301; with kind permission of Springer Science and Business Media.)

blood pressure have little to no effect on ICP. However, after brain injury and associated vasoparalysis, blood pressure increases mechanically produce cerebral vasodilatation, which increases ICP (**Fig. 8**).[24] Both elevations and decrements in blood pressure can increase ICP, suggesting the presence of a CPP optimum for ICP. In addition to preventing and treating plateau waves, it may be also be important to maintain MAP in the 80 to 100 mm Hg range in patients with high ICP. This concept is summarized in **Fig. 9**.

Recently, the relationship between ICP and blood pressure has been quantified in the form of a simple correlation coefficient, the so-called pressure reactivity index.[25–27] This measure and other continuous measures of autoregulation also suggest the presence

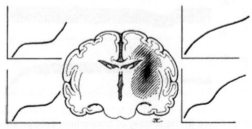

Fig. 7. Heterogeneous injury with some areas of retained autoregulation provides physiologic conditions conducive to the development of plateau waves. (*From* Kofke WA, Wechsler L. Neurointensive care. In: Albin M, editor. Textbook of neuroanesthesia. New York: McGraw-Hill; 1997. p. 1247–348; with permission.)

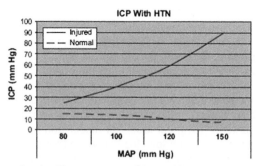

Fig. 8. In the context of a significant amount of injured brain with accompanying dysautoregulation, systemic hypertension produces intracranial hypertension, presumably from distension of injured, poorly autoregulating blood vessels. (*Adapted from* Matakas F, et al. Increase in cerebral perfusion pressure by arterial hypertension in brain swelling. A Mathematical model of the volume-pressure relationship. J Neurosurg 1975;42(3):282–9.)

of an optimum blood pressure for ICP. Retrospective observations suggest an association with better outcomes when the blood pressure is closer to this optimum.[26,27]

TREATMENT OF INTRACRANIAL HYPERTENSION

The general goal in treating intracranial hypertension is to promote nutritive blood flow in the brain by maintaining adequate CPP and tissue oxygenation and also preserving the nutrient supply via appropriate glucose management (without hypoglycemia or hyperglycemia). Clinically, the goals are to diagnose and treat the underlying causes, avoid exacerbating and noxious factors, and reduce ICP. Some underlying causes include masses, such as tumors and hematomas, hydrocephalus, cerebral edema,

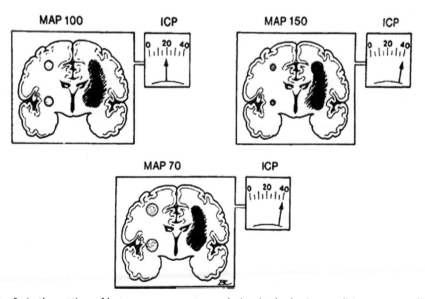

Fig. 9. In the setting of heterogeneous autoregulation in the brain, conditions may predispose to CBV-mediated increases in ICP, with either increases or decreases in blood pressure. (*From* Kofke WA, Wechsler L. Neurointensive care. In: Albin M, editor. Textbook of neurosanesthesia. New York: McGraw-Hill; 1997. p. 1247–348; with permission.)

and cerebrovascular dilatation. The therapy for intracranial hypertension is primarily targeted toward eliminating the cause. When this is not possible, therapy becomes aimed at controlling ICP, with the expectation that the primary cause of the intracranial hypertension will resolve. Controlling ICP is, therefore, a supportive maneuver intended to preserve viable neuronal tissue until the condition causing the elevated ICP resolves. Therapeutic maneuvers involve 1 or more of 6 classes of therapy: (1) decrease CBV; (2) decrease CSF volume; (3) induce serum hyperosmolarity; (4) resect unviable damaged brain tissue or resect viable but clinically less important brain tissue (eg, frontal lobe or anterior temporal lobe); (5) resect non-neural masses, such as tumors and hematomas; and (6) remove the calvarium (decompressive craniectomy) to permit more area for the edematous brain to expand. Recent advances in the use of brain tissue oxygen (PbrO2) monitors occasionally affect the manner in which these maneuvers are used, which ensures continued optimal PbrO2.

CBV Reduction

CBV can be decreased with hyperventilation, CBF-decreasing drugs, mannitol, or hypothermia.

Hyperventilation

Hyperventilation can acutely reduce CBF and CBV to reduce ICP.[28–32] However, CBF returns to its original state within minutes to hours in a normal situation.[28,32] Therefore, it is unclear why sustained decreases in ICP can be achieved with hyperventilation alone. There are several adverse effects of hyperventilation, including the risk of decreasing CBF to a dangerous level (**Fig. 10**).[33,34] In a study of trauma patients, routine hyperventilation was associated with worse neurologic outcome at 3 and 6 months after the injury[35]; however, the underlying mechanisms of this finding are unclear. Nonetheless, hyperventilation can be an effective means to decrease ICP if patients have hyperemic intracranial hypertension or are in imminent danger of herniation. The presence of hyperemia can be determined by the use of direct brain CBF measurement or via jugular bulb oximetry.[14,36] Brain tissue PbrO2 may provide additional information; however, the relationship of this method to CBF remains to be definitively demonstrated. High ICP associated with a low arteriovenous oxygen content difference (AVDO2) across the brain (3 vol%–4 vol%) is thought to indicate that hyperventilation can be safely used. In an emergency situation, regardless of the underlying cause of the increased ICP, hyperventilation should be used to decrease ICP and to treat imminent herniation or plateau waves until more definitive diagnoses or therapies can be performed.

CBV-decreasing drugs

CBF-decreasing drugs (which are also CBV decreasing) that decrease ICP include barbiturates,[37–39] benzodiazepines,[40] etomidate,[41,42] and propofol.[39,43] Notably, these drugs all are central nervous system depressants. Therefore, there is a compromise between the use of these treatments for lowering ICP and the loss of a reliable neurologic examination. This consideration is secondary intraoperatively but becomes important postoperatively. Unlike hyperventilation, these agents that decrease CBF are coupled to a decreased cerebral metabolic rate (CMR). Therefore, CBF decreases with the use of these drugs should not provide a milieu for anaerobic metabolism. Lidocaine also decreases CBF and CMR to decrease ICP, although with a less-pronounced decline in neurologic function.[44,45] However, at high doses, lidocaine may cause seizures, which will result in an increase in CBF, CBF, and ICP. Mannitol's immediate effects are also thought to be mediated by a reduction in CBV,[29] although this mechanism of action is minor and temporary.

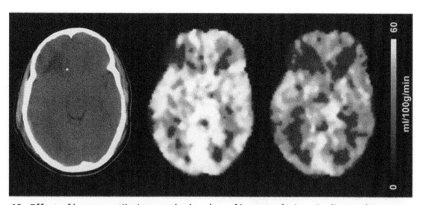

Fig. 10. Effect of hyperventilation on the burden of hypoperfusion. Radiographic computed tomography (*left*) and gray-scale positron emission tomographic imaging of CBF obtained from a 31-year-old man 7 days after injury at relative normocapnia (*middle*), Paco$_2$ 35 mm Hg (4.7 kPa), and hypocapnia (*right*), 26 mm Hg (3.5 kPa). Voxels with a CBF of less than 10 mL $\times$ 100g^{-1} $\times$ min^{-1} are shaded in black. Note the right frontal contusion and small parietal subdural hematoma. Baseline ICP was 21 mm Hg and baseline CPP was 74 mm Hg. Baseline Jugular venous oxygen saturation (Sjvo$_2$) values of 70% and AVDO2 of 3.7 mL/dL are consistent with hyperemia and support the use of hyperventilation for ICP control. Hyperventilation did result in a reduction in ICP to 17 mm Hg and an increase in CPP to 76 mm Hg, with maintenance of Sjvo$_2$ and AVDO2 within desirable ranges (58% and 5.5 mL/mL respectively). However, despite these Sjvo$_2$ and AVDO2 figures, baseline hypoperfused brain volume was 141 mL and increased to 428 mL with hyperventilation. These increases were observed in both perilesional and normal regions of brain tissue. AVDO2, arteriovenous oxygen content difference. (*From* Coles JP, Minhas PS, Fryer TD, et al. Effect of hyperventilation on cerebral blood flow in traumatic head injury: clinical relevance and monitoring correlates. Crit Care Med 2002;30(9):1950–9; with permission.)

CSF Drainage

CSF volume can be reduced by removing CSF via an external ventricular drain (EVD) (**Fig. 11**). Some risks of a constantly open EVD include excessive CSF drainage when patients cough, drain manipulation in the course of routine nursing procedures, increasing the height of the operating table, or with head elevation. Any of these circumstances can contribute to the collapse of the ventricles or the development of subdural hematomas, which is a sign of overdrainage.[46] An excessive and abrupt decrease in local pressure around the drain can produce intracranial gradients, which may lead to a herniation syndrome. Leaving the drain clamped and monitored, however, risks the development of untreated intracranial hypertension.

Hyperosmolar Therapy

Mannitol has become the traditional mainstay of hyperosmolar therapy. After the initial hypoviscosity-mediated autoregulatory vasoconstriction,[47] it may induce a further decrease in ICP through brain dehydration in areas with an intact blood brain barrier.[48–50] However, this effect may be limited through the generation of intracellular osmolytes, which equalizes the transmembrane osmolar gradients.[51,52] Theoretically, this effect may be limited through the concomitant administration of a loop diuretic.[53] Unfortunately, mannitol can have delayed effects that increase ICP, which occurs by 4 mechanisms. First, because mannitol is a potent diuretic, it can have a secondary effect of decreasing systemic blood volume, which decreases cardiac output and blood pressure. This effect can result in the normal reflex autoregulation that increases

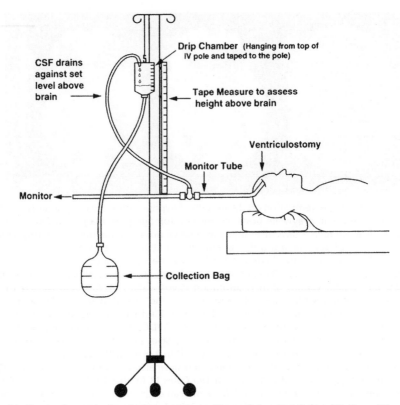

Fig. 11. External ventricular drainage system. (*From* Coles JP, Minhas PS, Fryer TD, et al. Effect of hyperventilation on cerebral blood flow in traumatic head injury: clinical relevance and monitoring correlates. Crit Care Med 2002;30(9):1950–9; with permission.)

CBV, which leads to an increase in ICP.[3] Second, if the increased urine output is not replaced with adequate intravenous fluid therapy, the hematocrit can become elevated, which opposes the initial hypoviscosity-mediated autoregulatory vasoconstriction.[54] Third, mannitol can cross the blood brain barrier in an unpredictable manner, which introduces the possibility of a rebound increase in ICP, similar to that observed with urea.[54,55] This effect is partly related to its reflection coefficient of 0.9, indicating that even in a normal state, mannitol can slowly diffuse into the brain.[56] Fourth, there is a theoretical possibility of increased intracellular osmolarity via the so-called idiogenic osmoles, which may predispose to a rebound increase in brain volume with the discontinuation of mannitol.[51,52] Urine output replacement with balanced crystalloid infusion and strict monitoring of blood osmolarity may help to avoid these potential complications of mannitol. In trauma, mannitol may be contraindicated because of the loss of blood volume from hemorrhage associated with many trauma patients. Hypertonic saline may be a viable alternative.

Hypertonic Saline

Hypertonic saline (HTS) is a recently revisited alternative to mannitol. With a reflection coefficient of 1.0 and no potential to produce undesired hypovolemia from diuresis, HTS has properties that make it an attractive hyperosmolar agent.[56] It is a useful niche agent to use in the group of patients who are refractory to mannitol or those in which mannitol is contraindicated. Hypertonic saline has undergone scrutiny in many laboratory and clinical studies, with virtually all indicating a beneficial effect to decrease ICP. The data on the efficacy of HTS are not a new observation because initial reports date back to 1919.[57] Studies in the more recent decades generally have used 3.0%, 7.5%, or 23.4% saline with or without a colloid (typically dextran or hetastarch). In clinical trials, the effect of HTS has been reported in numerous disease states, including ischemic stroke, intracerebral hemorrhage, subarachnoid hemorrhage (SAH), TBI, and hepatic encephalopathy. All studies show that HTS effectively and reproducibly reduces ICP with concomitant improvement in CPP.[58] Many randomized controlled trials comparing mannitol and varying concentrations of HTS in TBI or during elective supratentorial surgery found that HTS was more effective in treating intracranial hypertension.[59–64] One prospective randomized study did not show better ICP control with HTS compared with standard therapy. However, in this study, the sample size was small and the patients with HTS had more comorbidities than the control group on entry into the study.[65] Three studies report that HTS can be safely and effectively used in children to decrease ICP after TBI.[66–68] In the population of patients with SAH and ischemic stroke, several studies reported the HTS therapy effectively decreased ICP and increased CBF as compared with mannitol.[69–72] These studies also showed an important effect of 23.4% HTS: it is a therapy that effectively decreases ICP when all other medical therapies fail.[69,73] HTS clearly has the potential to exert a positive impact in the management of intracranial hypertension. However, HTS is not without potential complications. Deleterious effects, such as central pontine myelinolysis, have also been discussed in the literature.[70,74]

Optimizing Brain Oxygenation

The advent of brain tissue PO2 monitoring makes optimizing brain oxygenation an additional component in the management of elevated ICP. Hypoxemia, defined as PaO2 less than approximately 50 mm Hg to 60 mm Hg, is associated with cerebral vasodilation[75] and endangers neuronal survival. Studies on hyperoxia show that this increased systemic oxygenation state in normal healthy individuals produces vasoconstriction and hypocapnea.[76] However, in individuals with cerebrovascular disease, areas of the brain with impaired cerebrovascular reserve were not adversely affected by hyperoxia.[77] Nonetheless, Fiskum and colleagues[78–81] observed free radical–related negative effects with hyperoxia, and studies of hyperoxia reported negative outcome effects after cardiac arrest.[82] These findings suggest that hyperoxia may be deleterious. The optimal PaO2 to seek in patients with a brain injury remains unclear.[83–85] In addition, the bedside decision about PaO2 management is further complicated by the patient's cerebrovascular reserve. For example, a low PaO2 that would normally be tolerated through vasodilation may not be so well tolerated if the vasodilatory reserve is compromised in diseases, such as carotid occlusion, brain edema, or anemia.[86] Brain tissue PO2 monitoring demonstrates that brain hypoxia, which may occur in the presence of whole body normoxia, is associated with poor neurologic outcome in patients who have either suffered traumatic or SAH brain injury.[87–91] Studies advocate the treatment of brain hypoxia because this treatment is associated with decreased mortality in both adults and children.[92–94] In the absence of a PbrO2 monitor, the clinician bases therapy on assumptions about brain oxygenation and necessarily errs on the side of higher oxygen supply. In patients with mild brain injury, the clinician should provide high enough fraction of inspired oxygen (FiO2) to produce oxygen saturation greater than 95%. If there is an elevated ICP or areas of brain hypoperfusion, then a reasonable empiric approach would be to use an FiO2 of 60% with a positive end-expiratory pressure of 5 to 10 cm H2O. This practice maximizes PaO2 and PbrO2 without a significant risk of acute pulmonary injury.[95]

Resection of Brain Tissue

The resection of brain tissue is occasionally used for malignant intracranial hypertension. Because of its proximity to the brainstem and because it often compresses the brainstem in a herniation syndrome, the temporal lobe may be resected to aid in controlling ICP.[96,97] An alternative approach, suggested specifically for malignant intracranial hypertension caused by ischemic stroke, is to resect nonviable and edematous infarcted tissue, leaving noninfarcted tissue intact.[98] However, this strokectomy procedure could be difficult intraoperatively because there may be inadvertent resection of viable tissue.

Resection of Non-neural Masses or Hematomas

When elevated ICP is clinically diagnosed and imaging studies indicate the presence of a mass lesion, the initial response is to urgently remove the mass. The controversy lies with spontaneous intracerebral hematomas from nonvascular malformations. The literature tends toward reporting improved outcomes following aggressive surgical intervention.[99–102] More recent studies focus on ICH volume as the determining factor of choosing surgery over conservative treatment, especially in deep, noncortical ICH.[103] Surgical intervention can be life saving in patients suffering acute epidural hematomas with abrupt neurologic deterioration or cerebellar hematomas.[99,104] Efficacy of surgery for patients with subdural hematomas, especially chronic subdural hygromas, is less clear, although most surgeons would intervene on patients with acute subdural hematomas in the context of a recent trauma and neurologic deterioration.

Decompressive craniectomy

Many patients continue to have persistently elevated ICP or cerebral edema that is refractory to first-line therapies. In these cases of failed medical therapy, surgical decompressive craniectomy (DCH) has been advocated as a life-saving measure to prevent transtentorial herniation, decrease ischemic burden, decrease therapeutic intensity, and decrease mortality.[105–107] Surgical decompression has been tested in patients with severe TBI or stroke with varying results.[108–110] It is hypothesized that through decompressive surgery, the vicious cycle of extensive edema caused by elevated ICP, resulting in ischemia of neighboring brain tissue and further infarction, may be interrupted.[111] Decompressive surgery may then increase CPP and optimize perfusion, which allows a functionally compromised but viable brain to survive.[112] The use of DCH to control elevated ICP has been recognized since the beginning of the twentieth century. As early as 1905, Cushing[113,114] performed a subtemporal decompression to relieve elevated ICP from an inaccessible brain tumor and later reported the application of this operation to wartime trauma.

There are generally 2 forms of decompressive surgical operations: hemicraniectomy and bifrontal craniectomy. A hemicraniectomy is often performed in situations when there is unilateral injury or focal pathologic conditions. Briefly, decompressive hemicraniectomy is performed by removing a large bone flap with a diameter of at least 12 cm (including the frontal, parietal, temporal, and parts of the occipital squama).[115,116] The skull is removed so that the floor of the middle cerebral fossa can be exposed. The dura is opened in a cruciate fashion and left widely open without the removal of ischemic brain.[117] Dural substitutes may be applied over the dural defect. The bone is either placed into the patient's abdomen subcutaneously or stored sterile in a freezer.[118,119] Decompressive bifrontal craniectomy is effective for patients with bifrontal injury or in those patients with diffuse swelling with no focal pathologic condition.[120] A bifrontal craniectomy is performed with a bicoronal skin incision and reflection of the temporalis muscle. Burr holes are located at either side of the sagittal sinus at the posterior extent, bilaterally at the keyhole, and bilaterally at the roof of the zygoma. A large bifrontal cra-niectomy is created, extending posteriorly into the parietal bones approximately 3 to 5 cm posterior to the coronal sutures. A bone cut is made anteriorly over the sagittal sinus. The sagittal sinus and falx cerebri may be ligated and divided anteriorly to allow for further anterior expansion.[120] Regardless of the type of decompressive surgery, there continues to be controversy concerning the usefulness of DCH for intractable intracranial hypertension. Although DCH has been shown to be effective in reducing ICP, older retrospective studies disagreed on whether DCH improves overall outcome.[105,108,121–123] However, in the past few years, several prospective randomized controlled clinical trials have been published, most notably DECIMAL, DESTINY, HAMLET and DECRA.[116,120,124,125] One analysis[116] pooled 3 European clinical trials (DECIMAL, DESTINY, and HAMLET) that included data for patients who underwent a DCH within 48 hours of malignant infarction of the middle cerebral artery. The results from this study suggested that patients who underwent decompressive surgery after a malignant middle cerebral artery infarction had a more favorable functional outcome and decreased mortality. However, another randomized controlled trial examining adults who underwent a bifrontal decompressive craniectomy after severe TBI (DECRA) did not show such favorable results.[120] The conclusions from this trial showed that early bifrontal-temporal-parietal decompressive craniectomy was associated with decreased ICP but was also associated with a worse functional outcome. This trial was met with many criticisms, including limited follow-up time, small sample size, inap-propriate baseline prognostic criteria, imbalance of baseline characteristics, and a high rate of crossover.[126] In 2006, a clinical trial was started, RESCUEicp, that studied those patients with refractory elevated ICP after TBI. This trial is similar to DECRA but with an improved protocol, including a larger target population, broader age range, longer follow-up time, a more stringent definition of refractory elevated ICP, and exclusion criteria of fixed and dilated pupils. The trial is currently ongoing.[127] Decompressive cra-niectomy remains a valuable approach, supported by the literature, as a life-saving maneuver for moribund patients. Notwithstanding unavoidable morbidity related to the initial insult, patients can suggest support for having undergone the procedure. An excellent case report, authored by an anesthesiologist who underwent a decom-pressive craniectomy, supports this notion.[128]

ANESTHETIC MANAGEMENT WITH INTRACRANIAL HYPERTENSION

Patients presenting for surgery with intracranial hypertension, or for decompressive craniectomy, require careful consideration of the effects of anesthetic drugs on the neu-ropathophysiologic processes. There are little data describing the impact of anesthetic management on patient outcomes in this situation. Because of this, it becomes most appropriate to use anesthetic drugs associated with lower ICP. Such drugs usually decrease the cerebral metabolic rate with a coupled decrease in CBF and ICP. This decrease assumes the presence of appropriately reactive cerebral vasculature, even if heterogeneously present. Another consideration is whether hypnosis or analgesia is needed in the context of a patient who is unconscious from the underlying disease that is producing the elevated ICP. The extent of hypnotic or amnestic drugs to admin-ister becomes a matter of judgment. Given that there are situations when a patient can seem to be unconscious and yet have awareness would indicate that such drugs gener-ally should be used unless contraindicated by other physiologic concerns.

Volatile anesthetics all have a dose-related tendency to increase CBF or to induce cerebral vasodilation.[129] The most pronounced increase in CBF occurs with halothane but is also reported with isoflurane, sevoflurane, and desflurane.[130–136] There are some reports of metabolically coupled decreases in CBF with sevoflurane.[136] Based on potential increased CBF and CBV, it is expected that the use of these volatile anesthetics, at least around the minimum alveolar anesthetic concentration (MAC) dose or higher, will increase ICP. Nonetheless, several reports indicate that ICP does not increase appreciably in patients with brain tumors with isoflurane and desflurane[137] and that CO_2 reactivity is retained in patients being anesthetized with these agents,[135,138] such that any invoked hyperemia can be treated with hyperventilation. All of these drugs, in various contexts, have been shown to contain neuroprotective qualities that might support their use, perhaps in lower doses. There is little support for the use of nitrous oxide in patients who suffer from elevated ICP or brain injury. This drug clearly can increase ICP and CBF.[139–141] Without a neurosurgical procedure, nitrous oxide given to humans at a hyperbaric 1 MAC, produced severe systemic excitation with opisthotonos that one would expect to be associated with neuroexcitation, increased CBF, and increased ICP.[142] Given to humans in the context of preexisting high-dose isoflurane and a flat electroencephalogram, nitrous oxide produced increased CBF velocity, suggesting a direct vasodilatory effect.[129] Therefore, there is little support for the use of nitrous oxide in patients with elevated ICP and a brain injury. Barbiturates have been used for decades for the management of intracranial hypertension.[38,143] Although there is little doubt that they effectively reduce ICP, there remains controversy regarding their role in improving outcomes. In the context of this discussion, this category of drugs (eg, barbiturates, propofol, etomidate), should be an integral component of the anesthetic selection for patients with brain swelling caused by their ICP-decreasing qualities.[144] When choosing which drug in this group to use for a particular patient, the physician should take into consideration their differences in the extent of hemodynamic depression (barbiturates and propofol are stronger than etomidate)[144]; duration (barbiturates last longer than etomidate, which lasts longer than propofol); and adrenal suppression (etomidate).[145] Opioids are often used as the analgesic component of a general anesthetic. Mu opioids are the mainstay of antinociception during surgery. In patients with elevated ICP, preventing the systemic response to noxious stimuli can effectively prevent spikes in ICP.[14,146,147] Therefore, opioids have an important role in perioperative management of patients with elevated ICP. Opioids have an additional advantage of producing minor direct hemodynamic depression and can be reversed with a specific antagonist, naloxone. The administration of opioids that cause systemic release of histamine (eg, morphine, Demerol) may be associated with hypotension and increased ICP and, therefore, should be avoided in patients with intracranial hypertension. Limbic activation has been observed in humans at both high and low doses,[148] with occasional idiosyncratic reports of opioid-induced seizure and support for electroconvulsive seizure.[149] Nonetheless, there have been no reports that opioid use can produce neural injury in humans. Any theoretical risk of opioid neurotoxicity can be outweighed by the well-documented risk of ICP spikes associated with nociception.

SUMMARY

Intracranial hypertension can be caused by a complex interplay of numerous factors. The elevated ICP can be caused by hyperemia, in the context of abnormal intracranial compliance, edema, or other masses with concurrent oligemia. Changes in blood pressure can contribute to ICP elevations with significantly different outcomes. Several other physiologic and pharmacologic factors can exert a significant impact on ICP, largely because of the effects on CBV. Therapeutic maneuvers involve 1 or more of 6 classes of therapy: (1) decrease CBV; (2) decrease CSF volume; (3) induce serum hyperosmolarity; (4) resect unviable, damaged brain tissue or resect viable but clinically less important brain tissue (eg, frontal lobe or anterior temporal lobe); (5) resect non-neural masses, such as tumors and hematomas; and (6) remove the calvarium (decompressive craniectomy) to permit more area for the edematous brain to expand. These therapies can be introduced through a variety of physiologic, pharmacologic, and surgical approaches. Anesthetic management of patients with intracranial hypertension is superimposed on these considerations. In general, the most suitable anesthetic is one that produces decrements in CBF and CBV with matched decreases in the cerebral metabolic rate. Careful attention is noted to interactions with other ongoing ICP-reducing therapies and avoidance of factors that may exacerbate the primary disease process causing elevated ICP.

REFERENCES

1. Cushing H. Concerning a definite regulatory mechanism of the vaso-motor centre which controls blood pressure during cerebral compression. Johns Hopkins Hosp Bull 1900;126:290.
2. Risberg J, Lundberg N, Ingvar DH. Regional cerebral blood volume during acute transient rises of the intracranial pressure (plateau waves). J Neurosurg 1969;31:303–10.
3. Rosner MJ, Becker DP. Origin and evolution of plateau waves. Experimental observations and a theoretical model. J Neurosurg 1984;60:312–24.
4. Greenberg JH, Alavi A, Reivich M, et al. Local cerebral blood volume response to carbon dioxide in man. Circ Res 1978;43:324–31.
5. Sakai F, Nakazawa K, Tazaki Y, et al. Regional cerebral blood volume and hematocrit measured in normal human volunteers by single-photon emission computed tomography. J Cereb Blood Flow Metab 1985;5:207–13.
6. Strandgaard S, Olesen J, Skinhoj E, et al. Autoregulation of brain circulation in severe arterial hypertension. Br Med J 1973;1:507–10.
7. Drummond JC. The lower limit of autoregulation: time to revise our thinking? Anesthesiology 1997;86:1431–3.
8. Lundberg N, Troupp H, Lorin H. Continuous recording of the ventricular-fluid pressure in patients with severe acute traumatic brain injury. A preliminary report. J Neurosurg 1965;22:581–90.
9. Miller JD, Becker DP, Ward JD, et al. Significance of intracranial hypertension in severe head injury. J Neurosurg 1977;47:503–16.
10. Giulioni M, Ursino M, Alvisi C. Correlations among intracranial pulsatility, intracranial hemodynamics, and transcranial Doppler wave form: literature review and hypothesis for future studies. Neurosurgery 1988;22:807–12.
11. Hassler W, Steinmetz H, Gawlowski J. Transcranial Doppler ultrasonography in raised intracranial pressure and in intracranial circulatory arrest. J Neurosurg 1988;68:745–51.
12. Greitz T, Gordon E, Kolmodin G, et al. Aortocranial and carotid angiography in determination of brain death. Neuroradiology 1973;5:13–9.
13. Jalan R, Olde Damink SW, Deutz NE, et al. Moderate hypothermia prevents cerebral hyperemia and increase in intracranial pressure in patients undergoing liver transplantation for acute liver failure. Transplantation 2003;75:2034–9.
14. Kerr ME, Weber BB, Sereika SM, et al. Effect of endotracheal suctioning on cerebral oxygenation in traumatic brain-injured patients. Crit Care Med 1999;27:2776–81.
15. Kofke WA, Dong ML, Bloom M, et al. Transcranial Doppler ultrasonography with induction of anesthesia for neurosurgery. J Neurosurg Anesthesiol 1994;6: 89–97.

16. Aggarwal S, Kramer D, Yonas H, et al. Cerebral hemodynamic and metabolic changes in fulminant hepatic failure: a retrospective study. Hepatology 1994;19:80–7.
17. Aggarwal S, Obrist W, Yonas H, et al. Cerebral hemodynamic and metabolic profiles in fulminant hepatic failure: relationship to outcome. Liver Transpl 2005;11:1353–60.
18. Michenfelder JD. The 27th Rovenstine lecture: neuroanesthesia and the achievement of professional respect. Anesthesiology 1989;70:695–701.
19. Wilkins RH. Cerebral vasospasm. Crit Rev Neurobiol 1990;6:51–77.
20. Jaggi JL, Obrist WD, Gennarelli TA, et al. Relationship of early cerebral blood flow and metabolism to outcome in acute head injury. J Neurosurg 1990;72: 176–82.
21. Stocchetti N, Zanier ER, Nicolini R, et al. Oxygen and carbon dioxide in the cerebral circulation during progression to brain death. Anesthesiology 2005;103: 957–61.
22. Lundberg N. Continuous recording and control of ventricular fluid pressure in neurosurgical practice. Acta Psychiatr Scand Suppl 1960;36:1–193.
23. Rosner MJ, Becker DP. The etiology of plateau waves: a theoretical model and experimental observations. In: Ishii S, Nagai H, Brock M, editors. Intracranial pressure. New York: Springer-Verlag; 1983. p. 301.
24. Matakas F, Von Waechter R, Knupling R, et al. Increase in cerebral perfusion pressure by arterial hypertension in brain swelling. A mathematical model of the volume-pressure relationship. J Neurosurg 1975;42:282–9.
25. Czosnyka M, Smielewski P, Piechnik S, et al. Cerebral autoregulation following head injury. J Neurosurg 2001;95:756–63.
26. Steiner LA, Czosnyka M, Piechnik SK, et al. Continuous monitoring of cerebrovascular pressure reactivity allows determination of optimal cerebral perfusion pressure in patients with traumatic brain injury. Crit Care Med 2002;30:733–8.
27. Zweifel C, Lavinio A, Steiner LA, et al. Continuous monitoring of cerebrovascular pressure reactivity in patients with head injury. Neurosurg Focus 2008;25(4):E2.
28. Raichle ME, Posner JB, Plum F. Cerebral blood flow during and after hyperventilation. Arch Neurol 1970;23:394–403.
29. Lassen NA. Control of cerebral circulation in health and disease. Circ Res 1974; 34:749–60.
30. Shapiro HM. Intracranial hypertension: therapeutic and anesthetic considerations. Anesthesiology 1975;43:445–71.
31. Shenkin HA, Bouzarth WF. Clinical methods of reducing intracranial pressure. Role of the cerebral circulation. N Engl J Med 1970;282:1465–71.
32. Raichle ME, Plum F. Hyperventilation and cerebral blood flow. Stroke 1972;3: 566–75.
33. Stringer WA, Hasso AN, Thompson JR, et al. Hyperventilation-induced cerebral ischemia in patients with acute brain lesions: demonstration by xenon-enhanced CT. AJNR Am J Neuroradiol 1993;14:475–84.
34. Coles JP, Minhas PS, Fryer TD, et al. Effect of hyperventilation on cerebral blood flow in traumatic head injury: clinical relevance and monitoring correlates. Crit Care Med 2002;30:1950–9.
35. Muizelaar JP, Marmarou A, Ward JD, et al. Adverse effects of prolonged hyperventilation in patients with severe head injury: a randomized clinical trial. J Neurosurg 1991;75:731–9.
36. Cruz J, Miner ME, Allen SJ, et al. Continuous monitoring of cerebral oxygenation in acute brain injury: injection of mannitol during hyperventilation. J Neurosurg 1990;73:725–30.

37. Pierce EC Jr, Lambertsen CJ, Deutsch S, et al. Cerebral circulation and metabolism during thiopental anesthesia and hyper-ventilation in man. J Clin Invest 1962;41:1664–71.
38. Marshall LF, Shapiro HM, Rauscher A, et al. Pentobarbital therapy for intracranial hypertension in metabolic coma. Reye's syndrome. Crit Care Med 1978;6:1–5.
39. Hartung HJ. [Intracranial pressure in patients with craniocerebral trauma after administration of propofol and thiopental]. Anaesthesist 1987;36:285–7 [in German].
40. Larsen R, Hilfiker O, Radke J, et al. [The effects of midazolam on the general circulation, cerebral blood-flow and cerebral oxygen consumption in man (author's transl)]. Anaesthesist 1981;30:18–21 [in German].
41. Renou AM, Vernhiet J, Macrez P, et al. Cerebral blood flow and metabolism during etomidate anaesthesia in man. Br J Anaesth 1978;50:1047–51.
42. Prior JG, Hinds CJ, Williams J, et al. The use of etomidate in the management of severe head injury. Intensive Care Med 1983;9:313–20.
43. Vandesteene A, Trempont V, Engelman E, et al. Effect of propofol on cerebral blood flow and metabolism in man. Anaesthesia 1988;43(Suppl):42–3.
44. Sakabe T, Maekawa T, Ishikawa T, et al. The effects of lidocaine on canine cerebral metabolism and circulation related to the electroencephalogram. Anesthesiology 1974;40:433–41.
45. Yano M, Nishiyama H, Yokota H, et al. Effect of lidocaine on ICP response to endotracheal suctioning. Anesthesiology 1986;64:651–3.
46. Carmel PW, Albright AL, Adelson PD, et al. Incidence and management of subdural hematoma/hygroma with variable- and fixed-pressure differential valves: a randomized, controlled study of programmable compared with conventional valves. Neurosurg Focus 1999;7:e7.
47. Muizelaar JP, Lutz HA 3rd, Becker DP. Effect of mannitol on ICP and CBF and correlation with pressure autoregulation in severely head-injured patients. J Neurosurg 1984;61:700–6.
48. Reichenthal E, Kaspi T, Cohen ML, et al. The ambivalent effects of early and late administration of mannitol in cold-induced brain oedema. Acta Neurochir Suppl (Wien) 1990;51:110–2.
49. Rosenberg GA, Barrett J, Estrada E, et al. Selective effect of mannitol-induced hyperosmolality on brain interstitial fluid and water content in white matter. Metab Brain Dis 1988;3:217–27.
50. Bell BA, Smith MA, Kean DM, et al. Brain water measured by magnetic resonance imaging. Correlation with direct estimation and changes after mannitol and dexamethasone. Lancet 1987;1:66–9.
51. Chan PH, Fishman RA. Elevation of rat brain amino acids, ammonia and idiogenic osmoles induced by hyperosmolality. Brain Res 1979;161:293–301.
52. Pollock AS, Arieff AI. Abnormalities of cell volume regulation and their functional consequences. Am J Physiol 1980;239:F195–205.
53. McManus ML, Strange K. Acute volume regulation of brain cells in response to hypertonic challenge. Anesthesiology 1993;78:1132–7.
54. Kofke WA. Mannitol: potential for rebound intracranial hypertension? J Neurosurg Anesthesiol 1993;5:1–3.
55. Rudehill A, Gordon E, Ohman G, et al. Pharmacokinetics and effects of mannitol on hemodynamics, blood and cerebrospinal fluid electrolytes, and osmolality during intracranial surgery. J Neurosurg Anesthesiol 1993;5:4–12.
56. Zornow MH. Hypertonic saline as a safe and efficacious treatment of intracranial hypertension. J Neurosurg Anesthesiol 1996;8:175–7.

57. Weed L, McKibben P. Pressure changes in the cerebro-spinal fluid following intravenous injection of solutions of various concentrations. Am J Physiol 1919;48:512–30.

58. Qureshi AI, Suarez JI. Use of hypertonic saline solutions in treatment of cerebral edema and intracranial hypertension. Crit Care Med 2000;28:3301–13.

59. Cottenceau V, Masson F, Mahamid E, et al. Comparison of effects of equiosmolar doses of mannitol and hypertonic saline on cerebral blood flow and metabolism in traumatic brain injury. J Neurotrauma 2011;28:2003–12.

60. Ichai C, Armando G, Orban JC, et al. Sodium lactate versus mannitol in the treatment of intracranial hypertensive episodes in severe traumatic brain-injured patients. Intensive Care Med 2009;35:471–9.

61. Harutjunyan L, Holz C, Rieger A, et al. Efficiency of 7.2% hypertonic saline hydroxyethyl starch 200/0.5 versus mannitol 15% in the treatment of increased intracranial pressure in neurosurgical patients - a randomized clinical trial [ISRCTN62699180]. Crit Care 2005;9:R530–40.

62. Wu CT, Chen LC, Kuo CP, et al. A comparison of 3% hypertonic saline and mannitol for brain relaxation during elective supratentorial brain tumor surgery. Anesth Analg 2010;110:903–7.

63. Battison C, Andrews PJ, Graham C, et al. Randomized, controlled trial on the effect of a 20% mannitol solution and a 7.5% saline/6% dextran solution on increased intracranial pressure after brain injury. Crit Care Med 2005;33: 196–202 [discussion: 57–8].

64. Vialet R, Albanese J, Thomachot L, et al. Isovolume hypertonic solutes (sodium chloride or mannitol) in the treatment of refractory posttraumatic intracranial hypertension: 2 mL/kg 7.5% saline is more effective than 2 mL/kg 20% mannitol. Crit Care Med 2003;31:1683–7.

65. Shackford SR, Bourguignon PR, Wald SL, et al. Hypertonic saline resuscitation of patients with head injury: a prospective, randomized clinical trial. J Trauma 1998;44:50–8.

66. Simma B, Burger R, Falk M, et al. A prospective, randomized, and controlled study of fluid management in children with severe head injury: lactated Ringer's solution versus hypertonic saline. Crit Care Med 1998;26:1265–70.

67. Khanna S, Davis D, Peterson B, et al. Use of hypertonic saline in the treatment of severe refractory posttraumatic intracranial hypertension in pediatric traumatic brain injury. Crit Care Med 2000;28:1144–51.

68. Peterson B, Khanna S, Fisher B, et al. Prolonged hypernatremia controls elevated intracranial pressure in head-injured pediatric patients. Crit Care Med 2000;28:1136–43.

69. Suarez JI, Qureshi AI, Bhardwaj A, et al. Treatment of refractory intracranial hypertension with 23.4% saline. Crit Care Med 1998;26:1118–22.

70. Suarez JI. Hypertonic saline for cerebral edema and elevated intracranial pressure. Cleve Clin J Med 2004;71(Suppl 1):S9–13.

71. Horn P, Munch E, Vajkoczy P, et al. Hypertonic saline solution for control of elevated intracranial pressure in patients with exhausted response to mannitol and barbiturates. Neurol Res 1999;21:758–64.

72. Tseng MY, Al-Rawi PG, Pickard JD, et al. Effect of hypertonic saline on cerebral blood flow in poor-grade patients with subarachnoid hemorrhage. Stroke 2003; 34:1389–96.

73. Kerwin AJ, Schinco MA, Tepas JJ 3rd, et al. The use of 23.4% hypertonic saline for the management of elevated intracranial pressure in patients with severe traumatic brain injury: a pilot study. J Trauma 2009;67:277–82.

74. Patanwala AE, Amini A, Erstad BL. Use of hypertonic saline injection in trauma. Am J Health Syst Pharm 2010;67:1920–8.

75. Brown MM, Wade JP, Marshall J. Fundamental importance of arterial oxygen content in the regulation of cerebral blood flow in man. Brain 1985;108(Pt 1): 81–93.

76. Floyd TF, Clark JM, Gelfand R, et al. Independent cerebral vasoconstrictive effects of hyperoxia and accompanying arterial hypocapnia at 1 ATA. J Appl Physiol 2003;95:2453–61.

77. Nakajima S, Meyer JS, Amano T, et al. Cerebral vasomotor responsiveness during 100% oxygen inhalation in cerebral ischemia. Arch Neurol 1983;40: 271–6.

78. Fiskum G, Rosenthal R, Vereczki V, et al. Protection against ischemic brain injury by inhibition of mitochondrial oxidative stress. J Bioenerg Biomembr 2004;36(4): 347–52.

79. Danilov CA, Fiskum G. Hyperoxia promotes astrocyte cell death after oxygen and glucose deprivation. Glia 2008;56:801–8.

80. Richards EM, Fiskum G, Rosenthal RE, et al. Hyperoxic reperfusion after global ischemia decreases hippocampal energy metabolism. Stroke 2007;38:1578–84.

81. Richards EM, Rosenthal RE, Kristian T, et al. Postischemic hyperoxia reduces hippocampal pyruvate dehydrogenase activity. Free Radic Biol Med 2006;40: 1960–70.

82. Kilgannon JH, Jones AE, Shapiro NI, et al. Association between arterial hyperoxia following resuscitation from cardiac arrest and in-hospital mortality. JAMA 2010;303:2165–71.

83. Rao GS, Durga P. Changing trends in monitoring brain ischemia: from intracranial pressure to cerebral oximetry. Curr Opin Anaesthesiol 2011;24:487–94.

84. Chen HI, Stiefel MF, Oddo M, et al. Detection of cerebral compromise with multimodality monitoring in patients with subarachnoid hemorrhage. Neurosurgery 2011;69:53–63 [discussion: 63].

85. Pascual JL, Georgoff P, Maloney-Wilensky E, et al. Reduced brain tissue oxygen in traumatic brain injury: are most commonly used interventions successful? J Trauma 2011;70:535–46.

86. Levine S. Anoxic-ischemic encephalopathy in rats. Am J Pathol 1960;36:1.

87. Dings J, Meixensberger J, Jager A, et al. Clinical experience with 118 brain tissue oxygen partial pressure catheter probes. Neurosurgery 1998;43: 1082–95.

88. van den Brink WA, van Santbrink H, Steyerberg EW, et al. Brain oxygen tension in severe head injury. Neurosurgery 2000;46:868–76 [discussion: 76–8].

89. Valadka AB, Gopinath SP, Contant CF, et al. Relationship of brain tissue PO2 to outcome after severe head injury. Crit Care Med 1998;26:1576–81.

90. van Santbrink H, vd Brink WA, Steyerberg EW, et al. Brain tissue oxygen response in severe traumatic brain injury. Acta Neurochir (Wien) 2003;145: 429–38 [discussion: 38].

91. Meixensberger J, Vath A, Jaeger M, et al. Monitoring of brain tissue oxygenation following severe subarachnoid hemorrhage. Neurol Res 2003;25:445–50.

92. Bohman LE, Heuer GG, Macyszyn L, et al. Medical management of compromised brain oxygen in patients with severe traumatic brain injury. Neurocrit Care 2011;14:361–9.

93. Rohlwink UK, Zwane E, Fieggen AG, et al. The relationship between intracranial pressure and brain oxygenation in children with severe traumatic brain injury. Neurosurgery 2012;70(5):1220–31.

94. Stiefel MF, Spiotta A, Gracias VH, et al. Reduced mortality rate in patients with severe traumatic brain injury treated with brain tissue oxygen monitoring. J Neurosurg 2005;103:805–11.
95. Klein J. Normobaric pulmonary oxygen toxicity. Anesth Analg 1990;70:195–207.
96. Tseng SH. Reduction of herniated temporal lobe in patients with severe head injury and uncal herniation. J Formos Med Assoc 1992;91:24–8.
97. Lee EJ, Chio CC, Chen HH. Aggressive temporal lobectomy for uncal herniation in traumatic subdural hematoma. J Formos Med Assoc 1995;94:341–5.
98. Kalia KK, Yonas H. An aggressive approach to massive middle cerebral artery infarction. Arch Neurol 1993;50:1293–7.
99. Manno EM, Atkinson JL, Fulgham JR, et al. Emerging medical and surgical management strategies in the evaluation and treatment of intracerebral hemorrhage. Mayo Clin Proc 2005;80:420–33.
100. Lau D, El-Sayed AM, Ziewacz JE, et al. Postoperative outcomes following closed head injury and craniotomy for evacuation of hematoma in patients older than 80 years. J Neurosurg 2012;116:234–45.
101. Morioka J, Fujii M, Kato S, et al. Surgery for spontaneous intracerebral hemorrhage has greater remedial value than conservative therapy. Surg Neurol 2006;65:67–72 [discussion: 3].
102. Zuccarello M, Brott T, Derex L, et al. Early surgical treatment for supratentorial intracerebral hemorrhage: a randomized feasibility study. Stroke 1999;30:1833–9.
103. Cho DY, Chen CC, Lee HC, et al. Glasgow Coma Scale and hematoma volume as criteria for treatment of putaminal and thalamic intracerebral hemorrhage. Surg Neurol 2008;70:628–33.
104. Kirollos RW, Tyagi AK, Ross SA, et al. Management of spontaneous cerebellar hematomas: a prospective treatment protocol. Neurosurgery 2001;49:1378–86 [discussion: 86–7].
105. Delashaw JB, Broaddus WC, Kassell NF, et al. Treatment of right hemispheric cerebral infarction by hemicraniectomy. Stroke 1990;21:874–81.
106. Kjellberg RN, Prieto A Jr. Bifrontal decompressive craniotomy for massive cerebral edema. Journal of neurosurgery 1971;34:488–93.
107. Weiner GM, Lacey MR, Mackenzie L, et al. Decompressive craniectomy for elevated intracranial pressure and its effect on the cumulative ischemic burden and therapeutic intensity levels after severe traumatic brain injury. Neurosurgery 2010;66:1111–8 [discussion: 8–9].
108. Polin RS, Shaffrey ME, Bogaev CA, et al. Decompressive bifrontal craniectomy in the treatment of severe refractory posttraumatic cerebral edema. Neurosurgery 1997;41:84–92 [discussion: 4].
109. Elwatidy S. Bifrontal decompressive craniectomy is a life-saving procedure for patients with nontraumatic refractory brain edema. Br J Neurosurg 2009;23: 56–62.
110. Schwab S, Steiner T, Aschoff A, et al. Early hemicraniectomy in patients with complete middle cerebral artery infarction. Stroke 1998;29:1888–93.
111. Doerfler A, Engelhorn T, Forsting M. Decompressive craniectomy for early therapy and secondary prevention of cerebral infarction. Stroke 2001;32:813–5.
112. Forsting M, Reith W, Schabitz WR, et al. Decompressive craniectomy for cerebral infarction. An experimental study in rats. Stroke 1995;26:259–64.
113. Cushing H. The establishment of cerebral hernia as a decompressive measure for inaccessible brain tumor: with the description of intramuscular methods of making the bone defect in temporal and occipital regions. Surg Gynecol Obstet 1905;1:297–314.

114. Cushing HI. Subtemporal decompressive operations for the intracranial complications associated with bursting fractures of the skull. Ann Surg 1908;47: 641–4.1.
115. Aarabi B, Hesdorffer DC, Ahn ES, et al. Outcome following decompressive craniectomy for malignant swelling due to severe head injury. J Neurosurg 2006; 104:469–79.
116. Vahedi K, Hofmeijer J, Juettler E, et al. Early decompressive surgery in malignant infarction of the middle cerebral artery: a pooled analysis of three randomised controlled trials. Lancet Neurol 2007;6:215–22.
117. Michel P, Arnold M, Hungerbuhler HJ, et al. Decompressive craniectomy for space occupying hemispheric and cerebellar ischemic strokes: Swiss recommendations. Int J Stroke 2009;4:218–23.
118. Iwama T, Yamada J, Imai S, et al. The use of frozen autogenous bone flaps in delayed cranioplasty revisited. Neurosurgery 2003;52:591–6 [discussion: 5–6].
119. Movassaghi K, Ver Halen J, Ganchi P, et al. Cranioplasty with subcutaneously preserved autologous bone grafts. Plast Reconstr Surg 2006;117:202–6.
120. Cooper DJ, Rosenfeld JV, Murray L, et al. Decompressive craniectomy in diffuse traumatic brain injury. N Engl J Med 2011;364:1493–502.
121. Carter BS, Ogilvy CS, Candia GJ, et al. One-year outcome after decompressive surgery for massive nondominant hemispheric infarction. Neurosurgery 1997; 40:1168–75 [discussion: 75–6].
122. Kondziolka D, Fazl M. Functional recovery after decompressive craniectomy for cerebral infarction. Neurosurgery 1988;23:143–7.
123. Munch E, Horn P, Schurer L, et al. Management of severe traumatic brain injury by decompressive craniectomy. Neurosurgery 2000;47:315–22 [discussion: 22–3].
124. Hofmeijer J, Amelink GJ, Algra A, et al. Hemicraniectomy after middle cerebral artery infarction with life-threatening Edema trial (HAMLET). Protocol for a randomised controlled trial of decompressive surgery in space-occupying hemispheric infarction. Trials 2006;7:29.
125. Juttler E, Schwab S, Schmiedek P, et al. Decompressive surgery for the treatment of malignant infarction of the middle cerebral artery (DESTINY): a randomized, controlled trial. Stroke 2007;38:2518–25.
126. Honeybul S, Ho KM, Lind CR, et al. The future of decompressive craniectomy for diffuse traumatic brain injury. J Neurotrauma 2011;28:2199–200.
127. Hutchinson PJ, Corteen E, Czosnyka M, et al. Decompressive craniectomy in traumatic brain injury: the randomized multicenter RESCUEicp study (www. RESCUEicp.com). Acta Neurochir Suppl 2006;96:17–20.
128. Larach DR, Larach DB, Larach MG. A life worth living: seven years after craniectomy. Neurocrit Care 2009;11:106–11.
129. Matta BF, Lam AM. Nitrous oxide increases cerebral blood flow velocity during pharmacologically induced EEG silence in humans. J Neurosurg Anesthesiol 1995;7:89–93.
130. Reinstrup P, Ryding E, Algotsson L, et al. Distribution of cerebral blood flow during anesthesia with isoflurane or halothane in humans. Anesthesiology 1995;82:359–66.
131. Monkhoff M, Schwarz U, Gerber A, et al. The effects of sevoflurane and halothane anesthesia on cerebral blood flow velocity in children. Anesth Analg 2001;92:891–6.
132. Matta BF, Heath KJ, Tipping K, et al. Direct cerebral vasodilatory effects of sevoflurane and isoflurane. Anesthesiology 1999;91:677–80.

133. Kaisti KK, Langsjo JW, Aalto S, et al. Effects of sevoflurane, propofol, and adjunct nitrous oxide on regional cerebral blood flow, oxygen consumption, and blood volume in humans. Anesthesiology 2003;99:603–13.

134. Kolbitsch C, Lorenz IH, Hormann C, et al. Sevoflurane and nitrous oxide increase regional cerebral blood flow (rCBF) and regional cerebral blood volume (rCBV) in a drug-specific manner in human volunteers. Magn Reson Imaging 2001;19:1253–60.

135. Mielck F, Stephan H, Buhre W, et al. Effects of 1 MAC desflurane on cerebral metabolism, blood flow and carbon dioxide reactivity in humans. Br J Anaesth 1998;81:155–60.

136. Mielck F, Stephan H, Weyland A, et al. Effects of one minimum alveolar anesthetic concentration sevoflurane on cerebral metabolism, blood flow, and CO2 reactivity in cardiac patients. Anesth Analg 1999;89:364–9.

137. Fraga M, Rama-Maceiras P, Rodino S, et al. The effects of isoflurane and desflurane on intracranial pressure, cerebral perfusion pressure, and cerebral arteriovenous oxygen content difference in normocapnic patients with supratentorial brain tumors. Anesthesiology 2003;98:1085–90.

138. Nishiyama T, Matsukawa T, Yokoyama T, et al. Cerebrovascular carbon dioxide reactivity during general anesthesia: a comparison between sevoflurane and isoflurane. Anesth Analg 1999;89:1437–41.

139. Lorenz IH, Kolbitsch C, Hormann C, et al. Influence of equianaesthetic concentrations of nitrous oxide and isoflurane on regional cerebral blood flow, regional cerebral blood volume, and regional mean transit time in human volunteers. Br J Anaesth 2001;87:691–8.

140. Lorenz IH, Kolbitsch C, Hormann C, et al. The influence of nitrous oxide and remifentanil on cerebral hemodynamics in conscious human volunteers. Neuroimage 2002;17:1056–64.

141. Aono M, Sato J, Nishino T. Nitrous oxide increases normocapnic cerebral blood flow velocity but does not affect the dynamic cerebrovascular response to step changes in end-tidal P(CO2) in humans. Anesth Analg 1999;89:684–9.

142. Russell GB, Snider MT, Richard RB, et al. Hyperbaric nitrous oxide as a sole anesthetic agent in humans. Anesth Analg 1990;70:289–95.

143. Eisenberg HM, Frankowski RF, Contant CF, et al. High-dose barbiturate control of elevated intracranial pressure in patients with severe head injury. J Neurosurg 1988;69:15–23.

144. Schulte am Esch J, Pfeifer G, Thiemig I. [Effects of etomidate and thiopentone on the primarily elevated intracranial pressure (ICP) (author's transl)]. Anaesthesist 1978;27:71–5 [in German].

145. Preziosi P, Vacca M. Adrenocortical suppression and other endocrine effects of etomidate. Life Sci 1988;42:477–89.

146. Gemma M, Tommasino C, Cerri M, et al. Intracranial effects of endotracheal suctioning in the acute phase of head injury. J Neurosurg Anesthesiol 2002;14:50–4.

147. Jamali S, Archer D, Ravussin P, et al. The effect of skull-pin insertion on cerebrospinal fluid pressure and cerebral perfusion pressure: influence of sufentanil and fentanyl. Anesth Analg 1997;84:1292–6.

148. Kofke WA, Attaallah AF, Kuwabara H, et al. The neuropathologic effects in rats and neurometabolic effects in humans of large-dose remifentanil. Anesth Analg 2002;94:1229–36.

149. Sullivan PM, Sinz EH, Gunel E, et al. A retrospective comparison of remifentanil versus methohexital for anesthesia in electroconvulsive therapy. J Ect 2004;20: 219–24.

Neurophysiologic Monitoring in Neurosurgery

Leslie C. Jameson, MD*, Tod B. Sloan, MD, MBA, PhD

KEYWORDS

- Monitoring • Electroencephalography • Somatosensory-evoked potentials
- Electromyography • Motor-evoked potentials

KEY POINTS

- Neurophysiologic mapping and monitoring improve surgical decision making, refines procedures, and reduces undesired neural morbidity.
- Intraoperative monitoring (IOM) allows the neurosurgeon to better find the functional tissues put at risk by their procedures.
- IOM enhances the effectiveness of the surgery and reduces the risk of undesired morbidity.

INTRODUCTION

Neurophysiologic monitoring, often referred to as intraoperative monitoring (IOM), is commonly used in the operating room to improve surgical decision making and patient outcome. Recent articles and textbooks have extensively reviewed the methodology, patient physiology, anatomy, and impact of anesthesia drugs on neurophysiologic monitoring.[1–5] Most reviews and publications focus on spine surgery. In contrast, this article focuses on the application of monitoring in neurosurgical procedures. IOM for neurosurgery focuses on identifying and preserving functional areas of the central nervous system.

IOM combines with new developments in imaging to identify specific neurologic functions so the surgical approach to disease can avoid key areas, and identify specific target regions for tissue resection, lesioning, or stimulation. These monitoring techniques allow surgical procedures on neural structures previously avoided because the risk of disability outweighed the benefit of treatment. IOM contributes to prevention of surgical incursions into adjacent functional structures. These techniques depend on the unique tissue characteristics to allow neurophysiologic stimulation or recording. These techniques are useful for procedures on the brain, brainstem, spinal cord, and peripheral nervous system.

Department of Anesthesiology, University of Colorado, Anschutz Medical Campus, 12401 East 17th Avenue, Room 737, Aurora, CO 80045, USA
* Corresponding author.
E-mail address: leslie.jameson@ucdenver.edu

Anesthesiology Clin 30 (2012) 311–331
doi:10.1016/j.anclin.2012.05.005   anesthesiology.theclinics.com
1932-2275/12/$ – see front matter © 2012 Elsevier Inc. All rights reserved.

MONITORING IN THE CEREBRAL CORTEX

Electrocorticography (ECoG) was one of the first applications of IOM in neurosurgery. With ECoG, the recording electrodes are placed directly on or in the brain to record neuronal activity. This characteristic is in contrast to electroencephalography (EEG), in which the recording electrodes are located on the scalp. EEG and ECoG are often incorrectly used interchangeably. ECoG is commonly used to identify and then map the precise location of seizure foci or the edges of tumor. To remove a seizure locus, ECoG recordings can be performed in the operating room or postoperatively in specialized units designed to monitor seizure activity via ECoG grid recordings. Recording electrodes (cortical grids) are placed over brain areas that are suggested by magnetic resonance imaging (MRI), functional MRI, or positron emission tomography imaging to be the source of seizure activity (**Fig. 1**).[6] Over the next 3 to 5 days, continuous ECoG recording allows the neurologist and neurosurgeon to locate the area involved in the seizure activity. A repeat craniotomy is performed and seizure foci are removed. Depending on the location and the preference of the surgeon, the anesthetic management can either be a general anesthetic or awake with minimal sedation. In both situations, direct brain stimulation may be performed to induce

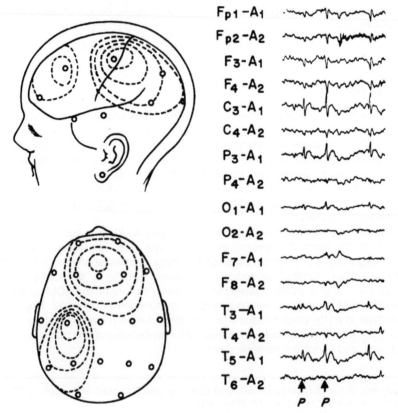

Fig. 1. Cortical mapping of a seizure focus. Dipole mapping on the scalp (*left*) shows upward deflection in locations C3, P3, and T5, downward deflection in locations Fp1, Fp2, F3, and F4, consistent with a seizure generator deep in the parasagittal region. (*Modified from* Daly DD. Epilepsy and syncope. In: Daly D, Pedley T, editors. Current practice of clinical electroencephalography. 2nd edition. New York: Raven Press; 1990. p. 277; with permission.)

seizurelike electrical activity, the classic spike and dome waveform seen on EEG or ECoG recordings. In awake patients, the stimulation can be used to identify symptoms similar to the seizure prodrome, areas with a low threshold to propagate seizures and areas that do not produce a response. This technique assists in identifying brain that can be removed without injury. Identification of abnormal brain improves the likelihood of a complete resection of the seizure focus (see **Fig. 1**).[7]

With tumor resection, direct stimulation of edge between tumor and normal brain is performed until there is disruption of the monitored response. During removal of lesions near the speech (Broca or Wernicke area), sensory, or motor cortex, the location of these regions is performed in awake patients. For surgery near the motor or sensory area, patients provide feedback on their perceptions (movement, sensation) in response to stimulation. In speech areas, mapping requires a listener to recognize errors in identifying pictures, words, or rote speech (counting). All awake cortical mapping carries the risk of stimulus-induced seizures, both local and generalized. With this technique, the anesthesiologist must be prepared to manage the patient's airway, abort seizures, and then manage a postictal, sedated patient.

In patients unsuitable for awake testing, functional MRI with fiducial placement can suggest functional areas to avoid. Specialized monitoring can supplement this MRI or computed tomography image-guided approach through the use of cortical–cortical-evoked potentials.[8–10] Stimulation of Broca or Wernicke areas produces an evoked response in the orofacial area of the motor cortex or vocalis muscles of the larynx, indicating a functional connection.[11] When motor or sensory mapping is necessary, direct cortical responses from peripheral sensory stimulation or direct motor stimulation with peripheral recording of electromyography (EMG) can be used. The sensory cortex is identified by locating the primary cortical peak of the somatosensory-evoked potential (SSEP) over the sensory area (**Fig. 2**). Sensory recordings show typical responses when electrodes are located on the cortical surface. A reversal of polarity occurs across the gyrus between the sensory and motor regions.[12,13] Stimulation of the probable motor cortex produces a motor-evoked potential (MEP). SSEP and MEP responses are reported to be successful for identifying sensory and motor cortex in 91% and 99% of patients.[13,14] Identifying the sensory-motor boundary can help the surgeon develop a safer approach for the removal of tumors involving sensory, motor and speech areas (see **Fig. 2**).

Monitoring using MEP and SEP has been used with tumors near the motor cortex and motor tracts (including in the brainstem) insula, including cavernous angiomas.[14] In these cases, the monitoring strategy is to continue resection until the MEP or SSEP is altered. Although not all motor deficits are avoided, combined MEP-SSEP monitoring is considered essential by some to limit unnecessary morbidity.[14]

Monitoring during stereotactic neurosurgery for movement disorders is standard.[15] The surgeon and IOM team follow recordings of EEG activity while the surgical probe is advanced. Because each area of brain has characteristic EEG recordings and sound, the microelectrode EEG recordings verify probe or electrode location. These EEG neuronal firing signatures change with movement-induced activity (especially with procedures for movement disorders) (**Fig. 3**). This process allows placement of deep brain stimulating electrodes or tissue lesions for treatment of Parkinson disease, essential tremor, and dystonia.[16] Other surgical targets that are deep, difficult to approach, and are not always clearly located by image-guided neuronavigation also use this technique. High-resolution MRI estimates the target boundaries with a resolution of between 1.5 mm and 5 mm by using anatomic reference atlases. Electrical stimulation of the electrode can test the clinical effectiveness and side effects of an implanted stimulation electrode at that location. Motor cortex stimulation has also

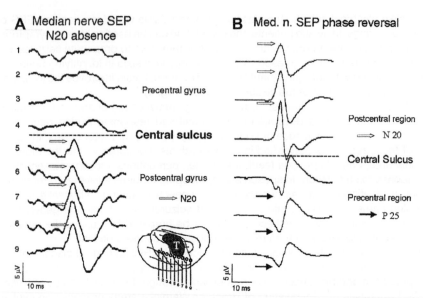

Fig. 2. SSEP mapping of the sensory strip is conducted by 2 methods. (*A*) A series of monopolar recordings moving anterior to the sulcus progressively posteriorly (note locations on brain figure); note the absence of a traditional N20 and SSEP recording when the electrode is anterior to the sensory strip. (*B*) Bipolar recordings in similar pairs of electrode positions; note the phase reversal when the electrode pair crosses the central sulcus between the sensory and motor areas. (*Modified from* Neuloh G, Schramm J. Intraoperative neurophysiological mapping and monitoring for supratentorial procedures. In: Deletis V, Shils JL, editors. Neurophysiology and neurosurgery. New York: Academic Press; 2002. p. [*A*] 355, [*B*] 357; with permission.)

been used for cortical basal degeneration, multiple sclerosis, and for management of some central pain syndromes (for example, postthalamic stroke). In these situations, signature EEG recordings are combined with direct cortical MEPs or SSEP to optimize electrode placement.

MONITORING IN NEUROVASCULAR SURGERY

Brain monitoring is frequently performed to assess for cerebral ischemia such as during intracranial and extracranial vascular surgery (eg, carotid endarterectomy [CEA]). Although a variety of techniques can be used, the classic method is EEG, although use of awake CEA and the use of transcutaneous cerebral oximetry are increasing in popularity.[17] The EEG allows monitoring of a large surface area of the cerebral cortex by using multiple scalp electrodes. Each EEG electrode provides a continuous view of a spherical region about 2 to 3 cm in diameter; this area consists of superficial pyramidal cells primarily in cortical layers 3, 5, and 6.[18] These pyramidal layers are extremely sensitive to both hypoxia and ischemia, with detectable change occurring within 30 seconds to 5 minutes.[19] Characteristic changes in EEG occur with decreases in cerebral blood flow (**Table 1**). Regions that have the highest metabolic rate or are farthest from the major supply arteries (ie, boundary regions) are most sensitive to changing perfusion, making the best electrode locations dependent on the specific area at risk for ischemia.

EEG monitoring during CEA is particularly effective because the anterior cerebral artery (ACA) and middle cerebral artery (MCA) perfuse the monitored area. The EEG

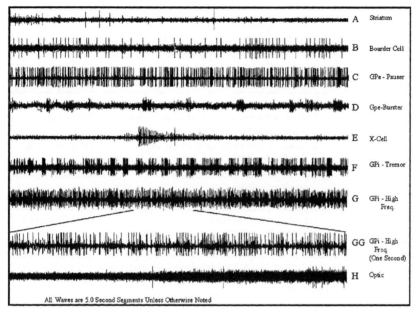

Fig. 3. Representative tracings from a microelectrode recording probe used for targeting the globus pallidus interna (GPi) for deep brain stimulator placement. Note the different electronic signatures of each region assist in the optimal electrode location. (*Modified from* Shils JL, Tagliati M, Alterman RL. Neurophysiological monitoring during neurosurgery for movement disorders. In: Deletis V, Shils JL, editors. Neurophysiology in neurosurgery. Boston: Academic Press; 2002. p. 405–8; with permission.)

montage varies from 6 frontal leads, with its emphasis on the perfusion area of the MCA, to a full 32-lead montage. Because many patients undergoing CEA have cerebrovascular disease involving the posterior circulation and circle of Willis, monitoring the 32-lead montage is most desirable.

Rapid flattening of the EEG (**Fig. 4**) is seen with hypoperfusion. Ischemic changes (see **Table 1**) that do not rapidly respond to increases in blood pressure are indications for carotid artery shunt placement. Shunt placement should be carefully considered because its use increases the risk of embolic stroke. EEG and other IOM techniques assist in determining when shunt placement is indicated to treat hypoperfusion. EEG can reduce ischemic time and risk of clinical stroke.[20] EEG monitoring may explain why ischemic stroke has been replaced by embolic stroke as the cause of an immediate postoperative neurologic injury. Two-thirds of postoperative strokes are focal embolic events and are not detected by IOM. In 1 study with 658 patients with CEA, all monitored with EEG, only 34 developed a postoperative neurologic deficit and only 7 (20%) of this group had computed tomography findings that supported hypoperfusion as the cause.[21]

Although EEG monitoring is a standard of care for CEA during general anesthesia in many practices, it is associated with a significant number of false-positive results.[22] Several studies have used neurologic changes detected during a regional anesthetic for CEA to estimate the incidence of false-positive and false-negative results. For example, 1 large study compared EEG changes in the patients during general anesthesia with the functional changes seen in comparable patients with a cervical block during CEA. Approximately 7% of patients with cervical block had true-positive results

Table 1
Effect of decreasing cerebral blood flow (CBF) on normal EEG activity in patients during a general anesthetic. Depth of anesthetic influences the EEG response because of the change normally seen with the administration of hypnotic drugs

Estimated CBF (mL/100 g/min)	Expected EEG Effect	Severity of Injury
35–70	Normal	None
25–35	Loss of fast β frequencies; often not seen during general anesthesia	Mild reversible
18–35	Increase in θ to <25% or decrease in amplitude >50%	Mild reversible
12–18	Increase in θ >25% or δ <25% and amplitude >50%	Moderate reversible
8–10	Suppression of all frequencies	Severe cell death
<8	No activity or isoelectric ECG may be present	Loss of neurons

Data from Illig KA, Sternbach Y, Zhang R, et al. EEG changes during awake carotid endarterectomy. Ann Vasc Surg 2002;16(1):6–11; and Malek BN, Mohrhaus CA, Sheth AK. Use of multi-modality intraoperative monitoring during carotid endarterectomy surgery: a case study. Am J Electroneurodiagnostic Technol 2011;51(1):42–53.

(both neurologic and EEG change indicating ischemia); 15% of general anesthesia patients had EEG changes supporting ischemia, suggesting an 8% false-positive rate. Patients in the general anesthesia group also often had bilateral changes, suggesting that the anesthetic could be putting the patient at additional real risk, detecting

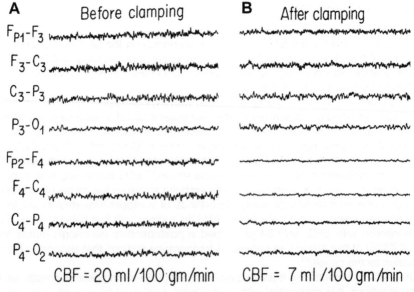

Fig. 4. EEG recording during CEA. (*A*) EEG under general anesthesia before cross clamping the carotid artery. (*B*) EEG changes after carotid cross clamping. Note flattening in the hemisphere where the cerebral blood flow was reduced after carotid cross clamping (7 mL/min/100 g). (*Modified from* Daube J, Harper CM, Litchy W. Intraoperative monitoring. In: Daly D, Pedley T, editors. Current practice of clinical electroencephalography. 2nd edition. New York: Raven Press; 1990. p. 743; with permission.)

real events that do not occur during regional anesthesia, or detecting real events that resolve during general anesthesia. EEG change is more difficult to interpret during general anesthesia.[23] After a recent stroke (>6 weeks old), EEG identification of new ischemic change is often not possible.[24]

The cost of EEG monitoring and the expertise needed for interpretation have led to research into the use of commercially processed EEG monitors. Pattern changes in the α, β, and δ frequencies suggest that algorithms could be developed to allow effective processed EEG analysis designed to indicate major and minor ischemia.[25] None of the currently available single channel monitors has been found to be reliable at detecting ischemia, even in awake patients.[26] No data are available to confirm that processed EEG monitors that monitor right and left frontal areas provide an accurate indication of ischemic change. Transcranial Doppler (TCD) monitoring can detect emboli and perfusion and could be used to alert the surgeon when technical changes are necessary to reduce ischemic injury.[19,24] Executing TCD monitoring during surgery is challenging and can prove unreliable or impossible.[27-29]

The SSEP can also be used for the detection of cerebral ischemia. Because of signal averaging and reduced sensitivity to ischemia, SSEP changes appear more slowly than EEG changes. SSEP is effective only when the neural tissue at risk includes sensory cortex. MEP monitoring is more sensitive to hypoperfusion and is gradually replacing SEP as a monitor for global or focal hypoperfusion.[30] Meta-analysis of EEG, MEP, and SSEP monitoring suggests that when used together, they are useful to identify ischemia with CEA, and neurologic outcome is improved when action is taken based on changes in these modalities.[31] Combined uses of EEG and SSEP have included testing the effects of vessel occlusion during carotid artery angioplasty and deliberate occlusion of various arterial vessels during aneurysm and arteriovenous malformation (AVM) management.[32] Because it can require up to 15 minutes for an ischemic effect to be detected using SSEP, effectiveness is limited. With aneurysms, 1 study stated that SSEP monitoring changed the procedure in 11.3% of the surgeries and the author found them indispensable.[33] The SSEP is not useful in surgery of the posterior circulation.

SSEP and MEP studies detect ischemia during intracerebral surgery when there is a risk of reduced blood flow during supratentorial procedures. These procedures include inadvertent vessel occlusion, vasospasm, ischemia from retractor pressure, suboptimal aneurysm clip application, and relative hypotension. In these situations, detection of ischemia has prompted changing the technical approach, applying papaverine to arteries, and reconsidering the procedure.[14] SSEP and MEP have been found useful in surgery for AVMs and cavernous malformations in the pericentral region of the brain. The MEP is particularly valuable with vascular surgery involving deep brain and brainstem structures near the motor pathways. When direct cortical MEPs are repeated as often as every minute, they are more effective than SSEP and EEG at detecting inadequate perfusion, when deep brain areas are involved.[34]

Because most aneurysm surgery involves the anterior circulation, MEP and SSEP monitoring should be effective when MCAs and ACAs are involved. For ACA aneurysms, the lower extremity is at risk, whereas surgery on the MCA is best monitored by the upper extremity SSEP or MEP. Because the MCA has a large perfusion area, upper extremity SSEP is preferred with aneurysms of the internal carotid artery unless the aneurysm is at the bifurcation of the carotid artery. During the clipping of an MCA aneurysm, the SSEP appears more specific and but less sensitive than the EEG, particularly when the ischemia includes the subcortical areas.

MEP is also useful in intracranial aneurysm surgery, in which perforating arteries may selectively put the motor pathways in the corona radiata, internal capsule, cerebral peduncle, basis pontis, and pyramids at risk.[35] Direct cortical MEP stimulation can produce seizure activity, which can be immediately treated by irrigation with iced saline. EEG monitoring is important to detect after discharge signals or spread of the MEP stimulation to adjacent areas. Because multiple vascular territories can be affected with AVM procedures, both SSEP and MEP monitoring are useful for the detection of ischemia. This situation is particularly true with resection or embolization with AVMs located near the central region or close to the sensory-motor pathways. Here, test occlusion of AVM feeders can be assessed (using EEG, SSEP, and MEP) for compromise of nearby normal tissue before permanent manipulation.

MONITORING ANESTHETIC DRUG EFFECT

Although not strictly used in neurosurgery alone, the use of standard EEG and process EEG monitoring should be addressed. EEG detects loss of synaptic activity caused by hypoglycemia, hypoperfusion, or drug effect. Most anesthetic agents in clinical use (eg, volatile, propofol, dexmedetomidine) depress synaptic activity in a reliable pattern beginning with an initial excitatory stage characterized by desynchronization and with increased relative power (fast β activity) prominently in the frontal regions.[36] As depth of anesthesia increases, fast β activity moves posteriorly, whereas EEG synchronization in the α range (8–13 Hz) develops over the posterior regions and moves to the frontal regions. With loss of consciousness from anesthetic and sedative agents, there is a marked decrease in γ-band activity (25–50 Hz), increase in slower frequency patterns (θ, δ), a large increase in power in the frontal lobes, a marked increase in synchrony of the EEG, and an uncoupling of interaction between frontal and parietal regions even across the midline.[37] Most anesthesiologists recognize the "fast and small awake, slow and tall asleep" pattern and can roughly gauge depth of anesthesia by observing the relative ratio of the 2 patterns. EEG achieves burst suppression (in which periods of EEG activity are interspersed with periods of a flat EEG) then electrical silence.[38] Volatile anesthetics produce burst suppression, usually at minimum alveolar concentration values of 1.5 or higher. This EEG pattern does not occur with administration of some anesthetic drugs, for example N_2O and ketamine, which increase activity.

Processed EEG equipment uses a complex mathematical analysis of amplitude, frequency, variability, and topography from frontal EMG to detect the awake state and general anesthesia. Each anesthetic agent (based on the receptor involved in its action) has a characteristic EEG profile for the transition from the awake to unconscious state. All processed EEG monitors have attempted to develop a proprietary depth of anesthesia algorithm that quantifies this complex series of events into a single dimensionless numeric index to represent the continuum from awake to deeply anesthetized. This value does not address drug-specific differences.[39]

BIS (Covidien, Boulder, CO, USA) has the longest clinical experience and the most peer-reviewed publications. It uses a combination of power spectrum and bispectrum from a single frontal EEG channel to calculate the BIS value. Recent changes may have changed this algorithm to use bilateral information. The Danmeter Cerebral State Monitor (Goalwick, Odense, Denmark), a small handheld wireless device, calculates a CSI using analysis of 4 calculated parameters derived from the single EEG channel. Entropy (GE Healthcare, Worldwide) describes the degree of asynchrony or variability of the EEG. The algorithm for calculation of entropy in the EEG signal has been published.[40] The monitor determines 2 separate entropy values. State entropy (SE) is an index ranging from 0 to 91 (awake), using EEG frequencies from 0.8 Hz to 32 Hz, and response entropy (RE) is an index ranging from 0 to 100 (awake). The Narcotrend

(Aither Medical, Makati, Philippines) uses the discontinuous nature of the EEG analysis, and defined EEG stages are calculated using unspecified multivariate algorithm. It is calculated based on 1 EEG channel. The SEDLine (Masimo, Irvine, CA, USA) algorithm is based on a 4-lead EEG recorded from a 5-forehead electrode array. The SEDLine analysis depends on the shift in power between the frontal and occipital areas that occurs during loss of consciousness and increasing hypnotic drug effect. The algorithm has been published.[41]

The literature is silent in defining the efficacy of these processed EEG monitors over a broad range of clinical uses. Practitioners use them to guide anesthetic dosing for management of cardiovascular perturbation and reducing intraoperative awareness. Their value as a monitor of anesthetic effect continues to evolve; they are an index of sedation/hypnosis rather than analgesia and measure analgesia only in relation to the arousal that occurs with painful stimuli. They may have a particular application in neurosurgery to gauge anesthetic management during the total intravenous anesthesia needed for some of the electrophysiologic monitoring (eg, MEPs).

MONITORING THE BRAINSTEM

Mapping and monitoring of the brainstem allows meticulous surgical techniques avoiding unplanned injury to neural structures.[42] A variety of safe entry zones have been identified in relation to normal brainstem structures; these are based on anatomic landmarks, which often become distorted, making mapping techniques critical (**Fig. 5**). These techniques are primarily but not exclusively based on recording EMG responses produced during stimulation of motor nuclei, VII, X-XI, and XII on

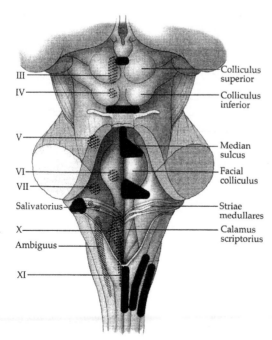

Fig. 5. Positions of the cranial nerve motor nuclei in the brainstem and relatively safe entry zones (*black regions*) for surgical access to deep structures. (*Modified from* Bricolo A, Sala F. Surgery of brainstem lesions. In: Deletis V, Shils JL, editors. Neurophysiology in neurosurgery. Boston: Academic Press; 2002. p. 267–89; with permission.)

the floor of the fourth ventricle (MEP) or stimulation of the cranial nerve in the brainstem.[43–45]

Monitoring during brainstem surgery can reduce the risk of unintended neural morbidity. Cranial nerves are susceptible to damage because of their small size, limited epineurium, and complicated course. Injury to brainstem motor nuclei/nerves cause severe disability that can be modified by MEP and EMG monitoring of the appropriate muscle groups (**Table 2**). Brainstem mapping of the corticospinal tract (CT) is accomplished with a handheld stimulator and then recording the compound muscle action potential (CMAP) or EMG response.[43,44] This technique has been found helpful in midbrain tumors, in which the CT is often dislocated, or in surgery near the cerebral peduncle and ventral medulla.[42,46] Other mapping techniques include localizing structures, usually nerves, which may be in the operative field. Classic examples are identifying the facial nerve when it is intertwined in or obscured by an acoustic neuroma or recording from the auditory nerve to locate the vestibular nerve while recording from the trigeminal nerve during surgery for trigeminal neuralgia.[47]

EMG is more resistant to the depressant effects of anesthetics and other physiologic variables (temperature, blood pressure), which makes it a good monitor of functional integrity.[48] Neurotonic discharges are high-frequency intermittent or continuous bursts of motor unit potentials (MUP) and usually indicate mechanical (compression, contusion, rubbing, manipulation, irrigation, stretching) or metabolic (ischemia) stimuli (**Fig. 6**) and are to be avoided.[45] Bursts may last less than 200 milliseconds, with single or multiple MUP firing at 30 to 100 Hz, or the bursts can be long trains of continuous

Table 2
Nerve roots and muscles commonly monitored

Spinal Cord	Nerve Root	Muscle
Cervical	C2–4	Trapezoids, sternocleidomastoid
	C5, 6	Biceps, deltoid
	C6, 7	Flexor carpi radialis
Thoracic	C8–T1	Adductor pollicis
	T2–6	Specific intercostals
	T5–12	Specific area of rectus abdominus
Lumbar	L2	Adductor longus
	L2–4	Vastus medialis
Sacral	L4–S1	Tibialis anterior
	L5–S1	Peroneus longus
	S1–2	Gastrocnemius
	S2–4	Anal sphincter
Cranial Nerves		
Oculomotor	III	Superior, medial, inferior rectus
Trochlear	IV	Superior oblique
Trigeminal	V	Masseter
Abducens	VI	Lateral rectus
Facial	VII	Obicularis oculi, oris; mentalis, temporalis
Glossopharyngeal	IX	Pharyngeal muscles
Vagus	X	Vocal cords
Spinal accessory	XI	Trapezius, sternocleidomastoid
Hypoglossal	XII	Tongue

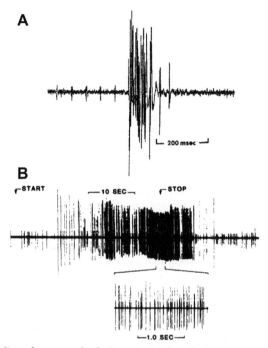

A

L 200 msec ⌐

B

⌐START   ⌐10 SEC⌐   ⌐STOP

⌐1.0 SEC⌐

Fig. 6. EMG recordings from muscle during monitoring during surgery near motor nerves. The upper trace (*A*) shows a single, brief burst of muscle activity from nerve irritation. The lower trace (*B*) shows sustained neurotonic activity from injurious nerve irritation. Note the difference in time scales. (*From* Prass RL, Luders H. Acoustic (loudspeaker) facial electromyographic monitoring: Part 1. Evoked electromyographic activity during acoustic neuroma resection. Neurosurgery 1986;19:392–400; with permission.)

discharges lasting 1 to 30 seconds.[48] Eliciting a response is best accomplished with a monopolar probe to minimize the chance of subthreshold stimulation or spread of the current. Nerves or cranial nerve nuclei are stimulated proximal to the site of potential operative injury, allowing assessment of nuclei and nerve functional integrity. Amplitude reduction in a facial nerve (CN VII) CMAP correlates with short-term and long-term paralysis.[49] After sharp transaction of a nerve, stimulation of the distal segment may still evoke an EMG response. This technique is used to facilitate repair of nerves outside the brainstem, but can lead to false-negative reports.

Monitoring can be accomplished in all motor cranial nerves (**Table 2**). Damage to lower cranial nerve nuclei (IX–XII) leads to dyspnea, severe dysphagia, and chronic aspiration. Oculomotor nerves (III, IV, VI) are not commonly monitored, but may be of value during tumor removal in the region of the cavernous sinus or intraventricular tumors.[50] EMG monitoring is useful in surgery with hyperactive cranial nerves and cranial nerve compression syndromes like trigeminal neuralgia (V), hemifacial spasm (VII), and vagoglossal-pharyngeal neuralgia (IX, X).[50] EMG monitoring of the facial nerve during surgery in the cerebellopontine angle (CPA) has become a standard of care because of the frequent risk of facial nerve injury.[51–53] In addition to neurotonic discharges, monitoring the latency from intentional stimulation to the muscle response can help differentiate between the different cranial nerves. The close proximity of nerve fibers and cranial nerve nuclei can lead to accidental stimulation of more than 1 cranial nerve, causing a motor response in several muscle groups. This situation is particularly notable for temporalis (CN VII) and masseter (CN V) muscle stimulation when EMG is recorded in the orbicularis oculi and oris (CN VII) muscles.[54] In posterior fossa surgery, use of EMG monitoring to guide the surgeon has been shown to correlate with postoperative neurologic status. In a study of pediatric patients undergoing surgery for removal of a brainstem tumor involving cranial nerves (IX, X, XII), a positive EMG event in one of the monitored nerves resulted in a postoperative deficit in 73% of patients, and temporary increases in EMG activity in all 3 nerves was always associated with a deficit. Postoperative aspiration or need for a tracheotomy was always associated with intraoperative EMG activity in at least one of these nerves.[55]

Auditory brainstem response (ABR) monitoring during acoustic neuroma surgery reduces risk of damage to the acoustic nerve and improves the probability of hearing preservation.[56] An ABR is the sensory response produced by a standard sound stimulus with recording from the mastoid process/ear lobes and a midline cranial electrode (F_{pz}). Traditional ABR recordings require a relatively long averaging period (1000 repetitions at 11.7 Hz) of approximately 90 seconds for each ear. ABR always predicts intact hearing if the ABR was present at the end of the procedure, but ABR loss does not always predict hearing loss.[52,53,57] Recording directly on the brainstem distal to the area at risk (from the auditory nerve or the cochlear nucleus) is effective when the extracranial portion of the nerve, the cochlea, or the labyrinthine artery is at risk. With a schwannoma, direct nerve recordings distal to the tumor provide the most rapid response, and loss of signal reliably predicts sound loss. The ability to hear sound does not equate with useful hearing. CPA recordings are also rapid and can monitor the distal and proximal portions of the nerve.

Cranial nerve function can be monitored outside posterior fossa. Vocal cord monitoring (recurrent laryngeal, superior laryngeal) acts as a surrogate for the vagus nerve (CN X). EMG monitoring is performed by placing needle electrodes in the cricothyroid or vocalis muscles or the use of contact electrodes on a specialized tracheal tube. The published literature supporting this is limited to radical neck dissections and thyroid surgery. If that experience is accepted, then the reported incidence of recurrent laryngeal nerve injury after neck surgery is 2.3% to 5.2%. The literature is equivocal regarding effectiveness of vocal cord EMG monitoring, but it is currently considered a standard of care.[53,58] EMG is reliable only if stimulation results in a positive response, because negative responses may be caused by altered nerve function, stimulation of nonnerve tissue, or equipment malfunction.[53,59]

ABR, SSEP, and EMG are used to assess the general integrity of the brainstem structures near the surgical site or under retractors. Spontaneous EMG activity may be helpful, but a correlation with outcome is not established.[60,61] SSEP and ABR can also monitor the functional integrity of about 20% of the brainstem.[61] Changes in ABR are more sensitive than vital signs in detecting brainstem injury.[62] With surgery close to the cerebral peduncles or the ventral medulla, injury to the CTs is a concern and monitoring with MEP is important.[63–65] Monitoring MEPs of the face and hand musculature can assess the CT and corticobulbar tract, in the posterior fossa.[46]

MONITORING THE SPINAL CORD

For surgery within the spinal cord, the identification of the midline for an entrance myelotomy is usually key to minimizing damage to the cord. Because the SSEP tracts follow the dorsal columns, which lie adjacent to the midline, stimulation of the lower extremity and recording from a series of electrodes or marked sites with a handheld device across the posterior aspect of the cord allow the identification of the dorsal median sulcus when it is distorted (**Fig. 7**).[66] SSEP monitoring may not be possible

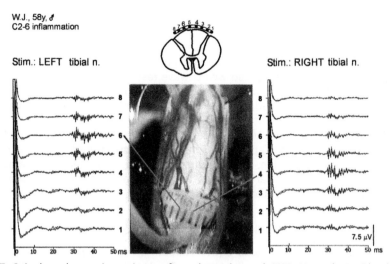

W.J., 58y, ♂
C2-6 inflammation

Stim.: LEFT tibial n.

Stim.: RIGHT tibial n.

7.5 μV

Fig. 7. Spinal cord mapping using surface electrodes and SSEP. Note the epidural SSEP recording shows a maximal amplitude from the left-sided and right-sided stimulation at electrodes 6 and 4 (respectively), suggesting the midline for myelotomy is under electrode 5. (*Modified from* Krza MJ. Intraoperative neurophysiological mapping of the spinal cord's dorsal columns. In: Deletis V, Shils JL, editors. Neurophysiology in neurosurgery. New York: Academic Press; 2002. p. 158; with permission.)

after myelotomy in up to 30% of patients. A neurologic examination to identify loss of position, vibration, and light touch is necessary to assess the feasibility of the technique. The problem is less frequent in children younger than 9 to 10 years because sensory pathways are more laterally located.[67]

Spine procedures can put the spinal cord at risk. Many articles have examined the effectiveness of SSEP, MEP, and EMG monitoring during corrective spine procedures,[1,68–71] which is outside the scope of this article. Similar monitoring techniques are applicable during neurosurgery for external spinal cord compression. There is little in the literature evaluating the efficacy of IOM in this specific situation. If one accepts the findings from the spine literature, then SSEP, EMG, and MEP monitoring has become the standard of care for external spinal cord compression. Some advocate for MEP-only monitoring because in spine surgery it has been shown to have nearly 100% specificity, 96% sensitivity, and a positive predictive value of 96%.[72,73] The evidence for this assertion is based on large case series and meta-analysis (level 2, 3 evidence), in which MEP changes predicted immediate postsurgical neurologic findings.[71,74–77] In one of the largest studies, 11.3% of patients had MEP change; in the 5 patients with permanent MEP change, all had partial or permanent neurologic injury.[78] Cervical spine surgery usually for spinal cord stenosis or traumatic injury is often the purview of the neurosurgeon. MEP is a de facto standard of care in this situation and is believed to decrease morbidity, in part because it may allow differentiation between cervical cord myelopathy and peripheral neuropathy.[79–81]

During spinal cord surgery, motor function can also be monitored using a D-wave response in the CT. It is less frequently used than the traditional EMG/CMAP technique. The amplitude of the D wave is believed to be a semiquantitative assessment of the number of preserved fibers in the fast conducting fibers of the CT[46] and it may correlate better with long-term motor outcome than EMG alone.[67] When the D-wave amplitude is unchanged or reduced less than 50%, the patient recovers motor function. Transient postoperative paralysis, lasting several hours to days, is believed to be caused by a loss of accessory motor pathways (eg, propriospinal systems that facilitate the CT pathway).[82] The MEP is most effective at evaluating these accessory pathways. Consequently, the combination of D wave and MEP is often attempted. In centers that are experienced with D-wave testing, a D-wave change of 30% to 50% loss is the warning criterion to halt or abandon surgery[46,83] MEP and D-wave monitoring in intramedullary spinal cord surgery has 100% sensitivity and 91% specificity.[46,83]

The use of both SSEP and MEP is recommended when surgery involves risks to specific vascular structures or specific regions within the spinal cord because of differences in spinal cord perfusion. Combined monitoring is used during the removal of spinal cord tumors or vascular anomalies[67] Studies report an excellent correlation with monitoring and clinical outcome.[84,85]

MONITORING THE CAUDA EQUINA

In surgery at or below the cauda equina, direct nerve stimulation is used.[86] The response is a motor response or the H reflex. The H reflex is a monosynaptic reflex usually obtained by electrically stimulating the tibial nerve, generally in the popliteal fossa, then recording from the gastrocnemius-soleus muscle group. It is best monitored in the flexors of the upper extremity and the extensors of the lower extremity, although it has been recorded in more than 20 muscles throughout body.[87] Although it is most commonly used in EMG laboratories to diagnose S1 radiculopathies and polyneuropathies, it can be used to monitor motor function below the cauda equina (Fig. 8). The H reflex measures the excitability of the motoneurons and is influenced

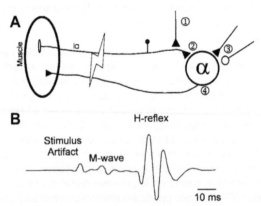

Fig. 8. (A) Schematic depiction of the neuronal components of the H-reflex arc. Shown are a Ia afferent with a monosynaptic projection to an homonymous _-motoneuron, a presynaptic connection onto the Ia afferent terminal, an excitatory postsynaptic connection, and an inhibitory postsynaptic connection. Each of the factors which can contribute to modulation of the amplitude of the H-reflex are indicated by numbers: 1, presynaptic inhibition; 2, homosynaptic depression; 3, fluctuations in motoneuronal excitability due to excitatory and inhibitory postsynaptic influences; and 4, changes in motoneuron membrane properties. (B) Sample trace of the electromyographic record of an H-reflex recorded in soleus depicting the H-reflex, M-wave (from direct activation of the _-motoneurons by the electrical stimulus), and stimulus artifact. In other muscles, for which the conduction distance is shorter, the H-reflex may overlap with the M-wave making dissociation of the two waveforms difficult. (From Misiaszek JE. The H-reflex as a tool in neurophysiology: its limitations and uses in understanding nervous system function. Muscle Nerve 2003;28(2):145; with permission.)

by descending pathways of the CT, rubrospinal, vestibulospinal, and reticulospinal systems.[88] A sustained, significant loss of the response strongly correlates with a new-onset motor deficit.[89]

EMG has also proved useful in monitoring the nerve roots, which collectively form the cauda equina. Procedures such as release of tethered cord and tumor excision carry the risk of damage to nerve roots innervating the muscles of the leg, as well as anal and urethral sphincters. Every effort is sought to avoid this loss of sphincter tone. The cauda equina monitoring includes evoked EMG, peripheral sensory stimulation with surgical field recording, MEPs, SSEPs, and the bulbocavernosus reflex.[90] The multimodality approach includes monitoring spontaneous and evoked EMG in anal sphincter, urethral sphincter, bladder detrusor muscle, tibial nerve SSEP, and MEP. Urethral sphincter EMG may be recorded using a bladder catheter with electrodes attached 2 cm from the inflating balloon.[91] Although bladder pressure is simple to measure, it measures primarily stimulated responses, and does not provide immediate and continuous feedback. It can be argued that anal sphincter EMG provides the needed information about the bladder because the innervation of both arises from the second to fourth sacral segments.[92]

Dorsal rhizotomy still remains a therapy for severe spasticity, especially in children, although supplemental therapy with botulism toxin is currently used. The spasticity is a result of hyperactivity of sensory rootlets that spreads to adjacent myotomes and results in excessive lower extremity tone and reflex muscle activity. Stimulation of the sensory nerve roots and recoding the EMG response identifies the rootlets to be sectioned.[46,77] When S2 may be involved, pudendal mapping of rootlets to the anal sphincter and urogenital system is necessary to minimize bowel and bladder complications.

MONITORING PERIPHERAL NERVES

Monitoring the peripheral nervous system includes spinal nerve roots as well as the plexus and individual nerves of the limbs; it is typically performed to prevent surgical injury or guide surgical repair. Injury may occur during procedures on the spinal column with or without in situ instrumentation, and removal of tumors. EMG monitoring follows the principles outlined for cranial nerve monitoring, namely, that either spontaneous or evoked activity is correlated to surgical events. The activity is either neurotonic discharges or CMAP. Neurotonic discharges alert the neurophysiologist and hence the surgeon to irritation of neural tissue, and the CMAP allows identification of individual nerve roots. When monitoring the EMG of the spinal nerve roots, it is important to select muscles that are enervated predominantly by the nerve roots or nerve at risk.

IOM for repair of nerves damaged by trauma can guide the surgeon's decision to graft, reapproximate the nerve, or do nothing. Blunt trauma typically leaves nerves in continuity with varying degrees of internal disruption. If the damage is neuropraxic or axonotmetic, then the nerve can be expected to recover over time by remyelination or axon growth. The presence of a nerve action potential recording over the injured segment of such a nerve that has been surgically exposed indicates the presence of regeneration, making a grafting procedure unnecessary. Absence of recordable action potentials indicates more severe disruption and neurotmetic injury; grafting is required for some recovery. In the case of a nerve root avulsion, action potentials can still be recorded because the injury is proximal to the dorsal root ganglion. Recording of cortical SSEP responses after stimulation of the proximal segment indicates that the injury is distal to the ganglion.[93] Mapping has been used in evaluation of neuroma-in-situ and in brachial plexus lesions to identify neural sections that maintain some motor or sensory continuity in which time improves function, or if no continuity exists, in which surgical reanastomosis or neural graft improves outcome.

SUMMARY

Neurophysiologic mapping and monitoring have become commonplace in neurosurgery to improve surgical decision making, refine procedures, and reduce undesired neural morbidity. Similar to the introduction of the operating microscope and stereotactic imaging procedures, IOM has allowed the neurosurgeon to better find the functional tissues put at risk by their procedures. IOM then allows continuous functional assessment of these structures. These procedures enhance the effectiveness of the surgery and reduce the risk of undesired morbidity. IOM has assisted in the development of neurosurgical procedures in ways not possible before their introduction.

REFERENCES

1. Koht A, Sloan TB, Toleikis JR, editors. Monitoring the nervous system for anesthesiologist and other health care professionals. New York: Springer; 2012.
2. Sala F, Manganotti P, Grossauer S, et al. Intraoperative neurophysiology of the motor system in children: a tailored approach. Childs Nerv Syst 2010;26(4): 473–90.
3. Moller A. Intraoperative neurophysiological monitoring. 3rd edition. New York: Springer; 2011.
4. Lopez JR. Neurophysiologic intraoperative monitoring of pediatric cerebrovascular surgery. J Clin Neurophysiol 2009;26(2):85–94.
5. Galloway GM, Nuwer MR, Lopez JR, et al. Intraoperative neurophysiologic monitoring. New York: Cambridge University Press; 2010.
6. Yamaguchi F, Takahashi H, Teramoto A. Navigation-assisted subcortical mapping: intraoperative motor tract detection by bipolar needle electrode in combination with neuronavigation system. J Neurooncol 2009;93(1):121–5.
7. MacDonald DB, Pillay N. Intraoperative electrocorticography in temporal lobe epilepsy surgery. Can J Neurol Sci 2000;27(Suppl 1):S85–91 [discussion: S92–86].
8. Greenlee JD, Oya H, Kawasaki H, et al. A functional connection between inferior frontal gyrus and orofacial motor cortex in human. J Neurophysiol 2004;92(2): 1153–64.
9. Gallentine WB, Mikati MA. Intraoperative electrocorticography and cortical stimulation in children. J Clin Neurophysiol 2009;26(2):95–108.
10. Matsumoto R, Nair DR, LaPresto E, et al. Functional connectivity in the human language system: a cortico-cortical evoked potential study. Brain 2004;127 (Pt 10):2316–30.
11. Rodel RM, Olthoff A, Tergau F, et al. Human cortical motor representation of the larynx as assessed by transcranial magnetic stimulation (TMS). Laryngoscope 2004;114(5):918–22.
12. Berger MS, Kincaid J, Ojemann GA, et al. Brain mapping techniques to maximize resection, safety, and seizure control in children with brain tumors. Neurosurgery 1989;25(5):786–92.
13. Cedzich C, Taniguchi M, Schafer S, et al. Somatosensory evoked potential phase reversal and direct motor cortex stimulation during surgery in and around the central region. Neurosurgery 1996;38(5):962–70.

14. Neuloh G, Schramm J. Intraoperative neurophysiological mapping and monitoring for supratentorial procedures. In: Deletis V, Shils JL, editors. Neurophysiology and neurosurgery. New York: Academic Press; 2002. p. 339–401.
15. Bootin M. Deep brain stimulation: overview and update. J Clin Monit Comput 2006;20:341–6.
16. Shils JL, Tagliati M, Alterman RL. Neurophysiological monitoring during neurosurgery for movement disorders. In: Deletis V, Shils JL, editors. Neurophysiology in neurosurgery. Boston: Academic Press; 2002. p. 405–48.
17. Tambakis CL, Papadopoulos G, Sergentanis TN, et al. Cerebral oximetry and stump pressure as indicators for shunting during carotid endarterectomy: comparative evaluation. Vascular 2011;19(4):187–94.
18. Ebersole JS, Ebersole JS. EEG source modeling. The last word. J Clin Neurophysiol 1999;16(3):297–302.
19. Jordan KG. Emergency EEG and continuous EEG monitoring in acute ischemic stroke. J Clin Neurophysiol 2004;21(5):341–52.
20. Deriu GP, Milite D, Mellone G, et al. Clamping ischemia, threshold ischemia and delayed insertion of the shunt during carotid endarterectomy with patch. J Cardiovasc Surg (Torino) 1999;40(2):249–55.
21. Krul JM, van Gijn J, Ackerstaff RG, et al. Site and pathogenesis of infarcts associated with carotid endarterectomy. Stroke 1989;20(3):324–8.
22. Findlay JM, Marchak BE, Pelz DM, et al. Carotid endarterectomy: a review. Can J Neurol Sci 2004;31(1):22–36.
23. Illig KA, Sternbach Y, Zhang R, et al. EEG changes during awake carotid endarterectomy. Ann Vasc Surg 2002;16(1):6–11.
24. Allain R, Marone LK, Meltzer J, et al. Carotid endarterectomy. Int Anesthesiol Clin 2005;43(1):15–38.
25. Visser GH, Wieneke GH, van Huffelen AC, et al. Carotid endarterectomy monitoring: patterns of spectral EEG changes due to carotid artery clamping. Clin Neurophysiol 1999;110(2):286–94.
26. Deogaonkar A, Vivar R, Bullock RE, et al. Bispectral index monitoring may not reliably indicate cerebral ischaemia during awake carotid endarterectomy [see comment]. Br J Anaesth 2005;94(6):800–4.
27. Moritz S, Kasprzak P, Arlt M, et al. Accuracy of cerebral monitoring in detecting cerebral ischemia during carotid endarterectomy: a comparison of transcranial Doppler sonography, near-infrared spectroscopy, stump pressure, and somatosensory evoked potentials. Anesthesiology 2007;107(4):563–9.
28. Edmonds HL. Monitoring of cerebral perfusion with transcranial Doppler ultrasound. In: Nuwer MR, editor. Intraoperative monitoring of neural function. handbook of clinical neurophysiology, vol. 8. Amsterdam: Elsevier; 2008. p. 909–23.
29. Sloan MA. Prevention of ischemic neurologic injury with intraoperative monitoring of selected cardiovascular and cerebrovascular procedures: roles of electroencephalography, somatosensory evoked potentials, transcranial Doppler, and near-infrared spectroscopy. Neurol Clin 2006;24(4):631–45.
30. Malek BN, Mohrhaus CA, Sheth AK. Use of multi-modality intraoperative monitoring during carotid endarterectomy surgery: a case study. Am J Electroneurodiagn Technol 2011;51(1):42–53.
31. Lopez JR. The use of evoked potentials in intraoperative neurophysiologic monitoring. Phys Med Rehabil Clin North Am 2004;15(1):63–84.
32. Sala F, Beltramello A, Gerosa M. Neuroprotective role of neurophysiological monitoring during endovascular procedures in the brain and spinal cord. Neurophysiol Clin 2007;37(6):415–21.

33. Schramm J, Zentner J, Pechstein U, et al. Intraoperative SEP monitoring in aneurysm surgery. Neurol Res 1994;16(1):20–2.

34. Neuloh G, Schramm J. Motor evoked potential monitoring for the surgery of brain tumours and vascular malformations. Adv Tech Stand Neurosurg 2004;29: 171–228.

35. MacDonald D. Intraoperative motor evoked potential monitoring: overview and update. J Monit Comput 2006;20:347–77.

36. Stockard J, Bickford R. The neurophysiology of anesthesia. In: Gordon E, editor. A basis and practice of neuroanesthesia. New York: Excerpta Medica; 1981. p. 3–50.

37. John ER, Prichep LS, Kox W, et al. Invariant reversible QEEG effects of anesthetics [see comment] [erratum appears in Conscious Cogn 2002 Mar;11(1):138]. Conscious Cogn 2001;10(2):165–83.

38. Rampil IJ. A primer for EEG signal processing in anesthesia [see comment]. Anesthesiology 1998;89(4):980–1002.

39. Hirota K. Special cases: ketamine, nitrous oxide and xenon. Best Pract Res Clin Anaesthesiol 2006;20(1):69–79.

40. Chen X, Tang J, White PF, et al. A comparison of patient state index and bispectral index values during the perioperative period. Anesth Analg 2002;95(6): 1669–74.

41. Drover DR, Lemmens HJ, Pierce ET, et al. Patient state index: titration of delivery and recovery from propofol, alfentanil, and nitrous oxide anesthesia. Anesthesiology 2002;97(1):82–9.

42. Bricolo A, Sala F. Surgery of brainstem lesions. In: Deletis V, Shils JL, editors. Neurophysiology in neurosurgery. Boston: Academic Press; 2002. p. 267–89.

43. Morota N, Ihara S, Deletis V. Intraoperative neurophysiology for surgery in and around the brainstem: role of brainstem mapping and corticobulbar tract motor-evoked potential monitoring. Childs Nerv Syst 2010;26(4):513–21.

44. Tanaka S, Takanashi J, Fujii K, et al. Motor evoked potential mapping and monitoring by direct brainstem stimulation. Technical note. J Neurosurg 2007;107(5): 1053–7.

45. Harper CM, Daube JR. Facial nerve electromyography and other cranial nerve monitoring [see comment]. J Clin Neurophysiol 1998;15(3):206–16.

46. Sala F, Lanteri P, Bricolo A, et al. Motor evoked potential monitoring for spinal cord and brain stem surgery. Adv Tech Stand Neurosurg 2004;29:133–69.

47. Stechison MT, Moller A, Lovely TJ, et al. Intraoperative mapping of the trigeminal nerve root: technique and application in the surgical management of facial pain. Neurosurgery 1996;38(1):76–81 [discussion: 81–2].

48. Harper CM. Intraoperative cranial nerve monitoring. Muscle Nerve 2004;29(3): 339–51.

49. Goldbrunner RH, Schlake HP, Milewski C, et al. Quantitative parameters of intraoperative electromyography predict facial nerve outcomes for vestibular schwannoma surgery. Neurosurgery 2000;46(5):1140–6 [discussion: 1146–8].

50. Moller AR. Intraoperative neurophysiologic monitoring. 2nd edition. Totowa (NJ): Humana Press; 2006.

51. Fukuda M, Oishi M, Hiraishi T, et al. Facial nerve motor-evoked potential monitoring during microvascular decompression for hemifacial spasm. J Neurol Neurosurg Psychiatry 2010;81(5):519–23.

52. Youssef AD, Downes AE. Intraoperative neurophysiological monitoring in vestibular schwannoma surgery: advances and clinical implications. Neurosurg Focus 2009;27(4):E9.

53. Randolph GW, Dralle H, International Intraoperative Monitoring Study Group. Electrophysiologic recurrent laryngeal nerve monitoring during thyroid and parathyroid surgery: international standards guideline statement. Laryngoscope 2011;121(Suppl 1):S1–16.

54. Daube JR. Intraoperative monitoring of cranial motor nerves. In: Schramm J, Moller A, editors. Intraoperative neurophysiologic monitoring in neurosurgery. New York: Springer-Verlag; 1991. p. 246–67.

55. Glasker S, Pechstein U, Vougioukas VI. Monitoring motor function during resection of tumours in the lower brain stem and fourth ventricle. Childs Nerv Syst 2006;22:1288–95.

56. Fischer C, Fischer G. Intraoperative brainstem auditory evoked potential (BAEP) monitoring in acoustic neuroma surgery. In: Schramm J, Moller A, editors. Intraoperative neurophysiologic monitoring in neurosurgery. New York: Springer-Verlag; 1991. p. 187–92.

57. James ML, Husain AM. Brainstem auditory evoked potential monitoring: when is change in wave V significant? Neurology 2005;65(10):1551–5.

58. Dralle H, Sekulla C, Lorenz K, et al, German IONM Study Group. Intraoperative monitoring of the recurrent laryngeal nerve in thyroid surgery. World J Surg 2008;32(7):1358–66.

59. Snyder SK, Hendricks JC. Intraoperative neurophysiology testing of the recurrent laryngeal nerve: plaudits and pitfalls. Surgery 2005;138(6):1183–91 [discussion: 1191–82].

60. Grabb PA, Albright AL, Sclabassi RJ, et al. Continuous intraoperative electromyographic monitoring of cranial nerves during resection of fourth ventricular tumors in children. J Neurosurg 1997;86(1):1–4.

61. Schlake HP, Goldbrunner R, Siebert M, et al. Intra-operative electromyographic monitoring of extra-ocular motor nerves (Nn. III, VI) in skull base surgery. Acta Neurochir (Wien) 2001;143(3):251–61.

62. Angelo R, Moller AR. Contralateral evoked brainstem auditory potentials as an indicator of intraoperative brainstem manipulation in cerebellopontine angle tumors. Neurol Res 1996;18(6):528–40.

63. Pechstein U, Cedzich C, Nadstawek J, et al. Transcranial high-frequency repetitive electrical stimulation for recording myogenic motor evoked potentials with the patient under general anesthesia. Neurosurgery 1996;39(2):335–43 [discussion: 343–4].

64. Deletis V, Sala F, Morota N. Intraoperative neurophysiological monitoring and mapping during brainstem surgery: a modern approach. Oper Techn Neurosurg 2000;3(2):109–13.

65. Deletis V, Kothbauer KF. Intraoperative neurophysiology of the corticospinal tract. In: Stalberg E, Sharma HS, Olsson Y, editors. Spinal cord monitoring. New York: Springer; 1998. p. 421–44.

66. Deletis V, Bueno De Camargo A. Interventional neurophysiological mapping during spinal cord procedures. Stereotact Funct Neurosurg 2001;77(1–4):25–8.

67. Sala F, Krzan MJ, Deletis V, et al. Intraoperative neurophysiological monitoring in pediatric neurosurgery: why, when, how? Childs Nerv Syst 2002;18(6-7): 264–87.

68. Sloan T, Jameson LC, Janik D. Evoked potentials. In: Cottrell J, Smith D, editors. Anesthesia and neurosurgery. 5th edition. New York: Elsevier; 2010. p. 115–30.

69. Park P, Wang AC, Sangala JR, et al. Impact of multimodal intraoperative monitoring during correction of symptomatic cervical or cervicothoracic kyphosis. J Neurosurg Spine 2011;14(1):99–105.

70. Vitale MG, Moore DW, Matsumoto H, et al. Risk factors for spinal cord injury during surgery for spinal deformity. J Bone Joint Surg Am 2010;92(1):64–71.

71. Sutter MA, Eggspuehler A, Grob D, et al. Multimodal intraoperative monitoring (MIOM) during 409 lumbosacral surgical procedures in 409 patients. Eur Spine J 2007;16(Suppl 2):S221–8.

72. Kelleher MO, Gamaliel T, Fehlings MG. Predictive value of intraoperative neurophysiological monitoring during cervical spine surgery: a prospective analysis of 1055 consecutive patients. J Neurosurg Spine 2008;8(3):215–21.

73. Hsu B, Cree AK, Lagopoulos J, et al. Transcranial motor-evoked potentials combined with response recording through compound muscle action potential as the sole modality of spinal cord monitoring in spinal deformity surgery. Spine 2008;33(10):1100–6.

74. Sutter M, Eggspuehler A, Grob D, et al. The validity of multimodal intraoperative monitoring (MIOM) in surgery of 109 spine and spinal cord tumors. Eur Spine J 2007;16(Suppl 2):S197–208.

75. Sala F, Palandri G, Basso E, et al. Motor evoked potential monitoring improves outcome after surgery for intramedullary spinal cord tumors: a historical control study. Neurosurgery 2006;58(6):1129–43 [discussion: 1129–43].

76. Eggspuehler A, Sutter MA, Grob D, et al. Multimodal intraoperative monitoring (MIOM) during cervical spine surgical procedures in 246 patients. Eur Spine J 2007;16(Suppl 2):S209–15.

77. Abbott R. Sensory rhizotomy for the treatment of childhood spasticity. In: Deletis V, Shils JL, editors. Neurophysiology in neurosurgery. Boston: Academic Press; 2002. p. 219–30.

78. Langeloo DD, Lelivelt A, Louis Journee H, et al. Transcranial electrical motor-evoked potential monitoring during surgery for spinal deformity: a study of 145 patients. Spine 2003;28(10):1043–50.

79. Freedman B, Potter B. Managing neurologic complications in cervical spine surgery. Curr Opin Orthop 2005;16:169–77.

80. Christakos A. The value of motor and somatosensory evoked potentials in evaluation of cervical myelopathy in the presence of peripheral neuropathy. Spine J 2004;29:e239–47.

81. Takahashi J, Hirabayashi H, Hashidate H, et al. Assessment of cervical myelopathy using transcranial magnetic stimulation and prediction of prognosis after laminoplasty. Spine 2008;33(1):E15–20.

82. Deletis V. Intraoperative neurophysiology and methodologies used to monitor the functional integrity of the motor system. In: Deletis V, Shils JL, editors. Neurophysiology in neurosurgery. New York: Academic Press; 2002. p. 25–51.

83. Deletis V, Sala F. Intraoperative neurophysiological monitoring of the spinal cord during spinal cord and spine surgery: a review focus on the corticospinal tracts. Clin Neurophysiol 2008;119(2):248–64.

84. Lorenzini NA, Schneider JH. Temporary loss of intraoperative motor-evoked potential and permanent loss of somatosensory-evoked potentials associated with a postoperative sensory deficit. J Neurosurg Anesthesiol 1996;8(2):142–7.

85. Herdmann J, Lumenta CB, Huse KO, et al. Magnetic stimulation for monitoring of motor pathways in spinal procedures. Spine 1993;18(5):551–9.

86. Janik DJ, Witt P. Surgery for tethered cord. In: Koht A, Sloan TB, Toleikis JR, editors. Monitoring the nervous system for anesthesiologists and other health care professionals. New York: Springer; 2012. p. 635–50.

87. Misiaszek JE. The H-reflex as a tool in neurophysiology: its limitations and uses in understanding nervous system function. Muscle Nerve 2003;28(2):144–60.

88. Leis AA, Zhou HH, Mehta M, et al. Behavior of the H-reflex in humans following mechanical perturbation or injury to rostral spinal cord. Muscle Nerve 1996; 19(11):1373–82.
89. Leppanen RE. Intraoperative applications of the H-reflex and F-response: a tutorial. J Clin Monit Comput 2006;20:267–304.
90. Kothbauer KF, Novak K. Intraoperative monitoring for tethered cord surgery: an update. Neurosurg 2004;16(2):E8.
91. Paradiso G, Lee GY, Sarjeant R, et al. Multi-modality neurophysiological monitoring during surgery for adult tethered cord syndrome. J Clin Neurosci 2005; 12(8):934–6.
92. Kothbauer K, Schmid UD, Seiler RW, et al. Intraoperative motor and sensory monitoring of the cauda equina. Neurosurgery 1994;34(4):702–7 [discussion: 707].
93. Holland NR. Intraoperative electromyography. J Clin Neurophysiol 2002;19(5): 444–53.

Perioperative Management of Adult Traumatic Brain Injury

Deepak Sharma, MD, DM[a,b], Monica S. Vavilala, MD[a,b,c,d,e],*

KEYWORDS

- Traumatic brain injury • Anesthesia • Perioperative management • Pathophysiology
- Outcomes

KEY POINTS

- Traumatic brain injury (TBI) is a major public health concern.
- Secondary insults are common after TBI and include physiologic derangements such as hypotension, hypocarbia, hyperglycemia, and hypoxemia.
- The perioperative period is the window of opportunity for anesthesiologists to prevent and reduce the burden of secondary insults after TBI.
- The choice of anesthetic agent must consider the pathophysiologic processes after TBI, and the effects of the anesthetic agents.

INTRODUCTION

Traumatic brain injury (TBI) is a major public health problem and a leading cause of death and disability.[1] Approximately 1.7 million people sustain TBI annually in the United States, accounting for 275,000 hospitalizations and 52,000 deaths.[1] TBI is a contributing factor in approximately one-third of all trauma deaths, and affects primarily children aged 0 to 4 years, adolescents aged 15 to 19 years, and elderly adults aged 65 years or older, with men being more affected.[1] Falls and motor vehicle/traffic injuries are the leading causes of TBI in the United States.[1] Multidisciplinary research

Funding Support: 5R01NS072308-02.

Portions of this article were previously published in Curry P, Viernes D, Sharma D. Perioperative management of traumatic brain injury. SYMPOSIUM ON TRENDS IN TRAUMA, 2011;1(1):27–35.

[a] Department of Anesthesiology and Pain Medicine, University of Washington, 325 Ninth Avenue, Box 359724, Seattle, WA 98115, USA; [b] Department of Neurological Surgery, University of Washington, 325 Ninth Avenue, Box 359724, Seattle, WA 98115, USA; [c] Department of Pediatrics, University of Washington, 325 Ninth Avenue, Box 359724, Seattle, WA 98115, USA; [d] Department of Radiology, University of Washington, 325 Ninth Avenue, Box 359724, Seattle, WA 98115, USA; [e] Department of Anesthesiology, Harborview Medical Center, 325 Ninth Avenue, Box 359724, Seattle, WA 98104, USA

* Corresponding author. Department of Anesthesiology, Harborview Medical Center, 325 Ninth Avenue, Box 359724, Seattle, WA 98104.

E-mail address: vavilala@uw.edu

efforts have led to the development of evidence-based guidelines for prehospital and intensive care management of TBI.[2–13] However, guidelines specific for intraoperative and anesthetic management do not exist, and intraoperative recommendations are frequently based on extrapolation from these other guidelines, physiologic and pharmacologic data, and limited direct evidence.

PATHOPHYSIOLOGY OF TBI

In TBI, the primary injury to the brain is caused by the initial mechanical impact, resulting in skull fracture, brain contusion, and vascular and parenchymal injury causing intracranial bleed and increased intracranial pressure (ICP).[14] An inflammatory process, edema formation, and excitotoxicity follow, resulting in further increase in ICP and reduced cerebral perfusion pressure (CPP).[14,15] Although the severity of the primary injury is the major factor determining the outcome of patients with TBI, secondary damage to the brain tissue caused by physiologic perturbations (secondary insults) contribute to the worsening of outcomes.[14,15] The most important secondary insults are hypotension (systolic blood pressure [SBP] <90 mm Hg in adult patients) and hypoxemia (Pao_2 <60 mm Hg),[16] which are independently associated with increased morbidity and mortality from severe TBI.[17–19] Other common secondary insults include hypoglycemia, hyperglycemia, hypercarbia, hypocarbia, and increased ICP.[20–25] All these can manifest both early and late in the course of TBI (**Table 1**). Moreover, the consequences of TBI may be evident in other organ systems besides the brain and may require prompt attention (**Box 1**).

IMPORTANCE OF PERIOPERATIVE PERIOD

Current TBI management focuses on prevention of primary injury and avoidance of secondary injuries. The key elements of TBI management are early resuscitation

Table 1
Time course and mechanisms of secondary insults in TBI

Secondary Insult	Early Causes	Delayed Causes
Hypoxemia	Aspiration Apnea Pneumothorax Pulmonary contusion Endobronchial intubation Neurogenic pulmonary edema	Adult respiratory distress syndrome Ventilator-acquired pneumonia Transfusion-related acute lung injury Pulmonary embolism
Hypotension	Associated high spinal cord Injury Long bone fracture Thoracic/abdominal bleeding	Shock Sepsis
Hypercarbia	Apnea Brainstem injury Inadequate ventilation	Iatrogenic (opioids) Pneumonia
Hypocarbia	Unwanted hyperventilation	Unwanted hyperventilation
Hyperglycemia	Stress	Persistent/new onset
Seizures	Electrolyte abnormalities hypoglycemia	Syndrome of inappropriate antidiuretic hormone
Vasospasm	—	In patients with traumatic subarachnoid hemorrhage
Intracranial hypertension	Mass effect of hematoma Herniation	Cerebral edema

---

Box 1
Multisystem effects of TBI

Cardiopulmonary

- Abnormal breathing patterns/apnea/hypoventilation
- Neurogenic pulmonary edema
- Pulmonary embolism
- Adult respiratory distress syndrome
- Neurogenic stunned myocardium/myocardial ischemia
  - Abnormal electrocardiographic patterns
  - Elevated cardiac isoenzymes (creatine kinase MB and creatinine kinase)
  - Left ventricular dysfunction

Metabolic

- Hyperglycemia and insulin resistance
- Increased catecholamine levels
- Increased caloric demand and nitrogen loss

Autonomic dysfunction syndrome

- Hypertension, tachycardia
- Fever, tachypnea
- Pupillary dilatation
- Extensor posturing

Endocrine

- Anterior pituitary insufficiency
- Posterior pituitary insufficiency
- Diabetes insipidus
- Syndrome of inappropriate antidiuretic hormone secretion

Hematologic

- Coagulopathy (↓ platelet count and/or ↑ international normalized ratio and/or activated partial thromboplastin time)
- Disseminated intravascular coagulation

Gastrointestinal

- Cushing ulcers (stress ulcers)
- Gastrointestinal dysfunction and increased mucosal permeability

---

and hemodynamic optimization, emergent surgical evacuation of mass lesions, control of ICP, support of CPP, and optimization of physiologic milieu. The immediate perioperative period may be particularly important in the course of TBI management because, despite the aggressive interventions to rapidly correct hypoxemia, hypotension, hypocarbia, hypercarbia, hypoglycemia, and hyperglycemia in the emergency department, one or more of these complicating factors may persist or remain undetected as the patient is transported to the operating room. Hence, the perioperative period provides an opportunity to continue and refine ongoing resuscitation, and to correct preexisting secondary insults. Moreover, surgery and anesthesia may predispose to new onset secondary insults, which may contribute adversely to outcomes.

Because secondary injury is potentially preventable and treatable, the perioperative period may be a window to initiate interventions that may improve the outcome of TBI. Perioperative management involves rapid evaluation, continuation of resuscitation (cerebral and systemic), early surgical intervention, intensive monitoring, and anesthetic planning.

INITIAL ASSESSMENT AND ONGOING RESUSCITATION

The initial assessment and stabilization is usually achieved as soon as the patient arrives in the emergency department. Nevertheless, another rapid but relevant assessment should be performed as the patient is received in the operating room. This process should involve evaluation of airway, breathing, and circulation; a rapid assessment of neurologic status and associated extracranial injuries; and evaluation of anemia, coagulopathy, glycemia, and the presence of adequate vascular access. Information about time and mechanism of injury can be valuable. Brief neurologic assessment is performed using Glasgow Coma Scale (GCS)[26] score and pupillary responses. Associated thoracic, abdominal, spinal, and long bone injuries may be stable or evolve during the perioperative period, and must be considered in the differential diagnosis of new onset hypotension, anemia, hemodynamic instability, or hypoxemia during anesthesia and surgery.

AIRWAY MANAGEMENT

Although many patients arrive in the operating room already intubated, some, particularly those with extradural hematoma, may be conscious and breathing spontaneously. Airway management in TBI is complicated by several factors, including urgency of situation (because of preexisting or worsening hypoxia), uncertainty of cervical spine status, uncertainty of airway (caused by presence of blood, vomitus, debris in the oral cavity, or laryngopharyngeal injury or skull base fracture), full stomach, intracranial hypertension, and uncertain volume status. All patients with TBI requiring urgent surgery must be assumed to have full stomach, and airway management must account for possible underlying cervical spine injury.[27,28]

Technique: Best Practices

The choice of technique for tracheal intubation is determined by urgency, individual expertise, and available resources, and generally incorporates rapid sequence intubation with cricoid pressure and manual in-line stabilization.[29] The anterior portion of the cervical collar may be removed when manual in-line stabilization is established to allow greater mouth opening and facilitate laryngoscopy. Newer airway devises, particularly videolaryngoscopes, have gained popularity recently for use in trauma victims and may be useful in difficult airway scenarios.[30] Nasal intubation should be avoided in patients with skull base fracture, severe facial fractures, or bleeding diathesis. In any case, having a backup plan ready is advisable in case of difficult intubation, given the significant risk of intracranial hypertension resulting from increased cerebral blood volume because of hypoxemia and hypercarbia.

Appropriate pharmacologic selection is important for uncomplicated airway management. Sodium thiopental, etomidate, and propofol decrease cerebral metabolic rate for oxygen ($CMRO_2$) and attenuate increases in ICP with intubation. However, propofol and thiopental may cause cardiovascular depression, leading to hypotension. Etomidate offers the advantage of hemodynamic stability during induction but may cause adrenal insufficiency, leading to delayed hypotension.[31] Ketamine, which causes limited cardiovascular compromise, has been associated with increased cerebral blood flow (CBF) and increased ICP, and may be contraindicated for intubating patients with preexisting intracranial hypertension.[32] The choice of muscle relaxant for rapid sequence induction is between succinylcholine and rocuronium.[33] Succinylcholine may contribute to increased ICP,[34,35] the clinical significance of which is questionable.[36,37] More importantly, hypoxia and hypercarbia during airway interventions are more likely to cause clinically significant increases in ICP. Hence, in patients with TBI, succinylcholine may not be avoided if a difficult airway is anticipated.[37]

ANESTHETIC MANAGEMENT

The major goals of anesthetic management of TBI are to facilitate early decompression, provide adequate analgesia and amnesia, treat intracranial hypertension and maintain adequate cerebral perfusion, provide optimal surgical conditions, and avoid secondary insults, such as hypoxemia, hypercarbia, hypocarbia, hypoglycemia, and hyperglycemia.

ANESTHETIC TECHNIQUE

Intravenous anesthetic agents, including thiopental, propofol, and etomidate, cause cerebral vasoconstriction and reduce CBF, cerebral blood volume, $CMRO_2$, and ICP.[38] Opioids have no direct effects on cerebral hemodynamics when ventilation is controlled.[39] All volatile anesthetic agents (isoflurane, sevoflurane, desflurane) decrease $CMRO_2$ but may cause cerebral vasodilation, resulting in raised ICP. However, at less than 1 minimum alveolar concentration, the cerebral vasodilatory effects are minimal and hence inhaled anesthetics may be used in low concentrations in patients with TBI.[40] Nitrous oxide should be avoided because it increases $CMRO_2$ and causes cerebral vasodilation and increased ICP.[41] The effects of anesthetic agents on outcome of TBI have not been demonstrated, and inhaled and intravenous anesthetic agents may be used judiciously. More importantly, the principles of anesthetic management should adhere to the guidelines for the management of severe TBI (**Table 2**).[2–13]

VENTILATION

Ventilation should be adjusted to ensure adequate oxygenation (Pao_2 >60 mm Hg) and normocarbia ($Paco_2$ 35–45 mm Hg). Monitoring arterial $Paco_2$ is recommended and hypercarbia-induced ($Paco_2$ >45 mm Hg) increases in CBF resulting in further increased ICP should be avoided.[12] Hyperventilation should be used judiciously for short-term control of ICP and to facilitate surgical exposure during craniotomy. Excessive and prolonged hyperventilation may cause cerebral vasoconstriction leading to ischemia. Normocarbia should be restored before dural closure. It is ideal to monitor cerebral oxygenation and CBF during prolonged hyperventilation. In the intraoperative period, this may be accomplished through jugular venous oximetry[9,42] and brain tissue oxygenation ($P_{BT}O_2$) or CBF monitoring (eg, using transcranial Doppler ultrasonography) in the postoperative period.[9]

MONITORING

In addition to standard American Society of Anesthesiology monitors, arterial catheterization is recommended for continuous blood pressure monitoring, blood gas analysis, and glucose sampling in patients who require surgical intervention. Central venous catheterization may be useful for resuscitation, but it is advisable not to delay

Table 2
Recommendations from the 2007 guidelines for management of severe traumatic brain injury

Parameters	Recommendations
Blood pressure	• Monitor and avoid hypotension (SBP <90 mm Hg) (level II)
Oxygenation	• Monitor and avoid hypoxia (Pao_2 <60 mm Hg or oxygen saturation <90%) (level III)
Hyperventilation	• Prophylactic hyperventilation ($Paco_2$ ≤25 mm Hg) is not recommended (level II) • Hyperventilation is recommended as a temporizing measure for the reduction of elevated intracranial pressure (level III)
Hyperosmolar therapy	• Mannitol (0.25–1.0 g/kg) is effective for control of raised intracranial pressure. Hypotension should be avoided (level II) • Restrict mannitol use before intracranial pressure monitoring to patients with signs of transtentorial herniation or progressive neurologic deterioration not attributable to extracranial causes (level III)
ICP	• ICP should be monitored in patients with severe TBI and abnormal CT scan (level II) and in patients with normal CT scan if two or more of following are present: age >40 years, motor posturing, systolic blood pressure <90 mm Hg (level III) • Treatment should be initiated if intracranial pressure is >20 mm Hg (level II)
Temperature	• Prophylactic hypothermia is not significantly associated with decreased mortality (level III) • Hypothermia may have higher chances of reducing mortality when cooling is maintained for more than 48 hours (level III)
CPP	• Maintain cerebral perfusion pressure between 50–70 mm Hg • Avoid aggressive treatment with fluid and pressors to maintain CPP >70 mm Hg (level II) • Avoid CPP <50 mm Hg (level III)
Brain oxygenation	• Treat when jugular venous oxygen saturation <50% or brain tissue oxygen tension <15 mm Hg (level III)
Steroids	• In patients with moderate or severe TBI, high-dose methylprednisolone is associated with increased mortality and is contraindicated (level I)

Data from Refs.[2–13]

surgical evacuation of expanding intracranial hematoma for the institution of invasive monitoring. According to the current guidelines, ICP monitoring is recommended in all salvageable patients with a severe TBI (GCS <9) and an abnormal CT scan (hematomas, contusions, swelling, herniation, or compressed basal cistern), and in patients with severe TBI with a normal CT scan if two or more of the following features are present: age older than 40 years, unilateral/bilateral motor posturing, or SBP less than 90 mm Hg.[5] The use of multimodal monitoring for postoperative and intensive care of patients with TBI is increasing, and monitoring cerebral oxygenation (global or focal) or CBF and metabolism parameters may be helpful in making important treatment decisions.[9]

Jugular venous oximetry is often useful in assessing adequacy of global cerebral oxygenation.[43] The indications are generally the same as those for ICP monitoring, and jugular venous oxygen saturation values less than 50% may indicate the need to optimize ventilation, improve systemic hemodynamics, or institute ICP-lowering measures.[43] Brain tissue oxygen monitors have the advantage of identifying focal areas of ischemia that may not be picked up by jugular venous oximetry.[43] Brain tissue Po_2 less than 15 mm Hg indicates ischemia.[43] Near infrared spectroscopy offers the capacity to conveniently and noninvasively monitor cerebral oxygen in the intensive care unit.[43] Transcranial Doppler ultrasonography is a noninvasive, nonradioactive, bedside monitor that can provide useful instantaneous cerebrovascular information, including changes in cerebral blood flow velocity, cerebral vasospasm, and autoregulation.[44]

INTRAVENOUS FLUIDS, BLOOD PRESSURE MANAGEMENT, AND VASOPRESSOR USE

Hypotension after TBI is well known to adversely affect outcomes. Therefore, blood pressure management, including choice of fluids and vasopressors, is of paramount importance. Brain Trauma Foundation guidelines for the management of TBI recommend avoiding hypotension (SBP <90 mm Hg) and maintaining CPP between 50 and 70 mm Hg.[2,8] Hypotension during craniotomy also contributes to adverse outcomes and is frequently encountered at the time of dural opening.[45] This "decompression hypotension" may be predicted from low GCS score, absence of mesencephalic cisterns on CT scan, and bilateral dilated pupils.[45] Moreover, the presence of multiple CT lesions, subdural hematoma, maximum thickness of CT lesion, and longer duration of anesthesia increase the risk for intraoperative hypotension, and anesthesiologists can use the presence of these factors to anticipate and expediently address these complications.[46] Perioperative hypotension should be treated promptly.

Warm, non–glucose-containing isotonic crystalloid solution is preferable for intravenous administration in patients with TBI. The role of colloid, however, is controversial. A post hoc analysis of the Saline versus Albumin Fluid Evaluation (SAFE) study showed that resuscitation with albumin was associated with higher mortality and unfavorable neurologic outcome at 24 months.[47] Hypertonic saline may be beneficial resuscitation fluid for patients with TBI because it increases intravascular fluid and decreases ICP. However, a double-blind randomized controlled trial comparing prehospital resuscitation of hypotensive patients with a TBI with hypertonic saline versus standard fluid resuscitation protocols found no difference in neurologic outcome at 6 months.[48] Data comparing the effectiveness of commonly used vasopressors in TBI are limited and indicate that the effects of norepinephrine and dopamine on cerebral blood flow velocity[49,50] and cerebral oxygenation or metabolism[51] are comparable, but the former produces more predictable and consistent effect,[50] whereas the later may lead to higher ICP.[49] A recent single-center retrospective study of patients with severe TBI who received phenylephrine, norepinephrine, or dopamine reported maximum increase in mean arterial pressure and CPP from baseline with phenylephrine use with no difference in ICP.[52] Current evidence does not show superiority of vasopressor over another in increasing cerebral perfusion, and the choice may need to be individualized to patient characteristics.

BLOOD TRANSFUSION

Anemia is associated with increased in-hospital mortality[53] and poor outcome in TBI.[54,55] Yet, little evidence supports red blood cell transfusion to correct anemia in TBI. Anemia may cause cerebral injury via various possible mechanisms, including tissue hypoxia, reactive oxygen species–induced damage, inflammation, disruption of blood-brain barrier (BBB) function, vascular thrombosis, and anemic cerebral hyperemia.[56] It may also impair cerebral autoregulation.[57] However, several cerebroprotective physiologic mechanisms become effective with anemia, including aortic chemoreceptor activation; increased sympathetic activity leading to increased heart rate, stroke volume, and cardiac index; reduced systemic vascular resistance; and enhanced oxygen extraction. Moreover, several cellular mechanisms of cerebral protection become effective, including increased hypoxia inducible factor; nitric oxide synthase and nitric oxide in the brain (nNOS/NO); erythropoietin; and vascular endothelial growth factor–mediated angiogenesis and vascular repair.[56] Besides increasing the oxygen carrier capacity of blood, red blood cell transfusion increases the circulating volume and can increase CBF in patients with impaired cerebral autoregulation secondary to the TBI. However, most studies have failed to demonstrate a consistent improvement in brain tissue oxygenation ($P_{BT}O_2$) with blood transfusion.[58,59] In fact, the increased hematocrit after red cell transfusion may potentially decrease CBF and increase the risk of cerebral ischemia.[60] The overall effects of anemia on the brain may depend on the relative balance between the competing protective and harmful factors of anemia and blood transfusion, and whether transfusion trigger in patients with TBI should be any different from that in other critically ill patients is unclear. Although the optimal hemoglobin level in TBI patients is unclear, a liberal transfusion strategy (transfusion when hemoglobin <10 g/dL) has no benefit in patients with moderate to severe TBI, and therefore is not recommended.[55]

COAGULOPATHY AND FACTOR VII

Coagulation disorders may be present in approximately one-third of patients with TBI and is associated with an increased mortality and poor outcome.[61] Brain injury leads to the release of tissue factor. Later, procoagulant factors are activated, resulting in thrombin formation and conversion of fibrinogen to fibrin. Disseminated intravascular coagulation inhibits the antithrombotic mechanism, causing imbalance of coagulation and fibrinolysis. Patients with GCS of 8 or less, Injury Severity Score (ISS) of 16 or higher, associated cerebral edema, subarachnoid hemorrhage, and midline shift are likely to have coagulopathy.[62] Currently, no guidelines exist for the management of coagulopathy in TBI, although hemostatic agents are sometimes used, including antifibrinolytic agents such as tranexamic acid and procoagulant drugs such as recombinant activated factor VII (rFVIIa). A Cochrane review found two randomized controlled trials that evaluated the effects of rFVIIa, but both were too small to draw a conclusion regarding the effectiveness of rFVIIa for patients with TBI.[63] The Clinical Randomization of Antifibrinolytics in Significant Hemorrhage (CRASH-2) trial, a large international placebo-controlled trial evaluating the effect of tranexamic acid on death, vascular occlusion events and blood transfusion in adult trauma patients, showed that tranexamic acid was associated with a reduction of mortality.[64]

HYPEROSMOLAR THERAPY

Mannitol is commonly used for hyperosmolar therapy and no level I evidence supports the use of one agent over another. The recommended dose of mannitol is 0.25 to 1 g/kg body weight. Because of osmotic diuresis, which can result in hypovolemia and hypotension, it is recommended only in presence of signs of transtentorial herniation or progressive neurologic deterioration not attributable to extracranial causes.[3] In patients with severe TBI and elevated ICP refractory to mannitol treatment, 7.5% hypertonic saline administered as second-tier therapy can increase cerebral oxygenation and improve cerebral and systemic hemodynamics.[65]

GLYCEMIC CONTROL

Hyperglycemia after TBI is associated with increased morbidity and mortality.[20,21,23] It is unclear to what extent it reflects the injury severity[66] or contributes to worse outcomes by itself.[66,67] Nevertheless, hyperglycemia can cause secondary brain injury, leading to increased glycolytic rates evidenced by increased lactate/pyruvate ratio, resulting in metabolic acidosis within brain parenchyma, overproduction of reactive oxygen species, and ultimately neuronal cell death.[66–69] Some early studies reported lower mortality associated with intensive insulin therapy (target blood glucose 80–110 mg/dL) in critically ill patients.[70] However, more recent studies not only failed to demonstrate the mortality benefit of intensive insulin therapy but also found an increased risk of hypoglycemia.[69,71] Hence, tight glucose control with intensive insulin therapy remains controversial. Although several studies have investigated hyperglycemia in adult TBI in different contexts (eg, admission vs intensive care unit; transient vs persistent; early vs late), the intraoperative data are scarce. Nonetheless, intraoperative hyperglycemia is common in adults undergoing urgent/emergent craniotomy for TBI, with up to 15% patients experiencing new onset hyperglycemia, which may be predicted by severe TBI, the presence of subdural hematoma, preoperative hyperglycemia, and age of 65 years or older. Similarly, perioperative hyperglycemia during craniotomy for TBI is common in children, hypoglycemia in the absence of insulin treatment is not rare, and TBI severity and the presence of subdural hematoma predict intraoperative hyperglycemia.[23] Given the current evidence for glucose control for TBI in perioperative period, a target glucose range of 80 to 180 mg/dL seems reasonable.

THERAPEUTIC HYPOTHERMIA AND STEROIDS

Hypothermia reduces cerebral metabolism during stress, reduces excitatory neurotransmitters release, attenuates BBB permeability, and has been used for brain protection in patients with TBI for decades. Yet, clinical evidence in terms of mortality and functional outcomes is still inconclusive. A recent meta-analysis reported statistically insignificant reduction in mortality and increased favorable neurologic outcome with hypothermia in TBI.[72] The benefits of hypothermia were greater when cooling was maintained for more than 48 hours, but the potential benefits of hypothermia may likely be offset by a significant increase in the risk of pneumonia.[72] These observations support previous findings that hypothermic therapy constitutes a beneficial treatment of TBI in specific circumstances. Accordingly, the Brain Trauma Foundation/American Association of Neurological Surgeons guidelines task force has issued a level III recommendation for optional and cautious use of hypothermia for adults with TBI.[4]

Steroids have not been shown to improve outcomes or lower ICP in TBI.[13] In fact, findings from a randomized multicenter study on the effect of corticosteroids (Medical Research Council CRASH trial) showed that administration of methylprednisolone within 8 hours of TBI was associated with higher risk of death, and the risk of death or severe disability was greater compared with placebo.[73] Therefore, the use of high-dose methylprednisolone is contraindicated in patients with moderate or severe TBI.[13]

SUMMARY

The perioperative period is critical for TBI management and outcomes. Although it may predispose the patient to new onset secondary injuries that may contribute adversely to outcomes, it is also an opportunity to detect and correct undiagnosed preexisting secondary insults. It may also be a potential window to initiate interventions that may improve the outcome of TBI. Additional research focused specifically on intraoperative and perioperative management of TBI is awaited; in the meantime, clinical management should continue to be based on physiologic optimization.

REFERENCES

1. Faul M, Xu L, Wald MM, et al. Traumatic brain injury in the United States: emergency department visits, hospitalizations, and deaths. Atlanta (GA): Centers for Disease Control and Prevention, National Center for Injury Prevention and Control; 2010.
2. Bratton SL, Chestnut RM, Ghajar J, et al, Brain Trauma Foundation; American Association of Neurological Surgeons; Congress of Neurological Surgeons; Joint Section on Neurotrauma and Critical Care, AANS/CNS. Guidelines for the management of severe traumatic brain injury Blood pressure and oxygenation. J Neurotrauma 2007;24:S7–13.
3. Bratton SL, Chestnut RM, Ghajar J, et al, Brain Trauma Foundation; American Association of Neurological Surgeons; Congress of Neurological Surgeons; Joint Section on Neurotrauma and Critical Care, AANS/CNS. Guidelines for the management of severe traumatic brain injury II. Hyperosmolar therapy. J Neurotrauma 2007;24:S14–20.
4. Bratton SL, Chestnut RM, Ghajar J, et al, Brain Trauma Foundation; American Association of Neurological Surgeons; Congress of Neurological Surgeons; Joint Section on Neurotrauma and Critical Care, AANS/CNS. Guidelines for the management of severe traumatic brain injury III Prophylactic hypothermia. J Neurotrauma 2007;24:S21–5.
5. Bratton SL, Chestnut RM, Ghajar J, et al, Brain Trauma Foundation; American Association of Neurological Surgeons; Congress of Neurological Surgeons; Joint Section on Neurotrauma and Critical Care, AANS/CNS. Guidelines for the management of severe traumatic brain injury. VI. Indications for intracranial pressure monitoring. J Neurotrauma 2007;24:S37–44.
6. Bratton SL, Chestnut RM, Ghajar J, et al, Brain Trauma Foundation; American Association of Neurological Surgeons; Congress of Neurological Surgeons; Joint Section on Neurotrauma and Critical Care, AANS/CNS. Guidelines for the management of severe traumatic brain injury. VII. Intracranial pressure monitoring technology. J Neurotrauma 2007;24:S45–54.
7. Bratton SL, Chestnut RM, Ghajar J, et al, Brain Trauma Foundation; American Association of Neurological Surgeons; Congress of Neurological Surgeons; Joint Section on Neurotrauma and Critical Care, AANS/CNS. Guidelines for the management of severe traumatic brain injury. VIII. Intracranial pressure thresholds. J Neurotrauma 2007;24:S55–8.
8. Bratton SL, Chestnut RM, Ghajar J, et al, Brain Trauma Foundation; American Association of Neurological Surgeons; Congress of Neurological Surgeons; Joint Section on Neurotrauma and Critical Care, AANS/CNS. Guidelines for the management of severe traumatic brain injury. IX. Cerebral perfusion thresholds. J Neurotrauma 2007;24:S59–64.
9. Bratton SL, Chestnut RM, Ghajar J, et al, Brain Trauma Foundation; American Association of Neurological Surgeons; Congress of Neurological Surgeons; Joint Section on Neurotrauma and Critical Care, AANS/CNS. Guidelines for the management of severe traumatic brain injury. X. Brain oxygen monitoring and thresholds. J Neurotrauma 2007;24:S65–70.
10. Bratton SL, Chestnut RM, Ghajar J, et al, Brain Trauma Foundation; American Association of Neurological Surgeons; Congress of Neurological Surgeons; Joint Section on Neurotrauma and Critical Care, AANS/CNS. Guidelines for the management of severe traumatic brain injury. XI. Anesthetics, analgesics, and sedatives. J Neurotrauma 2007;24:S71–6.

11. Bratton SL, Chestnut RM, Ghajar J, et al, Brain Trauma Foundation; American Association of Neurological Surgeons; Congress of Neurological Surgeons; Joint Section on Neurotrauma and Critical Care, AANS/CNS. Guidelines for the management of severe traumatic brain injury. XIII. Antiseizure prophylaxis. J Neurotrauma 2007;24:S83–6.

12. Bratton SL, Chestnut RM, Ghajar J, et al, Brain Trauma Foundation; American Association of Neurological Surgeons; Congress of Neurological Surgeons; Joint Section on Neurotrauma and Critical Care, AANS/CNS. Guidelines for the management of severe traumatic brain injury. XIV. Hyperventilation. J Neurotrauma 2007;24:S87–90.

13. Bratton SL, Chestnut RM, Ghajar J, et al, Brain Trauma Foundation; American Association of Neurological Surgeons; Congress of Neurological Surgeons; Joint Section on Neurotrauma and Critical Care, AANS/CNS. Guidelines for the management of severe traumatic brain injury. XV. Steroids. J Neurotrauma 2007;24: S91–5.

14. Greve MW, Zink BJ. Pathophysiology of traumatic brain injury. Mt Sinai J Med 2009;76:97–104.

15. Werner C, Engelhard K. Pathophysiology of traumatic brain injury. Br J Anaesth 2007;99:4–9.

16. Chesnut RM, Marshall LF, Klauber MR, et al. The role of secondary brain injury in determining outcome from severe head injury. J Trauma 1993;34:216–22.

17. Marshall LF, Becker DP, Bowers SA, et al. The National Traumatic Coma Data Bank. Part 1: design, purpose, goals, and results. J Neurosurg 1983;59:276–84.

18. McHugh GS, Engel DC, Butcher I, et al. Prognostic value of secondary insults in traumatic brain injury: results from the IMPACT study. J Neurotrauma 2007;24: 287–93.

19. Pietropaoli JA, Rogers FB, Shackford SR, et al. The deleterious effects of intraoperative hypotension on outcome in patients with severe head injuries. J Trauma 1992;33:403–7.

20. Liu-DeRyke X, Collingridge DS, Orme J, et al. Clinical impact of early hyperglycemia during acute phase of traumatic brain injury. Neurocrit Care 2009;11: 151–7.

21. Jeremitsky E, Omert LA, Dunham CM, et al. The impact of hyperglycemia on patients with severe brain injury. J Trauma 2005;58:47–50.

22. Griesdale DE, Tremblay MH, McEwen J, et al. Glucose control and mortality in patients with severe traumatic brain injury. Neurocrit Care 2009;11:311–6.

23. Sharma D, Jelacic J, Chennuri R, et al. Incidence and risk factors for perioperative hyperglycemia in children with traumatic brain injury. Anesth Analg 2009;108: 81–9.

24. Warner KJ, Cuschieri J, Copass MK, et al. The impact of prehospital ventilation on outcome after severe traumatic brain injury. J Trauma 2007;62:1330–6.

25. Dumont TM, Visioni AJ, Rughani AI, et al. Inappropriate prehospital ventilation in severe traumatic brain injury increases in-hospital mortality. J Neurotrauma 2010; 27:1233–41.

26. Teasdale G, Jennett B. Assessment of coma and impaired consciousness. A practical scale. Lancet 1974;2:81–4.

27. Holly LT, Kelly DF, Counelis GJ, et al. Cervical spine trauma associated with moderate and severe head injury: incidence, risk factors, and injury characteristics. J Neurosurg (Spine 3) 2002;69:285–91.

28. Demetriades D, Charalambides K, Chahwan S, et al. Nonskeletal cervical spine injuries: epidemiology and diagnostic pitfalls. J Trauma 2000;48:724–7.

29. Crosby ET. Airway management in adults after cervical spine trauma. Anesthesiology 2006;104:1293–318.

30. Platts-Mills TF, Campagne D, Chinnock B, et al. A comparison of GlideScope video laryngoscopy versus direct laryngoscopy intubation in the emergency department. Acad Emerg Med 2009;16:866–71.

31. Cohan P, Wang C, McArthur DL, et al. Acute secondary adrenal insufficiency after traumatic brain injury: a prospective study. Crit Care Med 2005;33:2358–66.

32. Schulte am Esch J, Pfeifer G, Thiemig I, et al. The influence of intravenous anaesthetic agents on primarily increased intracranial pressure. Acta Neurochir (Wien) 1978;45:15–25.

33. Perry JJ, Lee JS, Sillberg VA, et al. Rocuronium versus succinylcholine for rapid sequence induction intubation. Cochrane Database Syst Rev 2008;2:CD002788.

34. Minton MD, Grosslight K, Stirt JA, et al. Increases in intracranial pressure from succinylcholine: prevention by prior nondepolarizing blockade. Anesthesiology 1986;65:165–9.

35. Stirt JA, Grosslight KR, Bedford RF, et al. Defasciculation with metocurine prevents succinylcholine-induced increases in intracranial pressure. Anesthesiology 1987;67:50–3.

36. Kovarik WD, Mayberg TS, Lam AM, et al. Succinylcholine does not change intracranial pressure, cerebral blood flow velocity, or the electroencephalogram in patients with neurologic injury. Anesth Analg 1994;78:469–73.

37. Clancy M, Halford S, Walls R, et al. In patients with head injuries who undergo rapid sequence intubation using succinylcholine, does pretreatment with a competitive neuromuscular blocking agent improve outcome? A literature review. Emerg Med J 2001;18:373–5.

38. Turner BK, Wakim JH, Secrest J, et al. Neuroprotective effects of thiopental, propofol, and etomidate. AANA J 2005;73:297–302.

39. Schregel W, Weyerer W, Cunitz G. Opioids, cerebral circulation and intracranial pressure. Anaesthesist 1994;43:421–30.

40. Engelhard K, Werner C. Inhalational or intravenous anesthetics for craniotomies? Pro inhalational? Curr Opin Anaesthesiol 2006;19:504–8.

41. Schulte am Esch J, Thiemig I, Pfeifer G, et al. The influence of some inhalation anaesthetics on the intracranial pressure with special reference to nitrous oxide. Anaesthesist 1979;28:136–41.

42. Schaffranietz L, Heinke W. The effect of different ventilation regimes on jugular venous oxygen saturation in elective neurosurgical patients. Neurol Res 1998; 20:S66–70.

43. Haitsma IK, Maas AI. Monitoring cerebral oxygenation in traumatic brain injury. Prog Brain Res 2007;161:207–16.

44. Dagal A, Lam AM. Cerebral blood flow and the injured brain: how should we monitor and manipulate it? Curr Opin Anaesthesiol 2011;24(2):131–7.

45. Kawaguchi M, Sakamoto T, Ohnishi H, et al. Preoperative predictors of reduction in arterial blood pressure following dural opening during surgical evacuation of acute subdural hematoma. J Neurosurg Anesthesiol 1996;8(2):117–22.

46. Sharma D, Brown MJ, Curry P, et al. Prevalence and Risk factors for Intraoperative Hypotension During Craniotomy for Traumatic Brain Injury. J Neurosurg Anesthesiol 2012. [Epub ahead of print].

47. Myburgh J, Cooper DJ, Finfer S, et al, SAFE Study Investigators; Australian and New Zealand Intensive Care Society Clinical Trials Group; Australian Red Cross Blood Service; George Institute for International Health. Saline or albumin for fluid resuscitation in patients with traumatic brain injury. N Engl J Med 2007;357:874–84.

48. Cooper DJ, Myles PS, McDermott FT, et al. Prehospital hypertonic saline resuscitation of patients with hypotension and severe traumatic brain injury: a randomized controlled trial. JAMA 2004;291:1350–7.

49. Ract C, Vigué B. Comparison of the cerebral effects of dopamine and norepinephrine in severely head-injured patients. Intensive Care Med 2001;27: 101–6.

50. Steiner LA, Johnston AJ, Czosnyka M, et al. Direct comparison of cerebrovascular effects of norepinephrine and dopamine in head-injured patients. Crit Care Med 2004;32:1049–54.

51. Johnston AJ, Steiner LA, Chatfield DA, et al. Effect of cerebral perfusion pressure augmentation with dopamine and norepinephrine on global and focal brain oxygenation after traumatic brain injury. Intensive Care Med 2004;30:791–7.

52. Sookplung P, Siriussawakul A, Malakouti A, et al. Vasopressor use and effect on blood pressure after severe adult traumatic brain injury. Neurocrit Care 2011; 15(1):46–54.

53. Alvarez M, Nava JM, Rué M, et al. Mortality prediction in head trauma patients: performance of Glasgow Coma Score and general severity systems. Crit Care Med 1998;26:142–8.

54. Carlson AP, Schermer CR, Lu SW. Retrospective evaluation of anemia and transfusion in traumatic brain injury. J Trauma 2006;61:567–71.

55. Salim A, Hadjizacharia P, DuBose J, et al. Role of anemia in traumatic brain injury. J Am Coll Surg 2008;207:398–406.

56. Hare GM, Tsui AK, McLaren AT, et al. Anemia and cerebral outcomes: many questions, fewer answers. Anesth Analg 2008;107:1356–70.

57. Ogawa Y, Iwasaki K, Aoki K, et al. Central hypervolemia with hemodilution impairs dynamic cerebral autoregulation. Anesth Analg 2007;105:1389–96.

58. Leal-Noval SR, Rincón-Ferrari MD, Marin-Niebla A, et al. Transfusion of erythrocyte concentrates produces a variable increment on cerebral oxygenation in patients with severe traumatic brain injury: a preliminary study. Intensive Care Med 2006;32:1733–40.

59. Zygun DA, Nortje J, Hutchinson PJ, et al. The effect of red blood cell transfusion on cerebral oxygenation and metabolism after severe traumatic brain injury. Crit Care Med 2009;37:1074–8.

60. Pendem S, Rana S, Manno EM, et al. A review of red cell transfusion in the neurological intensive care unit. Neurocrit Care 2006;4:63–7.

61. Harhangi BS, Kompanje EJ, Leebeek FW, et al. Coagulation disorders after traumatic brain injury. Acta Neurochir (Wien) 2008;150:165–75.

62. Talving P, Benfield R, Hadjizacharia P, et al. Coagulopathy in severe traumatic brain injury: a prospective study. J Trauma 2009;66:55–61.

63. Perel P, Roberts I, Shakur H, et al. Haemostatic drugs for traumatic brain injury. Cochrane Database Syst Rev 2010;1:CD007877.

64. CRASH-2 trial collaborators, Shakur H, Roberts I, Bautista R, et al. Effects of tranexamic acid on death, vascular occlusive events, and blood transfusion in trauma patients with significant haemorrhage (CRASH-2): a randomised, placebo-controlled trial. Lancet 2010;376:23–32.

65. Oddo M, Levine JM, Frangos S, et al. Effect of mannitol and hypertonic saline on cerebral oxygenation in patients with severe traumatic brain injury and refractory intracranial hypertension. J Neurol Neurosurg Psychiatry 2009;80:916–20.

66. Young B, Ott L, Dempsey R, et al. Relationship between admission hyperglycemia and neurologic outcome of severely brain-injured patients. Ann Surg 1989;210:466–72.

67. Lipshutz AK, Gropper MA. Perioperative glycemic control: an evidence-based review. Anesthesiology 2009;110:408–21.
68. Rovlias A, Kotsou S. The influence of hyperglycemia on neurological outcome in patients with severe head injury. Neurosurgery 2000;46:335–42.
69. Bilotta F, Caramia R, Cernak I, et al. Intensive insulin therapy after severe traumatic brain injury: a randomized clinical trial. Neurocrit Care 2008;9:159–66.
70. van den Berghe G, Wouters P, Weekers F, et al. Intensive insulin therapy in the critically ill patients. N Engl J Med 2001;345:1359–67.
71. Finfer S, Chittock DR, Su SY, et al, NICE-SUGAR Study Investigators. Intensive versus conventional glucose control in critically ill patients. N Engl J Med 2009; 306:1283–97.
72. Peterson K, Carson S, Carney N. Hypothermia treatment for traumatic brain injury: a systematic review and meta-analysis. J Neurotrauma 2008;25:62–71.
73. Edwards P, Arango M, Balica L, et al. CRASH trial collaborators. Final results of MRC CRASH, a randomised placebo-controlled trial of intravenous corticosteroid in adults with head injury-outcomes at 6 months. Lancet 2005;365:1957–9.

Perioperative Pain Management in the Neurosurgical Patient

Lawrence T. Lai, MD[a],*, Jose R. Ortiz-Cardona, MD[b],
Audrée A. Bendo, MD[b]

KEYWORDS

- Perioperative • Neurosurgery • Analgesia • Craniotomy • Spine • Opioid • NSAID

KEY POINTS

- A multimodal approach to analgesia using various drugs and techniques is used to provide superior analgesia with minimum side effects.
- In addition to opioids, several classes of drugs are currently available or under investigation for use as adjuvants or alternative therapies.

The perioperative management of pain in neurosurgical patients is a controversial topic with management decisions based mainly on reports of anecdotal experiences. There is no consensus regarding the standardization of pain control in this patient population. The small number of evidence-based reports and conflicting conclusions found in the literature has resulted in inconsistent practice and, in many cases, suboptimal care.

In the last decade, improved awareness and advances in the practice of pain management have resulted in the implementation of diverse techniques to achieve adequate analgesia in this undertreated group of patients. This progress has led to an increased number and quality of studies and clinical trials to define optimal treatment approaches to prevent and treat pain in the neurosurgical patient.

This article provides information about the various techniques and approaches, based on the latest research and clinical trials conducted in this patient population. The physiology of pain in patients undergoing brain or spine surgery, the different modalities for pain control, and the diverse choice of drugs, with their associated risks and benefits, are reviewed.

---

[a] Department of Anesthesiology, State University of New York, Downstate Medical Center, 450 Clarkson Avenue, Box 6, Brooklyn, New York 11203, USA; [b] Department of Anesthesiology, University of Puerto Rico, Medical Sciences Campus, Anesthesiologia RCM, Suite 989, Edif Principal Ciencias Medicas, San Juan, Puerto Rico 00936-5067
* Corresponding author.
E-mail address: lawrence.lai@downstate.edu

Anesthesiology Clin 30 (2012) 347–367
doi:10.1016/j.anclin.2012.05.004
1932-2275/12/$ – see front matter © 2012 Elsevier Inc. All rights reserved.

UNDERTREATMENT OF PAIN IN NEUROSURGICAL PATIENTS: CAUSES AND CONSEQUENCES

Pain is a complex syndrome causing emotional and physical distress, which results in adverse physiologic impact to several organ systems (**Table 1**), ultimately affecting patient recovery and general well-being. There is evidence that pain after neurosurgical procedures is more severe than expected,[1,2] which may result in undertreatment by the perioperative team. Recent studies describe pain after craniotomy as moderate to severe and inadequately treated in approximately 50% of patients.[3–7] Postoperative pain management in patients having craniotomy is a challenge to the acute pain service provider. Because neurosurgical patients require frequent neurologic examinations, typical postoperative opioid therapy for analgesia is often inappropriate. Aggressive postoperative analgesia management may result in an unintended risk of producing an overly sedated patient, which could mask new neurologic deficits. The need to detect any change in mental status in a timely fashion may overshadow the timely treatment of pain. In addition, some neurosurgical patients may not be able to effectively communicate their need for analgesics because of altered mental status or neurologic deficits. The dilemma for the acute pain service providers is that inadequate analgesia may lead to agitation, hypertension, shivering, and vomiting, which may increase the risk of intracranial bleeding or other neurologic complications.[3]

In patients undergoing spine procedures, pain is often a source of significant preoperative distress. Most of these patients have become so-called chronic pain patients, requiring high, sometimes massive, doses of narcotics to achieve satisfactory analgesia. Postoperative pain management for these patients can be problematic if a one-dimensional approach for pain control is used. For example, if opioids are the sole agent administered, caregivers may be reluctant to order the high doses needed to achieve analgesia because of a fear of respiratory depression or other side effects.

Table 1 Physiologic sequelae of pain	
Organ System Response to Pain	
Respiratory	Increased skeletal muscle tension Decreased total lung compliance
Endocrine	Increased adrenocorticotropic hormone, cortisol, glucagon, epinephrine, aldosterone, antidiuretic hormone, catecholamines, and angiotensin II Decreased insulin and testosterone
Cardiovascular	Increased myocardial work (mediated by catecholamines, angiotensin II)
Immunologic	Lymphopenia Depression of reticuloendothelial system Leukocytosis Reduced killer T-cell cytotoxicity
Coagulation effects	Increased platelet adhesiveness Diminished fibrinolysis Activation of coagulation cascade
Gastrointestinal	Increased sphincter tone Decreased smooth muscle tone
Genitourinary	Increased sphincter tone Decreased smooth muscle tone

Data from Lubenow TR, Ivankovich AD, Barkin RL. Management of acute postoperative pain. In: Barash PG, Cullen BF, Stoelting RK, editors. Clinical anesthesia. 5th edition. Philadelphia: Lippincott Williams & Wilkins; 2006. p. 1411.

The implementation of a multimodal approach to manage pain is more often required in this patient population than in non–opioid-dependent patients.

PHYSIOLOGY OF PAIN

Pain, as defined by the International Association for the Study of Pain, is an unpleasant sensory and emotional experience associated with actual or potential tissue damage, or described in terms of such damage or both. It is an individual experience, with unique properties varying from patient to patient. The best way to assess whether a patient has pain and to what degree is simple: ask them. Because it is a subjective perception, the reliance on more physiologic objective measures, like changes in heart rate and blood pressure, or the absence of such, does not necessarily translate into adequate treatment.

Pain is sensed by nociceptors, free nerve endings located in the skin, muscles, joints, mucosa, and in visceral organs. Mechanical nociceptors respond to stimuli, such as sharp, pricking pain, and are supplied by myelinated A δ afferent nerve fibers. These are fast conducting, and possess a low threshold for activation. Polymodal nociceptors respond to high-intensity mechanical or chemical stimuli, and cold-hot stimuli, and are supplied by unmyelinated, slow C fibers.

Tissue injury triggers the release of inflammatory mediators, substance P, and calcitonin gene-related peptides, inducing vasodilatation, plasma extravasation at the site of injury, and activation of nociceptors.[8] Impulses generated at these peripheral receptors travel by the primary afferent neurons to the dorsal horn of the spinal cord. At this site, integration of peripheral nociceptive and descending modulatory input occurs, and synapsis with wide-dynamic-range second-order neurons occurs. First-order neurons also communicate with the cell bodies of the sympathetic nervous system and ventral motor nuclei, either directly or through internuncial neurons.[9] The second-order neurons transmit pain, temperature, and light touch to the central nervous system. They synapse at the thalamus, where third-order neurons relay information to the somatosensory cortex. Along the way to the thalamus, they also send axonal branches in the regions of the reticular formation, nucleus raphe magnus, periaqueductal gray, and other areas in the brainstem. Substance P, g-aminobutyric acid, glycine, dopamine, serotonin, somatostatin, norepinephrine, enkephalin, bradykinin, histamine, prostaglandins, L-glutamate, aspartate, corticotrophin-inhibiting peptide, and neuropeptide Y are among the numerous mediators that play a role in the complex modulation of nociceptive stimuli occurring peripherally and centrally, and, as such, provide potential targets for pharmacologic intervention.

Pain experienced by patients after craniotomy seems to be of somatic origin, most likely involving the scalp, pericranial muscles, and soft tissue, and from manipulation of the dura mater.[4,10] There is a strong correlation between the site of the surgical wound and the source of pain experienced by patients, with the subtemporal and suboccipital surgical routes yielding the highest incidence of postoperative pain.[4]

The scalp receives its innervations from branches originating at the cervical plexus and the trigeminal nerve. The anterior scalp is innervated by the supraorbital and supratrochlear nerves, divisions of the frontal nerve (ophthalmic division of the trigeminal nerve). The temporal scalp region is supplied by the zygomaticotemporal (maxillary division of the trigeminal nerve), temporomandibular, and auriculotemporal nerves (mandibular division of the trigeminal nerve). The occipital scalp region receives its sensory innervations from nerves originating in the cervical plexus: the greater auricular and the greater, lesser, and least occipital nerves. The dura mater is innervated by nerves that accompany the meningeal arteries.

METHODS OF ANALGESIC DELIVERY FOR POSTOPERATIVE PAIN AFTER CRANIOTOMY
Regional Analgesia

Scalp block

The scalp block, often performed before the insertion of cranial pins into the perios-teum in patients undergoing awake craniotomy procedures, has also been studied as an adjunct for treating pain after craniotomies (**Fig. 1**). It has been shown to be effective in providing transitional analgesia, similar to that of intravenous (IV) morphine, in the immediate postoperative period following a remifentanil-based anesthetic.[11] Scalp blocks decrease the amount of rescue pain medication requests, increase the time between the end of surgery and the first request for postoperative analgesics, and lower pain score values in the early postoperative period.[12] Lower pain scores lasting up to 48 hours have been described, and a preemptive analgesic mechanism has been hypothesized.[10] The technique, as described and modified by Pinosky and colleagues,[13] involves the injection of local anesthetic through the whole thickness of the scalp, onto the outer margin of the skull, in an area from the postauricular region, through the operative preauricular temporal site, and then crossing the glabella up to the preauricular and postauricular regions of the contralateral sites. Great care must be exercised at the preauricular site to avoid injection into the temporalis artery and to stay above the zygomatic arch, avoiding undesired anesthesia of the facial nerve. The choice of local anesthetic can be made by individual preference or availability. In general, bupivacaine 0.5% with epinephrine 1:200,000 is recommended because it is long acting. As always indicated, the total dose administered must be less than the recommended maximum dose for patient weight, and intravascular injection must be avoided. Because of the vascular nature of the scalp, it is common to observe cardiovascular evidence of epinephrine absorption following this block. Pharmacoki-netic studies on plasma levels after local anesthetic scalp infiltration suggest that systemic absorption occurs within minutes and in amounts of more than 50% of the infiltrated dose.[14,15] A maximum of 225 mg of ropivacaine with or without epinephrine is recommended.[14,15]

The major advantage of using scalp blocks is that they provide transitional analgesia without compromising neurologic examination. They do not affect the patient's mental status (except from the effects of systemic absorption of local anesthetic) or motor or sensory function, and provide ideal conditions for postoperative neurologic

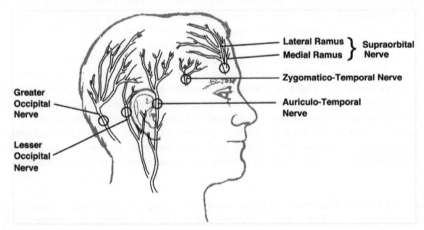

Fig. 1. Cutaneous nerves providing sensory innervation to the scalp. Open circles designate the points at which the nerves can be blocked most easily with local anesthetic injections.

assessment. The scalp block can be performed after skin closure, using the technique described previously, in patients undergoing supratentorial craniotomies with minimal side effects and a good safety profile.[10–13]

Wound infiltration

Preincision local anesthetic scalp infiltration is often used in neurosurgical practice to blunt the systemic responses to craniotomy and to minimize bleeding with skin incision (because of the epinephrine used with the local anesthetic). There is insufficient evidence either supporting or discouraging the use of local anesthetic wound infiltration after craniotomy as a means to improve postoperative analgesia, reduce opioid requirements, or reduce time to first pain medication request. Law-Koune and colleagues[16] studied wound infiltration with either 0.375% bupivacaine with epinephrine or 0.75% ropivacaine after skin closure, and found that both can decrease the morphine requirements during the first 2 postoperative hours, but with no significant effect on visual analogue scale (VAS) scores compared with placebo. A study using preincision wound infiltration of bupivacaine 0.25% showed no benefit in postoperative pain relief or decrease in postoperative analgesic requirements.[17]

Although more research is warranted, wound incision site infiltration does not seem to be as effective as the scalp block in improving postcraniotomy pain scores. In general, preincisional scalp infiltration should not be expected to provide postoperative analgesia in patients having craniotomy. However, local anesthetic wound infiltration after skin closure may prove beneficial in providing some transitional pain control in the immediate postoperative period.

Parenteral opioids

Parenteral opioids remain the cornerstone for managing moderate to severe pain, especially in the postoperative period after major surgery. The mechanism of action of opioids involves the stimulation of m and k receptors located centrally (brainstem, hypothalamus, limbic system, substantia gelatinosa of the spinal cord) and peripherally (gastrointestinal tract, peripheral histamine receptors). Activation of opioid receptors leads to inhibition of voltage-gated calcium channels and an increase in potassium influx, causing a reduction in neuronal excitability. More broadly, opioids inhibit the transmission of painful stimuli from the afferent first neuron to the second neuron at the dorsal horn of the spinal cord, both by presynaptic and postsynaptic mechanisms. They also activate the descending inhibitory pathways that go from the midbrain, rostral ventromedial medulla, ending in the dorsal horn of the spinal cord. There has also been evidence suggesting a peripheral action of opioids involving immune cells located at the inflammation site.[18]

Although intermittent systemic administration of opioids was a standard method for postoperative analgesia in the past, this strategy may result in periods of oversedation (peak opiate effect) followed by periods of inadequate analgesia (through opiate effect). Other methods, like patient-controlled analgesia (PCA) with morphine or oxycodone, have also been used effectively in patients after craniotomy.[19,20] Although sufficient to achieve adequate analgesia, opioids have side effects that can adversely affect patients' recovery from surgery. For example, nausea, vomiting, decreased gastrointestinal motility leading to constipation, pruritus, respiratory depression, and oversedation can all result in the need for additional pharmacologic intervention, and eventually an increased length of inpatient hospital stay. Jellish[19] concluded that, although the use of morphine PCA does not increase postoperative nausea and vomiting (PONV), the incidence of PONV was not reduced by the inclusion of ondansetron in the PCA.

The occurrence of postoperative sedation is especially troubling because of the need for frequent postoperative neurologic examinations. Concern about producing excessive postoperative sedation may lead to the clinician providing high-risk patients with inadequate analgesia. Some side effects caused by opioids are mediated primarily by receptors located in the periphery (nausea, vomiting, pruritus). These dose-dependent side effects, although not as problematic as respiratory depression and sedation, can limit the use of high-dose opioids. Peripheral opioid antagonists, such as nalmefene, have been shown to decrease significantly the need for anti-emetics and antipruritic medications in patients receiving IV morphine PCA.

Nalbuphine, an opioid agonist-antagonist, has been studied for postoperative pain control after supratentorial craniotomy by Verchere and colleagues.[3] They found 0.15 mg/kg to be effective in maintaining VAS score less than 30 mm when used in combination with paracetamol. Sudheer and colleagues[21] randomly allocated 60 patients having craniotomy to receive morphine PCA, tramadol PCA, or codeine 60 mg intramuscularly. There were no differences in arterial carbon dioxide tension or sedation between groups at any time, and morphine produced significantly better analgesia than tramadol and codeine. Recently, Morad and colleagues[22] randomized 64 patients having craniotomy to IV fentanyl PCA or fentanyl as needed. They found that fentanyl PCA more effectively treated supratentorial intracranial surgery pain than as-needed fentanyl, and the PCA group did not experience any untoward events related to the self-administration of opioids.

Nonsteroidal antiinflammatory drugs

These drugs can be divided into arylpropionic acids (ibuprofen, naproxen, flurbiprofen, ketoprofen); indole acetic acids (indomethacin, etodolac); heteroaryl acetic acids (diclofenac, ketorolac); enolic acids (piroxicam, phenylbutazone); and alkanones (nabumetone). Their mechanism of action involves the reversible, nonselective inhibition of the cyclooxygenase (COX) enzymes COX-1 and COX-2. COX acts on arachidonic acid to initiate a chain of reactions that result in the synthesis of prostaglandins (PGs; eg, PGD_2, PGE_2, PGI_2 [prostacyclin], PGF_2) and thromboxane. COX-1 is expressed constitutively in the brain and spinal cord. Among its various physiologic functions, it protects the gastric mucosa and provides vascular hemostasis. COX-2, induced by growth factors, cytokines, and tumor promoters, seems to be the dominant source of prostaglandins during inflammation and chronic disease. COX-2 enzyme has also been shown to be constitutively expressed in the brain and spinal cord with further upregulation after persistent noxious stimuli.[23] Analgesia is achieved by central and peripheral inhibition of prostaglandin-mediated amplification of chemical and mechanical irritants on the sensory pathways. There is also evidence supporting a spinal analgesic mechanism of nonsteroidal antiinflammatory drugs (NSAIDs).[23]

Although NSAIDs are effective in providing analgesia, they can lead to platelet dysfunction and increased bleeding times, which may be devastating in patients having neurosurgery.[1] They have limited use in the immediate postoperative period, especially in cases in which patients are at increased risk for bleeding, such as aneurysm repair, arteriovenous malformation resection, and hematoma evacuations. Hence, this may account for there being only 1 study investigating ketorolac, the only injectable option in the United States, in patients after craniotomy. Na and colleagues[24] randomly assigned 106 patients having craniotomy to either receive fentanyl and IV ketorolac PCA or intermittent fentanyl and ketorolac as needed. IV PCA with fentanyl and ketorolac was the more effective analgesic technique, without adverse events, than the intermittent administration of analgesics.

COX-2 inhibitors (rofecoxib, celecoxib, meloxicam, nimesulide) selectively inhibit the COX-2 enzyme, effectively achieving antiinflammatory and analgesic results, but sparing the side effects of nonselective COX inhibitors, such as prolonged postoperative bleeding, and gastrointestinal bleeding. They also spare the nausea, vomiting, respiratory depression, and sedation seen with opioid analgesics. Renal dysfunction characterized by sodium retention and decreased glomerular filtration rate warrants similar precautions to those followed with traditional NSAIDs.[25]

There has been concern about the risk of cardiovascular disease among patients receiving chronic COX-2 inhibitor therapy. This risk was first noted after rofecoxib caused a 4-fold increase in the incidence of myocardial infarction compared with naproxen in the Vioxx Gastrointestinal Outcomes Research trial. It seems that inhibition of prostacyclin synthesis, but not thromboxane synthesis, by these agents shifts the coagulation-anticoagulation balance toward the procoagulant effect of thromboxane. This study was performed on patients receiving the medication for a prolonged period of time (more than 18 months), leaving unanswered the question about COX-2 inhibitor safety for short-term use, as is the case in postoperative pain control. However, rofecoxib was voluntarily withdrawn from the worldwide market in 2004 and is no longer available. This withdrawal has led to the investigation of parecoxib, which is available in Europe but not approved by the US Food and Drug Administration (FDA) since 2005. However, Jones and colleagues[26] found only limited evidence to support parecoxib as an analgesic after craniotomy, and Williams and colleagues[27] found no added benefit of IV parecoxib. In both studies, only a single dose of parecoxib 40 mg was given, because of the coagulopathic concerns mentioned earlier.

Paracetamol (acetaminophen): N-acetyl-p-aminophenol

The analgesic mechanism of N-acetyl-p-aminophenol (acetaminophen) involves the central inhibition of COXs, with weak peripheral effects. It is nevertheless devoid of the side effects commonly observed with the use of NSAIDs.[28] Verchere and colleagues[3] studied the use of acetaminophen for postoperative pain after supratentorial craniotomy and concluded that acetaminophen alone (30 mg/kg IV 1 hour before the end of surgery and every 6 hours thereafter) is not sufficient to provide adequate analgesia for this kind of surgery. IV acetaminophen has recently become available in the United States for clinical use. When nalbuphine or tramadol were added to this regimen, VAS levels of less than 30 mm were achieved and maintained in the immediate postoperative period. Acetaminophen's opioid-sparing effect has not proved to be significant.[28]

Tramadol

Tramadol is a weak μ-opioid receptor agonist that releases serotonin and inhibits the reuptake of norepinephrine. It is available in Europe as an IV medication, but only available as an oral tablet in the United States. Vadivelu and colleagues[29] randomized 50 patients having craniotomy to receive IV tramadol with diclofenac or tramadol plus paracetamol. They concluded that the diclofenac-tramadol combination provided better pain relief than paracetamol-tramadol, and that neither combination caused sedation or respiratory depression after craniotomy. For the common opioid side effects of nausea and vomiting, Rahimi and colleagues[1] found that tramadol in addition to narcotics with acetaminophen may provide better pain control and decrease the side effects associated with narcotics. However, Verchere and colleagues[3] and Sudheer and colleagues[21] both found that the incidence of PONV was greater with the addition of tramadol.

α-2 Adrenergic agonists

The use of α-2 adrenergic agonists for pain management has gained popularity in recent years. Dexmedetomidine, a potent and highly selective α-2 agonist in presynaptic neurons in the spinal cord dorsal horn, provides sedation and analgesia without respiratory depression.[30] Clinical applications of dexmedetomidine for several procedures, such as awake craniotomy, preoperative sedation of patients with aneurysmal subarachnoid hemorrhage, and fiberoptic tracheal intubation, have been described.[31–33] The administration of dexmedetomidine before the completion of major inpatient surgical procedures has been associated with opioid-sparing effects, reducing morphine requirements by as much as 60%.[34] Another study has shown a potential preemptive analgesic effect.[35]

Further research with this interesting class of drugs is needed to assess the adequacy of pain control versus side effects following craniotomy. The ability to bring a patient from sedation to arousal immediately for neurologic examinations in the postanesthesia care unit is invaluable. This class of drugs may prove helpful in providing transitional analgesia from surgical anesthesia to the postanesthesia care unit.

N-methyl-D-aspartate receptor antagonists

N-methyl-D-aspartate antagonists are administered as adjuvant pain management drugs. N-methyl-D-aspartate receptors are ligand-gated ion channels that permit the passage of calcium, sodium, and potassium into the cell. These receptors are activated by glycine and glutamate and do not open at resting membrane potentials. Glutamate, a major excitatory neurotransmitter in the central nervous system, has a significant role in the modulation of pain at the level of the spinal cord, especially in the sensitization of nociceptors after exposure to noxious stimuli, increasing the magnitude and duration of neurogenic responses to pain, even after the initial peripheral input is stopped.[36] These agents do not possess intrinsic analgesic properties, but carry out their antinociceptive effects by inhibiting central sensitization to painful stimuli.

Low-dose ketamine (as an IV bolus, or infusion) and dextromethorphan by oral or intramuscular (IM) route have been studied as part of a multimodal pain management approach as adjuvants to opioid therapy and preemptive analgesics. The administration of IM dextromethorphan, 120 mg, 30 minutes before incision in patients undergoing abdominal surgery resulted in a longer time to the first request for analgesic medication in the immediate postoperative period, and a decrease in the amount of IV PCA opioid use with less incidence of hypoxemia.[37] In a systematic qualitative review of the literature by McCartney and colleagues,[38] the effect of preoperative N-methyl-D-aspartate antagonists on reducing postoperative pain and analgesic consumption beyond the clinical duration of action of the target drug was reviewed. Dextromethorphan and ketamine had significant immediate and preventive analgesic benefits in 67% and 58%, respectively, of studies reviewed. The use of ketamine in patients after craniotomy may be precluded by the undesirable increase in intracranial pressure that can be seen after administration of this drug. However, dextromethorphan when used as described by Helmy[37] may be a valuable adjuvant in the multimodal approach to pain management after craniotomy.

Other Analgesic Adjuvants and Advances in Pharmacotherapy

Gabapentin

Gabapentin is an anticonvulsant drug that has analgesic properties for acute postoperative pain. Gabapentin does not bind to γ-aminobutyric acid receptors, but to the α-2 δ subunit of the presynaptic voltage-gated calcium channels.[39] Ture and colleagues[39] found that addition of gabapentin to morphine PCA for patients undergoing craniotomy for supratentorial tumor resection was effective for prevention of acute postoperative pain. Even though it decreased analgesic consumption after surgery, gabapentin may lead to side effects such as delayed tracheal extubation and increased sedation.

Fentanyl iontophoretic transdermal system
Fentanyl iontophoretic transdermal (ITS) is a non–FDA-approved, needle-free, pre-programmed drug-delivery system that uses iontophoretic technology to deliver drug through the skin by application of a low-intensity electrical field.[29] In non-neurosurgical patients, Panchal and colleagues[40] found that fentanyl ITS was associated with a significantly lower incidence of analgesic gaps than morphine IV PCA. Adverse events associated with fentanyl ITS were similar to those reported with IV opioid administration. Although fentanyl ITS may decrease the risk of PCA programming errors, it is currently not being produced because of technical problems.

Local anesthetic delivery systems
To provide longer-lasting pain relief in scalp blocks, wound infiltrations, and epidural or intrathecal (IT) injections, liposome or polymer encapsulation of local anesthetics are being developed. Liposomes are microscopic phospholipid-bilayered vesicles that are biocompatible, biodegradable, and nonimmumnogenic.[29] Many local anesthetics have been loaded in liposomes or biodegradable polymer microspheres, and have the potential to decrease postoperative analgesic requirements.

However, these novel delivery systems are still not available because of problems such as shelf life, aggregation, leakage, and toxicity.[41]

Postoperative Pain Management After Spine Surgery

Considerations for postoperative pain management after spine surgery
Hundreds of thousands of spine surgeries are performed in the United States each year, and patients having spine surgery report high-severity postoperative pain.[42,43] Several studies have investigated risk factors for postoperative pain after spine surgery. These factors include psychological, social profile, and preoperative pain severity.[44–47] The use of minimally invasive neurosurgical techniques may decrease the occurrence of significant postoperative pain,[48,49] but these techniques are not widely performed. The typical patient having spine surgery has endured back pain chronically, with many of them on long-term pharmacologic analgesic therapy, sometimes requiring large doses of analgesics and narcotics. Patients presenting to the operating room for surgical revision after the so-called 'failed-back syndrome' may be challenging to provide with adequate postoperative analgesia because of high baseline opiate requirements and significant anxiety for having to go through the perioperative experience once again. In addition, these patients require frequent neurologic examinations to assess for any possible postoperative deterioration that may require immediate intervention. Patient cooperation and awareness are vital to ensure a positive surgical outcome.

It is not sufficient to provide pain relief that is adequate for patients only at rest. The importance of early ambulation on surgical outcomes, nonsurgical complications, and hospital length of stay is well known. Time to ambulation is frequently used when evaluating the adequacy of analgesia and is an important milestone on the way to postsurgical recovery. To facilitate early ambulation, adequate analgesia and patient safety are essential. With these considerations in mind, this article discusses the characteristics of pain after spine surgery and the various techniques available to provide postoperative analgesia.

Characteristics of back pain

A detailed description of the causes, diagnosis, and management of back pain, acute or chronic, in the perioperative setting may be obtained.[50–52] In brief, the sensation of back pain can originate in different structures, mediated by nociceptors and mechanoreceptors capable of eliciting a painful sensation, including the vertebrae, intervertebral disk, dura and nerve root sleeves, facet joint capsules, muscles, ligaments, and fascia. Innervation is by the posterior rami of the spinal nerve roots, which are linked to the sympathetic and parasympathetic nerves, and to the major somatic and motor nerves innervating the upper extremities (cervical spine), the thorax (thoracic spine), abdomen, pelvis, and the lower extremities (lumbar spine). Inflammation in these structures or mechanical compression of the nerves in this area causes pain. Given this interconnectivity, the occurrence of referred pain is common in these patients. Klimek and colleagues[44] observed that referred pain exceeded local and diffuse pain in the preoperative period in patients scheduled for spine surgery. After the surgery, pain was mostly local, and, in those patients in whom referred pain persisted, VAS scores were higher. Referred pain is mostly neuropathic pain, which does not respond well to conventional pain therapy, but is often relieved by treatment with anticonvulsants and antidepressant medications.[53–55]

There seems to be no significant difference in the severity of pain between cervical, thoracic, and lumbar spine surgeries.[44,56] Postoperative pain after spinal surgeries is proportional to the number of vertebrae included in the operation and to its invasiveness.[57]

METHODS OF PAIN MANAGEMENT AFTER SPINE SURGERY
Parenteral Administration

Opioids

Opioids have been used in combination with other analgesics or alone, sometimes with good results, sometimes with less than optimal results. Opioids are excellent drugs for pain control, but the dose is often not optimized because of fear of sedation and respiratory depression, or because patients do not tolerate the doses required for adequate analgesia without experiencing unpleasant side effects. Although in the past opioids were often administered as needed, superior postoperative analgesia occurs in patients treated with IV opioid PCA than with intermittent IM opioid administration.[58] Those who had previously received IM injections also reported that PCA was easy to use and provided better analgesia.[59] Although PCA is the preferred method for postoperative opioid-based analgesia, an opioid-only regimen can have many side effects and should not be seen as the only choice to achieve an appropriate level of analgesia. A multidrug approach may lead to better patient satisfaction and decreased doses of opioids (opioid-sparing effect), which should result in a decreased risk of side effects. This benefit was shown by Jirarattanaphochai and colleagues[60,61] when they found that administration of parecoxib with morphine PCA after lumbar spine surgery resulted in a reduction in opioid requirement and lower pain scores. Methadone has also been studied only once in this setting, but its benefits were considerable and extended well into the postoperative period.[61] In this study, administration of intraoperative methadone (0.2 mg/kg) compared with a continuous sufentanil infusion (0.25 μg/kg/h after a loading dose of 0.75 μg/kg) improved postoperative pain control for patients undergoing complex spine surgery.[61]

NSAIDs

Reports from several studies promote the use of NSAIDs in the perioperative period. Different routes of administration, different dosing regimens, and different drugs within this group have been studied. Some research has shown that the use of NSAIDs as the sole medication for pain control after spine surgery is not sufficient to provide adequate analgesia[62] but, when combined with opioids, the combination gives better results than either one alone.[63–66] In a systematic review of analgesia after spine surgery, Sharma and colleagues[67] concluded that, among the NSAIDs, parecoxib and the combination of paracetamol and ketoprofen were most effective in decreasing pain after spine surgery, as well as decreasing morphine consumption. Celecoxib, ibuprofen, and diclofenac suppositories were not found to be effective in reducing postoperative pain at 24 and 48 hours.[67] None of the studies reported bleeding complications.

Ketorolac, given intramuscularly or intravenously, is the most investigated drug among the NSAIDs. It has good analgesic potency and its opioid-sparing capacity has been well documented.[62–66] Because its onset of action is not immediate (about 30–60 minutes after IM injection), its use in severe acute pain in the postoperative period is best as an adjuvant to opioids, rather than as a sole agent. There is also a concern regarding the deleterious effects of NSAIDs on bone healing, because of the importance of PGE_2 in the early stages of bone healing.[68] High-dose (120–240 mg/d), but not low-dose, ketorolac has been associated with nonunion following spine fusion surgery.[69,70] Low-dose ketorolac, in the absence of contraindications, may be a safe and effective adjuvant to an opioid-based regimen for acute postoperative pain management after spine surgery.

Steroids

A small number of studies have assessed the use of IV corticosteroids to reduce postoperative pain. Steroids are antiinflammatory drugs that inhibit phospholipase A_2, but another mechanism of action involving a decrease in the expression of substance P at the dorsal root ganglion has been hypothesized.[71] The threshold of at least 1 type of peripheral nociceptors is lowered by certain endogenous chemicals liberated during the inflammatory process.[72] Some patients may still complain of radicular referred pain after the surgery, probably associated with nerve root inflammation. On that basis, the effect of IV dexamethasone after skin incision on postoperative pain has been studied. Intraoperative IV injection of 40 mg dexamethasone reduces postoperative radicular leg pain and narcotic use in patients after single-level herniated lumbar disk surgery.[73,74] Likewise, a lower dose of dexamethasone (10 mg IV during surgery) helped to reduce analgesic requirements in patients undergoing lumbar, but not cervical, diskectomy.[74] Larger trials are needed to confirm or refute these findings.

Acetaminophen

Propacetamol, an injectable prodrug of acetaminophen, has been studied to determine its analgesic efficacy and opioid-sparing effects in the postoperative period.[75,76] Its mechanism of action may involve centrally and peripherally located sites,[77,78] possibly involving inhibition of prostaglandins[79] and activation of descending serotoninergic inhibitory pathways.[80] In patients in whom NSAIDs may be contraindicated or if there is concern about postoperative hemostasis, paracetamol may be a useful alternative as an adjunct to opioid therapy. However, paracetamol alone was not effective in reducing postoperative pain at 48 hours.[81]

COX-2 inhibitors

Reports of adverse effects on bone healing by NSAIDs led to the investigation of the effects by COX-2 inhibitors on bone healing. COX-2–dependent PGE_2 produced at the early stage of bone healing is a prerequisite for efficient skeletal repair.[68] A study on healing bone fractures showed a decrease in osteogenesis potential after the cells were treated with celecoxib.[82] Reuben[69,83] studied the efficacy of the short-term use of COX-2 inhibitors for postoperative pain, opioid-sparing properties, and the effects on bone healing after spine fusion surgery. He concluded that the perioperative administration of celecoxib, given 1 hour before the induction of anesthesia and every 12 hours after surgery for the first 5 postoperative days, resulted in a significant reduction in postoperative pain and opioid use following spine fusion surgery. In addition, short-term administration had no apparent effect on the rate of nonunion. As mentioned earlier, these conflicting results from 2 different studies, make it difficult to formulate guidelines in the treatment of postoperative pain.

Similar to N-acetyl-p-aminophenol, COX-2 inhibitors do not affect platelets and bleeding time as do NSAIDs. These drugs can be used as alternatives for pain management in patients in whom hemostasis is an issue. However, until more evidence is gathered on long-term effects, their use remains controversial in surgeries involving bone healing because of the potential for adverse effects.

N-methyl-D-aspartate receptor antagonists

Ketamine has shown analgesic effects and decreased opioid consumption in both opioid-dependent and opioid-naive patients, although at times the duration of effect was limited.[67] Trials reported that a combination of ketamine and opioid (morphine or remifentanil) provides better postoperative pain relief than either drug alone and results in less cumulative morphine consumption.[67,84] A single study of dextromethorphan did not show any of these benefits.[85]

Gabapentinoids

Although gabapentin did not improve analgesia overall, it was effective in decreasing 24-hour cumulative opioid consumption in multiple trials.[86–88] Despite this, the acceptable adverse effect profile of gabapentin suggests that its use could be considered in this population.[67]

Neuraxial administration: IT

Opioids IT opioids are extensively used for the management of acute pain in the perioperative period. The pharmacokinetics of different IT administered opioids has been extensively studied.[89] Lipophilic opioids, such as fentanyl, alfentanil, and sufentanil, have a faster onset of action but shorter duration of action (2–4 hours) compared with morphine (18–24 hours with a delayed onset of analgesia). Achieving adequate analgesia from IT opioids depends on the rate and extent to which opioids distribute from the cerebrospinal fluid to opioid receptors in the spinal cord dorsal horn as opposed to competing extraspinal sites. Because of its extended duration of action and its lower incidence of neurotoxicity, preservative-free morphine could be the drug of choice if the use of an IT opioid is intended for pain relief in the postoperative period. The same side effect profile that accompanies the IV injection of morphine applies to IT administration. Nausea, vomiting, pruritus, urinary retention (up to 35% incidence), and respiratory depression (early and delayed) can be seen in most patients who receive doses in excess of 0.3 mg. The need for monitoring for oversedation and respiratory depression assumes that the patient has a hospital stay of at least 24 hours after administration of IT morphine. Compared with the more lipophilic opioids, this drug is not recommended for ambulatory procedures. In addition, prolonged continuous infusion of drug through an IT catheter is not recommended because of the risk of cauda equina syndrome.[90]

Studies evaluating the administration of IT morphine after spine surgery are limited. Urban and colleagues[91] studied the use of IT morphine (20 mg/kg) for postoperative analgesia after elective multilevel spine fusion surgery with good results. He reported that patients were comfortable immediately after surgery, remained pain free for a longer period, and required significantly less additional narcotic. Several studies also investigated the use of IT morphine as a single bolus, with doses ranging from 2 to 20 mg/kg, for pain relief after anterior or posterior spine fusion.[92,93] Postoperative analgesia was prolonged up to 36 hours after surgery, and there was a decrease in the need for supplemental analgesia. IT opioids can be easily administered by the surgeon when the thecal sac is exposed. Although this therapy provides effective analgesia, it is also associated with respiratory depression following spine surgery.[94]

Local anesthetics
Experience with the IT administration of local anesthetics for postoperative pain management is mostly in combination with opioids or other adjuvants. Various studies have analyzed with favorable results the postoperative continuous IT administration of bupivacaine and morphine in the treatment of pain after selective dorsal rhizotomy.[95,96] Doses of up to 0.6 mg/kg/h of morphine with bupivacaine (40 mg/kg/h) have been associated with good analgesic effect, a decrease in the need for parenteral narcotics, and minimum side effects.

Other agents
Other adjuncts to IT-administered local anesthetics have been studied mainly for orthopedic procedures. The addition of drugs like clonidine[97] and neostigmine[98] to IT local anesthetics has been shown to prolong sensory and motor block. Prolonged block is not desirable in the early postoperative period after spine surgery, because of the need to assess neurologic function of the lower extremities. Clinical studies evaluating the use for these medications in conjunction with IT morphine are needed to determine whether their known analgesic effects result in a decrease in opioid requirements and better pain scores after spine surgery. One study found that combining IT morphine (250 mg) with IT clonidine (25 or 75 mg) reduced the need for supplemental analgesics and improved pain control after total knee arthroplasty,[99] and similar results were also seen in a more recent study of IT neostigmine during lumbar disc surgery.[100]

Studies in experimental animals suggest that spinally administered ketorolac may be useful in treating postoperative pain caused by its inhibition of COX-1 enzyme.[101,102] The safety profile has been studied for up to 6 months after administration; no significant complications have been reported.[103] However, the study also reports that the IT administration of selective COX-2 inhibitors has minimal analgesic effects. To date, there are no human studies assessing the efficacy of these drugs after IT administration.

Neuraxial Administration: Epidural

Opioids, local anesthetics, and the combination of both
There are several clinical trials studying the efficacy and safety of epidural administration of drugs for postoperative pain control following different procedures. Compared with IT administration, epidural opioids have a better safety margin and a lower incidence of dose-dependent respiratory depression and urinary retention. There is controversy as to whether this more invasive procedure is superior to the standard IV or IM route after spine surgery.

Opioids affect the modulation of nociceptive input mainly by acting on receptors in the dorsal horn without producing motor or sympathetic blockade. Because of this, opioids are potentially useful in the treatment of patients having spine surgery in whom postoperative motor and sensory function are closely monitored. Compared with IM opioids, epidural opioids produce longer-lasting analgesia with smaller doses. A review of the literature reveals that the benefits of administering opioid-only solutions may not outweigh the risks associated with this procedure.[104] Side effects including nausea, vomiting, and pruritus are also commonly seen with this technique. The use of local anesthetic-only solutions also has disadvantages. The dose required for adequate analgesia can produce a motor block, interfering with lower extremity neurologic examination, and potentially can cause sympathectomy-mediated hypotension. The combination of local anesthetic and opioids may provide more advantages than administering either agent alone. Adding opioids to local anesthetic decreases the amount of local anesthetic and opioid necessary to achieve good results, thereby decreasing the incidence of side effects. It has also been documented that this combination improves the quality of dynamic pain relief[105] compared with opioid-only infusion.

The choice of opioid and local anesthetic varies among different practices. Ropivacaine seems to provide an advantage compared with bupivacaine with respect to safety index and the selectivity of ropivacaine toward sensory rather than motor blockade, although this may be apparent only at the higher dose range. Different techniques for epidural injection have been studied, including single and double catheters, intermittent boluses, patient-controlled epidural analgesia, and continuous infusion of medication. The placement of the epidural catheter during surgery can be done by the surgical team under direct vision with relative ease and high success rate. As with parenteral administration, intermittent bolus administration of epidural opioids may result in patients who are more likely to experience pain and unnecessary suffering, whereas patients being treated with epidural PCA experience overall lower pain scores and decreased side effects.[106] The advantages of epidural opioids and the combination of opioids and local anesthetics include low pain scores,[107,108] decreased parenteral opioid requirements,[109,110] a decrease in the incidence of pulmonary morbidity,[111] and better patient satisfaction. Other studies report that both patient-controlled epidural analgesia and IV PCA are equally effective,[43,110,112] with no difference observed in the epidural groups in time to oral intake of liquids or solids, ambulation, bowel sounds, or length of stay compared with placebo,[112] but a greater incidence of side effects has been reported with the patient-controlled epidural analgesia group.[110] Even more surprising, Sharma and colleagues[67] reviewed 14 trials and found that continuous epidural analgesia with opioid and local anesthetic did not provide significant benefit, and a few studies in which either opioids or local anesthetics were used alone did show benefit. The divergent conclusions can be explained because of the lack of a standardized method of infusion (intermittent bolus vs continuous infusion, vs patient-controlled epidural analgesia with or without baseline infusion) and the different drugs, doses, and combinations used. It is not clear at this time which method is most effective for postoperative analgesia in patients following spine surgery.

Other agents

α-2 Agonists have been used for epidural analgesia as adjuncts to opioids, local anesthetic, or the combination of both to potentiate their action. They produce minimal respiratory depression compared with opioids. Clonidine is effective in the treatment of neuropathic pain, especially when administered in the epidural space,[113] which theoretically makes it a good addition to the management of postoperative pain, because patients who still feel neuropathic, referred pain after surgery tend to have higher VAS scores and are more challenging to manage. In a study by Ekatodramis and colleagues,[114] a double-catheter approach of bupivacaine, fentanyl, and clonidine infusion was used with good results. Jellish and colleagues[115] concluded that epidural clonidine (150 mg), in addition to subcutaneous bupivacaine at the incision site, improved postoperative pain and hemodynamic stability in patients undergoing lower spine procedures. Epidural doses of clonidine greater than 4 mg/kg have been associated with reduced pain by more than 70% and effects lasting for 4 to 5 hours. Bradycardia, hypotension, and sedation were reported as the most common side effects.[116]

Tizanidine and dexmedetomidine have also been studied, but further randomized controlled trials involving spine procedures need to be performed. These agents provide a fast onset of analgesia and may provide a smooth transition between intraoperative anesthesia and epidural infusion of opioids with or without local anesthetics.

Extended-release epidural morphine

A new drug, a single-dose, extended-release epidural morphine (EREM) called DepoDur, has been found to have a duration of action up to 48 hours with long-lasting analgesia in the absence of large systemic concentrations of opioids as well as better patient activity levels.[117] EREM is formulated for a 1-time dose, given epidurally at the lumbar level. As expected, pruritus and respiratory depression were common side effects. DepoDur has only been evaluated in such surgeries as knee arthroplasty and cesarean section, but may be an alternative for the management of postoperative pain in spinal surgery.

SUMMARY

Until recently, perioperative pain management in neurosurgical patients has been inconsistently recognized and inadequately treated. An increased awareness of pain management in general, along with advances in understanding of pain modulation and pathophysiology, has led to improved practice and perioperative care of patients. The greatest challenge to managing neurosurgical patients is the need to assess neurologic function while providing superior analgesia with minimal side effects. To achieve this goal, a multimodal approach to analgesia using various drugs and techniques is used. In addition to opioids, several classes of drugs are currently available or under investigation for use as adjuvants or alternative therapies. There still remains a need to conduct randomized, controlled trials to determine the best combination of drugs or techniques for treating perioperative pain in this patient population. Improved awareness, assessment, and treatment of pain result in better care and overall patient outcome.

REFERENCES

1. Rahimi SY, Vender JR, Macomson SD, et al. Postoperative pain management after craniotomy: evaluation and cost analysis. Neurosurgery 2006;59(4):852–7.
2. Quiney N, Cooper R, Stoneham M, et al. Pain after craniotomy: a time for reappraisal? Br J Neurosurg 1996;10(3):295–9.
3. Verchere E, Grenier B, Mesli A, et al. Postoperative pain management after supratentorial craniotomy. J Neurosurg Anesthesiol 2002;14(2):96–101.
4. De Benedittis G, Lorenzetti A, Migliore M, et al. Postoperative pain in neurosurgery: a pilot study in brain surgery. Neurosurgery 1996;38(3):466–9.

5. Dunbar PJ, Visco E, Lam AM. Craniotomy procedures are associated with less analgesic requirements than other surgical procedures. Anesth Analg 1999;88: 335–40.

6. Stoneham MD, Walters FJ. Post-operative analgesia for craniotomy patients: current attitudes among neuroanaesthetists. Eur J Anaesthesiol 1995;12(6): 571–5.

7. Roberts GC. Post-craniotomy analgesia: current practices in British neurosurgical centres-a survey of post-craniotomy analgesic practices. Eur J Anaesthesiol 2005;22(5):328–32.

8. Julius D, Basbaum AI. Molecular mechanisms of nociception. Nature 2001;413: 203–10.

9. Kerr FW. The structured basis of pain: circulatory and pathway. In: Ng LW, Bonica JJ, editors. Pain, discomfort and humanitarian care. New York: Elsevier; 1980. p. 49.

10. Nguyen A, Girard F, Boudreault D, et al. Scalp nerve blocks decrease the severity of pain after craniotomy. Anesth Analg 2001;93(5):1272–6.

11. Ayoub C, Girard F, Boudreault D, et al. A comparison between scalp nerve block and morphine for transitional analgesia after remifentanil-based anesthesia in neurosurgery. Anesth Analg 2006;103(5):1237–40.

12. Bala I, Gupta B, Bhardwaj N, et al. Effect of scalp block on postoperative pain relief in craniotomy patients. Anaesth Intensive Care 2006;34(2):224–7.

13. Pinosky ML, Fishman RL, Reeves ST, et al. The effect of bupivacaine skull block on the hemodynamic response to craniotomy. Anesth Analg 1996;83:1256–61.

14. Rosenberg PH, Veering BT, Urmey WF. Maximum recommended doses of local anaesthetics: a multifactorial concept. Reg Anesth Pain Med 2004;29:564–75.

15. Costello TG, Cormack JR, Hoy C, et al. Plasma ropivacaine levels following scalp block for awake craniotomy. J Neurosurg Anesthesiol 2004;16:147–50.

16. Law-Koune JD, Szekely B, Fermanian C, et al. Scalp infiltration with bupivacaine plus epinephrine or plain ropivacaine reduces postoperative pain after supratentorial craniotomy. J Neurosurg Anesthesiol 2005;17(3):139–43.

17. Biswas BK, Bithal PK. Preincision 0.25% bupivacaine scalp infiltration and post-craniotomy pain: a randomized double-blind, placebo-controlled study. J Neurosurg Anesthesiol 2003;15(3):234–9.

18. Stein C. The control of pain in peripheral tissue by opioids. N Engl J Med 1995; 332:1685–90.

19. Jellish WS. Morphine/ondansetron PCA for postoperative pain, nausea, and vomiting after skull base surgery. Otolaryngol Head Neck Surg 2006;135(2): 175–81.

20. Stoneham MD, Cooper R, Quiney NF, et al. Pain following craniotomy: a preliminary study comparing PCA morphine with intramuscular codeine phosphate. Anaesthesia 1996;51(12):1176–8.

21. Sudheer PS, Logan SW, Terblanche C, et al. Comparison of the analgesic efficacy and respiratory effects of morphine, tramadol and codeine after craniotomy. Anaesthesia 2007;62:555–60.

22. Morad AH, Winters BD, Yaster M, et al. Efficacy of intravenous patient-controlled analgesia after supratentorial intracranial surgery: a prospective randomized controlled trial. J Neurosurg 2009;111(2):343–50.

23. Svensson CI, Yaksh TL. The spinal phospholipase-cyclooxygenase-prostanoid cascade in nociceptive processing. Annu Rev Pharmacol Toxicol 2002;42: 553–83.

24. Na HS, An SB, Park HP, et al. Intravenous patient-controlled analgesia to manage the postoperative pain in patients undergoing craniotomy. Korean J Anesthesiol 2011;60(1):30–5.
25. Brater DC. Renal effects of cyclooxygenase-2-selective inhibitors. J Pain Symptom Manage 2002;23:S15–20.
26. Jones SJ, Cormack J, Murphy MA, et al. Parecoxib for analgesia after craniotomy. Br J Anaesth 2009;102(1):76–9.
27. Williams DL, Pemberton E, Leslie K. Effect of intravenous parecoxib on postcraniotomy pain. Br J Anaesth 2011;107(3):398–403.
28. Remy C, Marret E, Bonnet F. State of the art of paracetamol in acute pain therapy. Curr Opin Anaesthesiol 2006;19(5):562–5.
29. Vadivelu N, Mitra S, Narayan D. Recent advances in postoperative pain management. Yale J Biol Med 2010;83(1):11–25.
30. Sakaguchi Y, Takahashi S. Dexmedetomidine. Masui 2006;55(7):856–63.
31. Souter MJ, Rozet I, Ojemann JG, et al. Dexmedetomidine sedation during awake craniotomy for seizure resection: effects on electrocorticography. J Neurosurg Anesthesiol 2007;19(1):38–44.
32. Grant SA, Breslin DS, MacLeod DB, et al. Dexmedetomidine infusion for sedation during fiberoptic intubation: a report of three cases. J Clin Anesth 2004; 16(2):124–6.
33. Sato K, Kamii H, Shimizu H, et al. Preoperative sedation with dexmedetomidine in patients with aneurysmal subarachnoid hemorrhage. Masui 2006; 55(1):51–4.
34. Arain SR, Ruehlow RM, Uhrich TD, et al. The efficacy of dexmedetomidine versus morphine for postoperative analgesia after major inpatient surgery. Anesth Analg 2004;98(1):153–8.
35. Unlugenc H, Gunduz M, Guler T, et al. The effect of pre-anaesthetic administration of intravenous dexmedetomidine on postoperative pain in patients receiving patient-controlled morphine. Eur J Anaesthesiol 2005;22(5):386–91.
36. Dickenson AH. Spinal cord pharmacology of pain. Br J Anaesth 1995;75: 193–200.
37. Helmy SA. The effect of the preemptive use of the NMDA receptor antagonist dextromethorphan on postoperative analgesic requirements. Anesth Analg 2001;92(3):739–44.
38. McCartney CJ, Sinha A, Katz J. A qualitative systematic review of the role of N-methyl-D-aspartate receptor antagonists in preventive analgesia. Anesth Analg 2004;98(5):1385–400.
39. Türe H, Sayin M, Karlikaya G, et al. The analgesic effect of gabapentin as a prophylactic anticonvulsant drug on postcraniotomy pain: a prospective randomized study. Anesth Analg 2009;109(5):1625–31.
40. Panchal S, Damaraju C, Nelson W, et al. System-related events and analgesic gaps during postoperative pain management with the fentanyl iontophoretic transdermal system and morphine intravenous patient controlled analgesia. Anesth Analg 2007;105(5):1437–41.
41. Shikanov A, Domb A, Weiniger C. Long acting local anesthetic-polymer formulation to prolong the effect of analgesia. J Control Release 2007;117(1): 97–103.
42. Bianconi M, Ferraro L, Ricci R, et al. The pharmacokinetics and efficacy of ropivacaine continuous wound installation after spine fusion surgery. Anesth Analg 2004;98:166–72.

43. Cohen BE, Hartman MB, Wade JT, et al. Postoperative pain control after lumbar spine fusion: patient-controlled analgesia versus continuous epidural analgesia. Spine 1997;22:1892–7.
44. Klimek M, Ubben J, Ammann J, et al. Pain in neurosurgically treated patients: a prospective observational study. J Neurosurg 2006;104:350–9.
45. Kalkman CJ, Visser K, Moen J, et al. Preoperative prediction of severe postoperative pain. Pain 2003;105(3):415–23.
46. Kotzer AM. Factors predicting postoperative pain in children and adolescents following spine fusion. Issues Compr Pediatr Nurs 2000;23:83–102.
47. Epker J, Block AR. Pre-surgical psychological screening in back pain patients: a review. Clin J Pain 2001;17(3):200–5.
48. Fessler RG. The development of minimally invasive spine surgery. Neurosurg Clin North Am 2006;17(4):401–9.
49. Oskouian RJ, Johnson JP. Endoscopic thoracic microdiscectomy. J Neurosurg Spine 2005;3(6):459–64.
50. Waddell G. The back pain revolution. 2nd edition. Edinburgh (UK): Churchill Livingstone; 2004.
51. McMahon S. Wall and Melzack's textbook of pain. 5th edition. Philadelphia: Elsevier, Churchill Livingstone; 2006.
52. Devereaux MW. Neck and low back pain. Med Clin North Am 2003;87:643–62.
53. Sumpton JE. Treatment of neuropathic pain with venlafaxine. Ann Pharmacother 2001;35(5):557–9.
54. Tremont-Lukats IW. Anticonvulsants for neuropathic pain syndromes: mechanisms of action and place in therapy. Drugs 2000;60(5):1029–52.
55. Backonja MM. Anticonvulsants (antineuropathics) for neuropathic pain syndromes. Clin J Pain 2000;16(Suppl 2):S67–72.
56. Jaffe RA, Samuels SI. Anesthesiologist's manual of surgical procedures. 3rd edition. Philadelphia: Lippincott Williams & Wilkins; 2004.
57. Bernard JM, Surbled M, Lagarde D, et al. Analgesia after surgery of the spine in adults and adolescents. Cah Anesthesiol 1995;43(6):557–64.
58. Bollish SJ, Collins CL, Kirking DM, et al. Efficacy of patient-controlled versus conventional analgesia for postoperative pain. Clin Pharm 1985;4(1):48–52.
59. Egbert AM, Parks LH, Short LM, et al. Randomized trial of postoperative patient-controlled analgesia vs intramuscular narcotics in frail elderly men. Arch Intern Med 1990;150(9):1897–903.
60. Jirarattanaphochai K, Thienthong S, Sriraj W, et al. Effect of parecoxib on postoperative pain after lumbar spine surgery: a bicenter, randomized, double-blinded, placebo-controlled trial. Spine (Phila Pa 1976) 2008;33(2):132–9.
61. Gottschalk A, Durieux ME, Nemergut EC. Intraoperative methadone improves postoperative pain control in patients undergoing complex spine surgery. Anesth Analg 2011;112:218–23.
62. Izquierdo E, Fabregas N, Valero R, et al. [Postoperative analgesia in herniated disk surgery: comparative study of diclofenac, lysine acetylsalicylate, and ketorolac]. Rev Esp Anestesiol Reanim 1995;42(8):316–9 [in Spanish].
63. Le Roux PD. Postoperative pain after lumbar disc surgery: a comparison between parenteral ketorolac and narcotics. Acta Neurochir (Wien) 1999;141(3):261–7.
64. Gwirtz KH, Kim HC, Nagy DJ, et al. Intravenous ketorolac and subarachnoid opioid analgesia in the management of acute postoperative pain. Reg Anesth 1995;20(5):395–401.

65. Sevarino FB, Sinatra RS, Paige D, et al. The efficacy of intramuscular ketorolac in combination with intravenous PCA morphine for postoperative pain relief. J Clin Anesth 1992;4(4):285–8.

66. Turner DM, Warson JS, Wirt TC, et al. The use of ketorolac in lumbar spine surgery: a cost-benefit analysis. J Spinal Disord 1995;8(3):206–12.

67. Sharma S, Balireddy RK, Vorenkamp KE, et al. Beyond opioid patient-controlled analgesia: a systematic review of analgesia after major spine surgery. Reg Anesth Pain Med 2012;37(1):79–98.

68. O'Keefe RJ, Tiyapatanaputi P, Xie C, et al. COX-2 has a critical role during incorporation of structural bone allografts. Ann N Y Acad Sci 2006;1068: 532–42.

69. Reuben SS. High dose nonsteroidal anti-inflammatory drugs compromise spinal fusion. Can J Anaesth 2005;52(5):506–12.

70. Li Q, Zhang Z, Cai Z. High-dose ketorolac affects adult spinal fusion: a meta-analysis of the effect of perioperative nonsteroidal anti-inflammatory drugs on spinal fusion. Spine (Phila Pa 1976) 2011;36(7):E461–8.

71. Wong HK, Tan KJ. Effects of corticosteroids on nerve root recovery after spinal nerve root compression. Clin Orthop Relat Res 2002;403:248–52.

72. King JS, Gallant P, Myerson V, et al. The effects of anti-inflammatory agents on the responses and the sensitization of unmyelinated (C) fiber polymodal nociceptors [Wenner-Gren Center International Symposium Series, vol. 28]. In: Zotterman Y, editor. Sensory functions of the skin in primates with special reference to man. Oxford (UK): Pergamon Press; 1976. p. 441–61.

73. Aminmansour B, Khalili HA, Ahmadi J, et al. Effect of high-dose intravenous dexamethasone on postlumbar discectomy pain. Spine 2006;31(21):2415–7.

74. King JS. Dexamethasone: a helpful adjunct in management after lumbar discectomy. Neurosurgery 1984;14:697–700.

75. Vuilleumier PA, Buclin T, Biollaz J, et al. Comparison of propacetamol and morphine in postoperative analgesia. Schweiz Med Wochenschr 1998;128(7): 259–63.

76. Delbos A, Boccard E. The morphine-sparing effect of propacetamol in orthopedic postoperative pain. J Pain Symptom Manage 1995;10:279–86.

77. Moore UJ. Effects of peripherally and centrally acting analgesics on somatosensory evoked potentials. Br J Clin Pharmacol 1995;40(2):111–7.

78. Piletta P, Porchet HC, Dayer P. Central analgesic effect of acetaminophen but not of aspirin. Clin Pharmacol Ther 1991;49:350–4.

79. Flower RJ, Vane JR. Inhibition of prostaglandin synthetase in brain explains the antipyretic activity of paracetamol. Nature 1972;240:410–1.

80. Tjolsen A, Lund A, Hole K. Antinociceptive effect of paracetamol in rats is partly dependent on spinal serotoninergic systems. Eur J Pharmacol 1991;193(2): 193–201.

81. Hans P, Brichant JF, Bonhomme V, et al. Analgesic efficiency of propacetamol hydrochloride after lumbar disc surgery. Acta Anaesthesiol Belg 1993;44: 129–33.

82. Daluiski A. Cyclooxygenase-2 inhibitors in human skeletal fracture healing. Orthopedics 2006;29(3):259–61.

83. Reuben SS. The effect of cyclooxygenase-2 inhibition on analgesia and spinal fusion. J Bone Joint Surg Am 2005;87(3):536–42.

84. Hadi BA, Al Ramadani R, Daas R, et al. Remifentanil in combination with ketamine versus remifentanil in spinal fusion surgery–a double blind study. Int J Clin Pharmacol Ther 2010;48:542–8.

85. Suski M, Bujak-Gizycka B, Madej J, et al. Co-administration of dextromethorphan and morphine: reduction of post-operative pain and lack of influence on morphine metabolism. Basic Clin Pharmacol Toxicol 2010;107:680–4.

86. Rusy LM, Hainsworth KR, Nelson TJ, et al. Gabapentin use in pediatric spinal fusion patients: a randomized, double-blind, controlled trial. Anesth Analg 2010;110:1393–8.

87. Turan A, Karamanlioglu B, Memis D, et al. Analgesic effects of gabapentin after spinal surgery. Anesthesiology 2004;100:935–8.

88. Pandey CK, Sahay S, Gupta D, et al. Preemptive gabapentin decreases postoperative pain after lumbar discoidectomy. Can J Anaesth 2004;51:986–9.

89. Ummenhofer WC. Comparative spinal distribution and clearance kinetics of intrathecally administered morphine, fentanyl, alfentanil, and sufentanil. Anesthesiology 2000;92(3):739–53.

90. Rigler ML, Drasner K, Krejcie TC, et al. Cauda equine syndrome after spinal anesthesia. Anesth Analg 1991;72:275–81.

91. Urban MK, Jules-Elysee K, Urquhart B, et al. Reduction in postoperative pain after spinal fusion with instrumentation using intrathecal morphine. Spine 2002;27(5):535–7.

92. Dalens B, Tanguy A. Intrathecal morphine for spinal fusion in children. Spine 1988;13:494–8.

93. Blackman RG, Reynolds J, Shively J. Intrathecal morphine dosage and efficacy in younger patients for control of postoperative pain following spinal fusion. Orthopedics 1991;14:555–7.

94. France JC. The use of intrathecal morphine for analgesia after posterolateral lumbar fusion: a prospective, double-blind, randomized study. Spine 1997;22(19):2272–7.

95. Hesselgard K, Stromblad LG, Romner B, et al. Postoperative continuous intrathecal pain treatment in children after selective dorsal rhizotomy with bupivacaine and two different morphine doses. Paediatr Anaesth 2006;16(4):436–43.

96. Hesselgard K, Stromblad LG, Reinstrup P. Morphine with or without a local anaesthetic for postoperative intrathecal pain treatment after selective dorsal rhizotomy in children. Paediatr Anaesth 2001;11(1):75–9.

97. Strebel S, Gurzeler JA, Schneider MC, et al. Small-dose intrathecal clonidine and isobaric bupivacaine for orthopedic surgery: a dose-response study. Anesth Analg 2004;99(4):1231–8.

98. Liu SS, Hodgson PS, Moore JM, et al. Dose-response effects of spinal neostigmine added to bupivacaine spinal anesthesia in healthy volunteers. Anesthesiology 1999;90:710–7.

99. Sites BD, Beach M, Biggs R, et al. Intrathecal clonidine added to a bupivacaine-morphine spinal anesthetic improves postoperative analgesia for total knee arthroplasty. Anesth Analg 2003;96:1083–8.

100. Khan ZH, Hamidi S, Miri M, et al. Post-operative pain relief following intrathecal injection of acetylcholine esterase inhibitor during lumbar disc surgery: a prospective double blind randomized study. J Clin Pharm Ther 2008;33:669–75.

101. Zhu X, Conklin D, Eisenach JC. Cyclooxygenase-1 in the spinal cord plays an important role in postoperative pain. Pain 2003;104:15–23.

102. Conklin DR, Eisenach JC. Intrathecal ketorolac enhances antinociception from clonidine. Anesth Analg 2003;96:191–4.

103. Eisenach JC, Curry R, Hood DD, et al. Phase I safety assessment of intrathecal ketorolac. Pain 2002;99:599–604.

104. Wheatley RG, Schug SA, Watson D. Safety and efficacy of postoperative epidural analgesia. Br J Anaesth 2001;87:47–61.
105. Dahl JB, Rosenberg J, Hansen BL, et al. Differential analgesic effects of low-dose epidural morphine and morphine-bupivacaine at rest and during mobilization after major abdominal surgery. Anesth Analg 1992;74:362–5.
106. Rockemann MG. Epidural bolus clonidine/morphine versus epidural patient-controlled bupivacaine/sufentanil: quality of postoperative analgesia and cost-identification analysis. Anesth Analg 1997;85(4):864–9.
107. Schenk MR, Putzier M, Kugler B, et al. Postoperative analgesia after major spine surgery: patient-controlled epidural analgesia versus patient-controlled intravenous analgesia. Anesth Analg 2006;103(5):1311–7.
108. Lowry KJ, Tobias J, Kittle D, et al. Postoperative pain control using epidural catheters after anterior spinal fusion for adolescent scoliosis. Spine 2001;26:1290–3.
109. Amaranth L, Andrish JT, Gurd AR, et al. Efficacy of intermittent epidural morphine following posterior spinal fusion in children and adolescents. Clin Orthop Relat Res 1989;249:223–6.
110. Fisher CG, Belanger L, Gofton EG. Prospective randomized clinical trial comparing patient-controlled intravenous analgesia with patient-controlled epidural analgesia after lumbar spinal fusion. Spine 2003;28(8):739–43.
111. Ballantyne JC, Carr DB, deFerranti S, et al. The comparative effects of postoperative analgesic therapies on pulmonary outcome: cumulative meta-analyses of randomized, controlled trials. Anesth Analg 1998;87(3):598–612.
112. O'Hara JF. The effect of epidural vs intravenous analgesia for posterior spinal fusion surgery. Paediatr Anaesth 2004;14(12):1009–15.
113. Eisenach J, Detweiler D, Hood D. Hemodynamics and analgesic actions of epidurally administered clonidine. Anesthesiology 1993;78:277–87.
114. Ekatodramis G, Min K, Cathrein P, et al. Use of a double epidural catheter provides effective postoperative analgesia after spine deformity surgery. Reg Anesth Pain Med 2002;49:173–7.
115. Jellish WS, Abodeely A, Fluder EM, et al. The effect of spinal bupivacaine in combination with either epidural clonidine and/or 0.5% bupivacaine administered at the incision site on postoperative outcome in patients undergoing lumbar laminectomy. Anesth Analg 2003;96(3):874–80.
116. Rockemann MG, Seeling W. Epidural and intrathecal administration of alpha 2-adrenoceptor agonists for postoperative pain relief. Schmerz 1996;10(2):57–64.
117. Carvalho B, Riley E, Cohen S, et al. Single-dose, sustained-release epidural morphine in the management of postoperative pain after elective cesarean delivery: results of a multicenter randomized controlled study. Anesth Analg 2005;100(4):1150–8.

Controversies in Neurosciences Critical Care

Tiffany R. Chang, MD, Neeraj S. Naval, MD,
J. Ricardo Carhuapoma, MD*

KEYWORDS

- Neurocritical care • Red blood cell transfusion • Platelet dysfunction
- Coagulopathy reversal • Seizure prophylaxis

KEY POINTS

- Patients with subarachnoid and intracerebral hemorrhage (ICH) should have different blood/packed red blood cell (RBC) transfusion goals than the general medical population.
- Platelet transfusion should be given to patients with intracranial bleeding and significant thrombocytopenia; platelet function assays may be helpful in guiding platelet transfusion for reversal of antiplatelet medication.
- For emergency reversal of warfarin, prothrombin complex concentrate (PCC) should be first-line therapy due to rapid onset of action, efficacy, and favorable adverse effect profile; reversal of coagulopathy secondary to direct thrombin inhibitors is less clear.
- Seizure prophylaxis may be indicated in the first week after traumatic brain injury (TBI); there is currently no indication for empiric seizure prophylaxis in ICH whereas prophylaxis in the setting of aneurysmal subarachnoid hemorrhage (SAH) should be based on risk stratification.
- Levetiracetam is a potentially effective alternative to phenytoin for seizure prophylaxis and has a favorable side-effect profile.
- Transfer to a dedicated neurocritical care unit should be considered in all patients with critical neurologic injury or illness.

INTRODUCTION

Neurocritical care is a rapidly growing and evolving subspecialty dedicated to the care of critically ill neurologic patients. Through evolving research in this field, neurointensivists are learning that the traditional management of many diseases can be improved. In addition, advanced neuroimaging and neuromonitoring can provide invaluable data to

Conflict of interest: None.
Funding sources: None.
Division of Neurosciences Critical Care Medicine, Department of Anesthesiology and Critical Care Medicine, The Johns Hopkins Hospital, The Johns Hopkins University, 600 North Wolfe Street, Meyer 8-140, Baltimore, MD 21287, USA
* Corresponding author.
E-mail address: jcarhua1@jhmi.edu

Anesthesiology Clin 30 (2012) 369–383
doi:10.1016/j.anclin.2012.05.006
1932-2275/12/$ – see front matter © 2012 Elsevier Inc. All rights reserved.

guide management using hitherto unavailable treatment options. Many controversies still exist in the care of patients with neurologic injury, discussions of several of which are outside the scope of this article. This article focuses on current practices in RBC transfusion, platelet dysfunction, and coagulopathy reversal with a brief review of the available evidence for those practices. Indications for seizure prophylaxis in brain injury and the available options are also reviewed. Finally, the role of dedicated neurocritical care units and specialists in management of neurocritical illness is examined.

TRANSFUSION THRESHOLDS IN THE CRITICALLY ILL NEUROLOGIC/NEUROSURGICAL PATIENT
Anemia and Packed Red Blood Cell Transfusion

Anemia is a common problem in all critical care settings. The World Health Organization defines anemia as hemoglobin less than 13 g/dL in men and 12 g/dL in women.[1] A common practice in critical care is a goal hemoglobin level between 7 g/dL and 9 g/dL. Higher goals may be indicated in certain populations, such as patients with acute coronary syndromes.[2] Although anemia can generally be corrected by RBC transfusion, liberal transfusion strategies in ICUs have been associated with worse outcomes in several studies.[2–4] In neurocritical care, cerebral blood flow dynamics and oxygen delivery are critical components of acute management. Treatment goals for anemia in the neurocritical care unit remain controversial and vary depending on the nature of the neurologic injury.

Aneurysmal SAH represents a unique group of stroke patients. Management involves both acute stroke care as well as the prevention and treatment of vasospasm, to prevent delayed cerebral ischemia. Traditional triple-H management of vasospasm includes hemodilution, hypervolemia, and hypertension.[5] This approach can lead to an increased incidence of anemia in this patient population. One study reported the development of anemia in 47% of patients after SAH.[6] Factors associated with the development of anemia were female gender, baseline hematocrit, hypertension, poor grade (ie, worse neurologic condition), and surgical treatment.

Anemia is of particular concern in SAH because it may decrease tissue oxygen delivery, placing patients at risk of neurologic injury in the setting of delayed cerebral ischemia. A prospective study of patients with poor-grade SAH found decreased brain tissue oxygen tension, increased lactate:pyruvate ratios, and increased brain hypoxia in patients with hemoglobin levels less than 9 g/dL.[7] Transfusion of packed RBCs has also been shown to improve brain oxygen delivery in the setting of SAH.[8,9] Therefore, targeting a higher hemoglobin goal may provide a therapeutic option to prevent secondary brain injury after SAH. The ideal hemoglobin level to improve outcomes and minimize transfusion-related complications, however, remains unclear.

Higher hemoglobin levels have been associated with improved outcomes in multiple studies. A retrospective study of patients with aneurysmal SAH found that patients with higher admission and mean hemoglobin values had decreased risk of cerebral infarction, poor outcome, and death.[10] A larger retrospective study of 611 patients reported that patients with functional independence (modified Rankin scale [mRS] 0–3) had higher mean and nadir hemoglobin values.[11] The mRS is shown in **Table 1**. Patients with lower hemoglobin values have been reported to have worse outcomes after controlling for the presence of vasospasm, Hunt and Hess grade, modified Fisher scale, and World Federation of Neurological Surgeons scale.[11,12]

RBC transfusions are not a benign therapy. Both anemia and transfusion have been associated with worse outcomes and increased mortality.[13] Higher rates of infection and other medical complications have been reported in patients who received

Grade	Description
Table 1	
The modified Rankin scale	
0	No symptoms at all
1	No significant disability despite symptoms; able to carry out all usual duties and activities
2	Slight disability; unable to carry out all previous activities but able to look after own affairs without assistance
3	Moderate disability; requiring some help, but able to walk without assistance
4	Moderately severe disability; unable to walk without assistance and unable to attend to own bodily needs without assistance
5	Severe disability; bedridden, incontinent, and requiring constant nursing care and attention

Adapted from van Swieten JC, Koudstaal PJ, Visser MC, et al. Interobserver agreement for the assessment of handicap in stroke patients. Stroke 1988;19(5):604–7.

transfusions.[14] Transfusion during the acute period has also been reported as a risk factor for cognitive impairment at 12 months after SAH.[15] Other studies, however, have failed to consistently demonstrate an independent association between transfusion and poor outcome.[16]

Transfusion goal in aneurysmal SAH continues to be under debate. There are few studies that have evaluated transfusion in a prospective fashion. One recent randomized prospective study examined the safety of packed RBC transfusion in SAH[17]; 44 patients at high risk for vasospasm were transfused to a goal hemoglobin value of 11.5 g/dL or 10 g/dL. There were no differences in adverse events between the 2 groups. There was a slight trend toward improved outcomes in the higher goal group, including 14-day National Institutes of Health Stroke Scale and functional independence at 14, 30, and 90 days; however, this did not reach statistical significance. Because this was primarily designed as a safety study, further trials are needed to evaluate the benefits of RBC transfusion and potential target hemoglobin concentrations.

Overall, patients with SAH seem to benefit from a higher hemoglobin goal than the general medical population. The Neurocritical Care Society has recommended packed RBC transfusion to target a hemoglobin concentration above 8 g/dL to 10 g/dL.[18] In practice, intensivists seem to favor a goal in the upper range, especially in the setting of cerebral vasospasm. An international survey of critical care physicians conducted by Stevens and colleagues[19] evaluated current opinion in SAH management. They found that a hematocrit goal of greater than 30% was an accepted therapeutic goal in the majority of responders.

The approach to anemia management and use of transfusion in spontaneous ICH has been less studied than in SAH. ICH comprises approximately 10% to 15% of all strokes, is associated with mortality rates between 30% and 50%, and often results in severe disability.[20] Although the same principles of brain oxygen delivery apply in ICH, patients are not generally at risk for delayed cerebral ischemia secondary to vasospasm. This may lead to a more conservative threshold. The presence of anemia is common in patients with ICH and has been shown an independent predictor of hematoma size[21]; the significance of this finding is unclear at this time. Hematoma volume significantly contributes to mortality. Mortality from ICH can be predicted using the ICH score, which includes patient age, ICH location, hematoma size, intraventricular extension, and Glasgow Coma Scale score at admission.[22]

Anemia has been directly associated with worse outcomes after ICH. Diedler and colleagues[23] retrospectively reviewed 196 patients with supratentorial ICH. Patients with poor neurologic outcomes (mRS 4–6) at discharge and at 3 months had lower average and nadir hemoglobin values during their hospital stay. Hemoglobin was not an independent predictor of in-hospital mortality, and there was no significant relationship between outcomes and packed RBC transfusion.

A recent study evaluated the relationship between packed RBC transfusion and ICH mortality in 546 patients.[24] Anemia was present at presentation or developed in 72% of patients. Transfusion was associated with decreased 30-day mortality after controlling for anemia, Glasgow Coma Scale score, hematoma size and location, warfarin use, and do-not-resuscitate or comfort care status. Patients with improved outcomes did not have significantly increased hemoglobin values after transfusion. The intervention in this study was applied on an ad hoc basis, making it possible that potential confounders may have influenced the results of the data obtained by retrospective analysis. In summary, it is unknown at this time if aggressive treatment of anemia can affect hematoma volume, hematoma expansion, or outcomes after ICH.

Transfusion in patients with TBI also continues to be controversial, and there is little consensus regarding the appropriate transfusion threshold in this population. Patients with TBI tend to be young, have few medical comorbidities, and may be exposed to large volumes of blood products for various reasons. In general, most neurointensivists agree that hemoglobin should be maintained above 7 g/dL to provide adequate cerebral oxygen delivery. The concern is that the injured brain may require greater oxygen delivery in the acute phase of trauma to maintain cellular function and promote healing. Transfusion has been shown to increase oxygen brain tissue oxygen in the setting of isolated TBI.[25,26] This has not been consistently shown to improve brain metabolism or outcomes.

Transfusion has been evaluated retrospectively in the setting of isolated TBI. George and colleagues[27] reviewed 82 patients with nadir ICU hemoglobin levels between 8 g/dL and 10 g/dL, of whom 42 (52%) received a transfusion. No difference in morbidity or mortality was found between the 2 groups. Patients with hemoglobin less than 8 g/dL were not included in this study because 96% of patients in this category received packed RBC transfusion. Duane and colleagues[28] reviewed 788 patients with isolated TBI. Anemia and total blood products administered were associated with increased in-hospital mortality. Hemoglobin less than 8 g/dL was more strongly associated with death than higher levels.

One prospective trial evaluated the use of transfusion in patients with TBI.[29] Patients were randomized to receive restrictive (7–9 g/dL) or liberal (10–12 g/dL) transfusion strategies. No significant differences were found in 30-day mortality, length of stay, or organ dysfunction between the 2 groups. The liberal group did receive more blood products. This study, however, was limited by a small sample size of 67 patients.

Anemia in TBI, as with SAH and ICH, is associated with worse outcomes. Although transfusion has not demonstrated a benefit and has been reported to be potentially harmful, studies have been limited by small sample size and other confounding variables General practice seems to favor a higher hemoglobin goal than is currently supported by the literature. A survey of physicians at trauma centers reported that among neurosurgeons, mean thresholds were 8.3 mg/dL for patients with normal intracranial pressure and 8.9 mg/dL for patients with increased intracranial pressure.[30] Neurosurgeons also had significantly higher thresholds than trauma surgeons and intensivists (7.5 g/dL and 8.4 g/dL, respectively). Further prospective study is needed to define the role of transfusion in TBI.

Platelet Dysfunction

Platelet function plays in important role in the development and outcome from intracranial bleeding. Patients with significant thrombocytopenia at ICH presentation should receive platelet transfusion according to American Heart Association guidelines.[31] Decreased platelet counts have been associated with hematoma growth in ICH.[32] Platelet counts do not take into account, however, platelet dysfunction that may arise secondary to systemic illness or medication effect. Platelet function was previously assessed by measuring bleeding times, which are now considered impractical and inaccurate. More recently, platelet function assays are commercially available and can provide a rapid, objective measurement of platelet function.

Platelet dysfunction may be common in patients with intracranial bleeding, especially considering the widespread use of antiplatelet medications, such as aspirin and clopidogrel. In a study of patients with subdural hematoma (SDH), 38% of patients had an abnormal platelet function test at baseline.[33] Platelet function has been most extensively studied in the setting of ICH. Naidech and colleagues[34] examined platelet activity in 68 patients with spontaneous ICH. Decreased platelet activity at admission, defined as fewer than 550 aspirin reaction units on a platelet function assay (VerifyNow, Aspirin Test, Accumetrics, San Diego, CA, USA), was associated with hematoma growth and worse neurologic outcomes at 3 months. Surprisingly, 16 patients with inhibited platelet function had no history of antiplatelet use. Other studies have also shown that ICH patients with platelet dysfunction have worse outcomes and increased intraventricular hemorrhage independent of hematoma volume or location.[35,36]

The most recent American Heart Association guidelines consider platelet transfusion for antiplatelet reversal an investigational treatment of ICH and do not make a recommendation for their use (class IIb, level B).[31] It is common in clinical practice, however, to give platelets to patients with a history of antiplatelet use presenting with intracranial hemorrhage. This should be considered in patients with evidence of active bleeding. Guidelines for antiplatelet agent reversal in intracranial bleeding are based on clinical experience and do not use platelet function results to guide transfusion practice.[37] This leads clinicians to transfuse a fixed volume or target a goal platelet count. The appropriate volume of transfusion has not been scientifically determined and likely varies between patients; one study found that a single unit of apheresis platelets may be sufficient to reverse the effect of aspirin.[38] Certain patients may benefit from a larger or repeat transfusion, such as those on multiple antiplatelet medications.

The practice of antiplatelet reversal relies heavily on reported medication history. Unfortunately, patients with intracranial bleeding are often incapable of providing a history. Abnormal platelet function has been discovered with higher frequency than reported antiplatelet use in patients with ICH.[39] Obtaining a platelet function test at the time of presentation may be a helpful screening tool to identify patients who may benefit from transfusion. Using platelet function assays, transfusions have been demonstrated to improve platelet activity in the setting of ICH and SDH.[33,34,38] The natural history of platelet function in ICH and the effect of transfusion on serial platelet function have not been studied.

Platelet transfusion should be considered in ICH with platelet dysfunction, regardless of platelet count. A careful history of antiplatelet use should be taken on all patients with intracranial bleeding. Because impaired platelet function cannot be accurately predicted by a history of antiplatelet use, consideration should be given to using a platelet function assay to guide therapy. Alternatives to platelet transfusion are under investigation. For example, desmopressin has been shown to improve platelet function in the setting of uremia,[40] but further study is needed to evaluate its efficacy in the setting of intracranial bleeding and antiplatelet therapy.

Reversal of Coagulopathy

ICH is a feared complication of oral anticoagulation therapy (OAT). Common indications for OAT include stroke prevention in atrial fibrillation, thromboembolic disease, and hypercoagulable states. The risk of ICH increases with the duration of anticoagulation therapy and more anticoagulated state (ie, higher international normalized ratio [INR] values).[41] As the widespread use of OAT has increased, OAT-associated ICH comprises approximately 17% of all ICH.[42] Reversal of anticoagulation in the setting of acute ICH represents a unique challenge in the management of stroke.

Administration of vitamin K promotes the replenishment of coagulation factors needed to permanently reverse coagulopathy. Vitamin K–dependent factors include II, VII, IX, and X. Although vitamin K should be given promptly, when given alone, it may take up to 24 hours for reversal.[43] Intravenous administration achieves correction more rapidly and is recommended in cases of life-threatening hemorrhage.

Fresh frozen plasma (FFP) is one of the most commonly used agents for emergency OAT reversal. FFP is a blood product that contains all clotting factors, although different products may contain variable factor concentrations. Because it is a blood product, patients are at risk for allergic and transfusion reactions, including acute lung injury. FFP administration may be delayed because availability to the patient requires that the product be processed (eg, cross-matched and thawed) and transported from the blood bank. Because of multiple delays in administration of FFP, it has been reported to take more than 24 hours to reverse OAT in the setting of ICH.[44] Another major limitation of FFP is that it may require a large volume of product for correction of the INR. Initial recommended dose is 15 mL/kg to 30 mL/kg, and repeat dosing is often necessary.[41] The large volume required limits the speed of administration and, in patients with cardiac comorbidities, may precipitate an episode of congestive heart failure.

PCC is an alternative to FFP for emergency anticoagulation reversal. PCC is derived from plasma and contains factors II, VII, IX, and X. It is not subject to the same time limitations and adverse reactions seen with FFP. Pabinger and colleagues[45] conducted a prospective study of the use of PCC in patients on OAT requiring emergent reversal. Patients received a median volume of 90 mL over a median infusion time of 12 minutes. INR decreased to target level of less than or equal to 1.3 within 30 minutes in 93% of patients; the remaining patients had an INR of 1.4 at 30 minutes. 88% of patients also received vitamin K, and INR remained stable over 48 hours. The ability to rapidly correct INR with PCC offers a significant advantage over FFP.

In addition to rapid onset of action, PCC has been associated with reduced hematoma enlargement and improved outcomes in ICH.[46] The International Normalised Ratio Normalisation in Patients with Coumadin-Related Intracranial Hemorrhages trial is currently under way to prospectively evaluate the efficacy of combined treatment with PCC and FFP in patients with OAT-related ICH or SDH.[47] The major limitation in the use of PCC is cost. Although PCC is significantly more expensive than FFP, a recent United Kingdom study found PCC overall more cost effective than FFP for the treatment of life-threatening bleeding, including intracranial hemorrhage.[48]

Recombinant activated factor VII (rFVIIa) has also been studied for the treatment of ICH and reversal of anticoagulation. A preliminary trial of rFVIIa in spontaneous ICH resulted in decreased hematoma growth and mortality.[49] This led to the phase 3 Factor Seven for Acute Hemorrhagic Stroke Trial, which included 841 patients with ICH not associated with anticoagulation therapy.[50] Although there was a significant reduction in hematoma growth, there was no beneficial effect on mortality. In addition, there was an increased incidence of arterial thrombotic events in the treatment group. This led to the American Heart Association recommendation against the use of rFVIIa for spontaneous ICH (class III, level A).[31] In patients on OAT, rFVIIa has been shown to effectively reverse coagulopathy.[51,52] The lack of evidence in OAT-associated ICH, however, does not support its use as monotherapy for coagulopathy reversal at this time. A recent study evaluated the combination of PCC and rFVIIa for the reversal of warfarin in ICH.[53] Although the combination was effective in reducing the INR, there was an increased risk of thrombotic events with the combination. Further studies are indicated to determine the role of rFVIIa in the treatment of OAT-associated ICH.

Direct thrombin inhibitors (eg, argatroban and hirudin) are a novel class of anticoagulants with increasing clinical use. There is currently no proved effective reversal agent for this class of medications. Activated charcoal can be used in cases of oral thrombin inhibitor overdose. In emergency situations, hemodialysis is an option to rapidly decrease serum drug concentrations.[54] Coagulation factors, such as FFP, PCC, and rFVIIa, have potential benefit, but their role is unclear at this time. In an experimental model of ICH, PCC decreased hematoma expansion in mice.[55] Further study is needed to determine the best reversal strategy in cases of intracranial bleeding.

SEIZURE PROPHYLAXIS
Indications

Seizure prophylaxis with antiepileptic drugs (AEDs) is a common practice in neurocritical care and neurosurgery. Prophylaxis is commonly administered in SAH, ICH, TBI, and postcraniotomy patients. As more about adverse effects of AED use has been learned, the potential benefits of this approach should be critically reviewed. In all conditions, clinical seizure activity should be treated with AEDs. Duration of therapy should be tailored to the individual patient and risk of recurrent seizure activity. Also, the increased risk of nonconvulsive seizures in this population should be kept in mind. Continuous electroencephalogram (EEG) should be considered in circumstances of suspected seizure activity, and electrographic seizures should be treated appropriately if there is a concern for clinical significance.

Seizures are common after SAH, the majority of which are seen during the acute period. A subset of patients go on to develop late epilepsy. One study found an overall incidence of seizures to be 21.2%, with 7.8% at onset, 2.3% preoperative, 1.8% postoperative, 9.7% in the first postoperative week, and late epilepsy in 6.8%.[56] All patients in this study, however, were treated with surgical clipping and were given empiric AED prophylaxis, usually with phenytoin. The incidence of seizures seems significantly lower in patients treated with endovascular coiling. A recent analysis of the International Subarachnoid Aneurysm Trial found an overall incidence of seizures of 8.3% after coiling and 13.6% after surgical clipping.[57] Significant predictors of seizure risk included surgical treatment, younger age, higher grade, and delayed cerebral ischemia secondary to vasospasm. With either endovascular or surgical approach, middle cerebral artery aneurysm location was independently associated with increased risk.

There are no randomized controlled trials to assess the efficacy of AED prophylaxis in SAH. Seizures occur more frequently in patients with higher disease severity and may serve as a marker rather than an etiology for poor outcome. There have been conflicting reports on whether seizures have an impact on outcome from SAH,[58,59] and treatment has not been conclusively shown beneficial. Perioperative seizures have not been correlated with the development of late epilepsy.[56] AED therapy, however, has been associated with significant morbidity. Rosengart and colleagues[60] reviewed 3552 patients with SAH in multiple countries between 1991 and1997. They reported increased risk of higher Glasgow Coma Scale score, vasospasm, infarction, and fever in patients treated with AEDs.

The incidence of seizures after SAH remains high, and the decision to start prophylaxis should be based on individual risk stratification. The American Heart Association guidelines state that seizure prophylaxis may be considered in the acute period (class IIb, level B) but recommend against routine long-term AED therapy (class III, level B).[61]

The Neurocritical Care Society makes similar recommendations, except they advise against the use of phenytoin as a prophylactic agent.[18] In the absence of clinical seizure activity, they recommend limiting the duration of therapy to 3 to 7 days. In a recent analysis, a 7-day course of phenytoin was compared with a 3-day course of levetiracetam after SAH.[62] Rates of early seizures were similar between the 2 groups, but in-hospital seizures were increased in the levetiracetam group. This suggests that a longer duration of therapy may be more effective in reducing seizure risk.

Seizures may also occur frequently after ICH. In a prospective study of stroke patients, seizures occurred in 10.6% of patients with ICH and 8.6% of patients with ischemic stroke.[63] Seizures most frequently occur at onset and are strongly associated with a cortical location of hemorrhage. Although prophylactic AED treatment has been reported to decrease the risk of seizure, this has not been demonstrated to influence outcome.[64] Messe and colleagues[65] found that patients treated prophylactically had no reported seizures, but AED use was an independent predictor of poor outcome (mRS 5–6). This remained significant after controlling for factors that may have prompted the initiation of AED therapy, such as neurologic worsening, lobar location, and neurosurgical intervention. The majority of patients in this study received phenytoin.

With growing evidence of long-term adverse effects of AED use, routine administration has now fallen out of favor in ICH. Previous American Heart Association guidelines recommended the short-term use of prophylactic AED in patients with lobar ICH.[20] The most recent 2010 update states that prophylactic use of AED therapy should not be used (class III, level B)[31] in spontaneous ICH.

TBI places patients at high risk for seizures in the acute period after injury and is also associated with the development of late epilepsy. The risk of epilepsy increases with the severity of TBI and may be as high as 50% in patients with penetrating injuries.[66,67] Prophylaxis has been shown to decrease the incidence of posttraumatic seizures, but has not been conclusively shown to have an impact on mortality.[68,69] In a landmark study, Temkin and colleagues[68] conducted a randomized controlled trial of phenytoin prophylaxis in 404 patients with severe TBI. In the first week, seizures occurred in 3.6% of patients in the phenytoin group compared with 14.2% in the placebo group. Treatment beyond the first week, however, showed no significant benefit in seizure incidence or mortality.

Because the risk seizure is particularly high in this population, patients with TBI have traditionally been treated with antiseizure prophylaxis. Brain Trauma Foundation guidelines support the use of prophylactic AED therapy to decrease the frequency of seizures in the first 7 days after trauma.[67] Because benefit has not been demonstrated beyond the first week, it is important to limit the duration of therapy in patients without clinical seizure activity. There have been no recent randomized controlled trials to re-evaluate the benefits of prophylactic treatment; most current clinical trials focus on AED selection.

Choice of Antiepileptic Agent

Once a decision has been made to start prophylactic therapy, the selection of an antiepileptic agent should always be individualized. Medical comorbidities, in particular, liver and kidney dysfunction, should be considered. It is also crucial to carefully review current medications for potential interactions. Phenytoin has historically been the agent of choice in ICU patients because it can be rapidly loaded, levels can be easily followed, and it is an effective AED. For this reason, phenytoin is the best studied in the literature. One study found similar rates of early post-TBI seizures using phenytoin or valproic acid, but there was a trend toward increased mortality in the valproic acid group.[70] Although valproic acid may be an effective agent for seizure prevention,[71] adverse effects limit its use as a prophylactic agent. Phenobarbital has similar limitations and has also not been shown to decrease the risk of developing late post-TBI epilepsy.[72] Newer antiepileptic agents have fewer side effects and fewer medication interactions. Levetiracetam has emerged as a competitive alternate to phenytoin in the ICU.

Phenytoin prophylaxis has been associated with worse outcomes in multiple studies. A study of SAH patients examined total phenytoin exposure, estimated from mean phenytoin levels and duration of treatment.[59] Increased exposure was associated with poor 14-day functional outcome and cognitive dysfunction at 3 months. In a prospective observational study on ICH, phenytoin was associated with fever, increased National Institutes of Health Stroke Scale, and worse neurologic outcomes at 14, 30, and 90 days.[73] No relationship was identified between levetiracetam use and outcome in this study. This interpretation of the results of this study is difficult given that the mean differences in ICH volume between patients receiving phenytoin for seizure prophylaxis and those receiving levetiracetam or no prophylaxis were 9 mL and 20 mL respectively, and hematoma volume has a significant impact on outcomes after ICH. When compared with levetiracetam, phenytoin use has, in other studies, been associated with more adverse effects, including depressed mental status, elevated liver enzymes, fever, rash, and gastrointestinal disturbance.[74]

Although levetiracetam has fewer side effects, one potential concern is if it has the same broad-spectrum efficacy seen with phenytoin. Szaflarski and colleagues[75] conducted a randomized trial comparing phenytoin with levetiracetam for seizure prophylaxis in patients with SAH and severe TBI. Patients received continuous EEG monitoring for the first 72 hours. No significant difference was found in seizure frequency during monitoring or at 6 months. In addition, patients treated with levetiracetam had improved functional outcomes at 3 and 6 months. A trend toward a higher mortality (41%) in the levetiracetam group compared with the phenytoin group (22%) suggests that arguments can be made in favor or against either drug. More importantly, a larger trial is necessary before any meaningful conclusions can be drawn. Another small study reviewed TBI patients treated with levetiracetam compared with historical phenytoin controls.[76] No difference in seizure frequency was detected; however, levetiracetam patients were reported to have increased epileptiform activity on routine EEG. Patients did not receive continuous EEG monitoring and no differences in outcome were found, so the significance of this epileptiform activity is unclear.

In summary, prophylactic treatment with levetiracetam seems a safe and possibly effective alternative to phenytoin. Phenytoin has been reported as more cost effective in for seizure prevention[77,78] but has been correlated with unfavorable outcomes in SAH, ICH, and TBI. In light of the majority of studies on seizure prophylaxis using phenytoin, re-evaluating the safety and efficacy of prophylaxis using an agent, such as levetiracetam, should be considered. Further trials are necessary to answer these questions, and insufficient evidence exists at this time to recommend levetiracetam as a superior alternative to phenytoin for prophylaxis in neurocritical care patients.

SPECIALIZED NEUROCRITICAL CARE UNITS

Care for the critically ill neurologic patient involves complex management distinct from the general medical population on many levels. Although neurocritical care is a growing field, access to specialized neurocritical care units (NCCUs) is limited throughout the United States. Only 21% of the population can reach an NCCU in 60 minutes by ground and 51% can by air.[79] NCCU care is most available in the Northeast, with the South having the most limited access. The cost and inherent risks of patient transfer are limiting factors in pursuing a higher level of care for neurologically injured patients.

Specialized units and the availability of a neurointensivist have demonstrated benefit in multiple studies. Implementation of a specialized care team may decrease overall in-hospital mortality and length of stay in critically ill neurologic patients.[80] Care by a neuro-intensivist has been associated with decreased length of stay and favorable discharge disposition in patients with stroke and TBI.[81,82] The benefits have been particularly robust in patients with SAH. NCCU care has been shown to improve functional outcomes and increase the likelihood of discharge to home.[83,84] These benefits may be the result of a more aggressive management approach and increased use of invasive monitoring and neurosurgical procedures. SAH patients admitted to NCCUs are more likely to receive definitive aneurysm treatment, invasive monitoring for intracranial pressure and hemodynamic status, and tracheostomy.[84,85] In cases where patients have poor neurologic outcomes despite optimal medical therapy, specialized centers may also offer the advantage of coordinating organ donation.

Transfer to a high-volume center, particularly one with a neurocritical care team, should be strongly considered. High-volume centers have consistently reported improved outcomes and decreased mortality from SAH.[86–89] In addition, a recent cost analysis found that transfer of SAH patients increased expected years of quality life with similar or decreased overall costs.[90] In this study, the mortality rate associated with patient transfer was estimated to be 2%.

The team required to optimally care for critically ill neurologic patients extends beyond neurointensivists and neurosurgeons. Skilled practitioners in nursing, physical and occupational therapy, speech and language pathology, respiratory therapy, and social work are vital to providing specialized care for neurologic patients. A dedicated neurocritical care team is invaluable to patients who suffer devastating neurologic injury, and transfer to a specialized high-volume center should always be considered (see **Table 1**).

REFERENCES

1. WHO/UNICEF/UNU. Iron deficiency anaemia: assessment, prevention, and control. Vol (WHO/NHD/01.3). Geneva (Switzerland): World Health Organization; 2001.
2. Hebert PC, Wells G, Blajchman MA, et al. A multicenter, randomized, controlled clinical trial of transfusion requirements in critical care. Transfusion Requirements in Critical Care Investigators, Canadian Critical Care Trials Group. N Engl J Med 1999;340(6):409–17.
3. Vincent JL, Baron JF, Reinhart K, et al. Anemia and blood transfusion in critically ill patients. JAMA 2002;288(12):1499–507.
4. Corwin HL, Gettinger A, Pearl RG, et al. The CRIT Study: anemia and blood transfusion in the critically ill—current clinical practice in the United States. Crit Care Med 2004;32(1):39–52.
5. Sen J, Belli A, Albon H, et al. Triple-H therapy in the management of aneurysmal subarachnoid haemorrhage. Lancet Neurol 2003;2(10):614–21.
6. Sampson TR, Dhar R, Diringer MN. Factors associated with the development of anemia after subarachnoid hemorrhage. Neurocrit Care 2010;12(1):4–9.
7. Oddo M, Milby A, Chen I, et al. Hemoglobin concentration and cerebral metabolism in patients with aneurysmal subarachnoid hemorrhage. Stroke 2009;40(4): 1275–81.

8. Smith MJ, Stiefel MF, Magge S, et al. Packed red blood cell transfusion increases local cerebral oxygenation. Crit Care Med 2005;33(5):1104–8.
9. Dhar R, Zazulia AR, Videen TO, et al. Red blood cell transfusion increases cerebral oxygen delivery in anemic patients with subarachnoid hemorrhage. Stroke 2009;40(9):3039–44.
10. Naidech AM, Drescher J, Ault ML, et al. Higher hemoglobin is associated with less cerebral infarction, poor outcome, and death after subarachnoid hemorrhage. Neurosurgery 2006;59(4):775–9 [discussion: 779–80].
11. Naidech AM, Jovanovic B, Wartenberg KE, et al. Higher hemoglobin is associated with improved outcome after subarachnoid hemorrhage. Crit Care Med 2007;35(10):2383–9.
12. Kramer AH, Zygun DA, Bleck TP, et al. Relationship between hemoglobin concentrations and outcomes across subgroups of patients with aneurysmal subarachnoid hemorrhage. Neurocrit Care 2009;10(2):157–65.
13. Kramer AH, Gurka MJ, Nathan B, et al. Complications associated with anemia and blood transfusion in patients with aneurysmal subarachnoid hemorrhage. Crit Care Med 2008;36(7):2070–5.
14. Levine J, Kofke A, Cen L, et al. Red blood cell transfusion is associated with infection and extracerebral complications after subarachnoid hemorrhage. Neurosurgery 2010;66(2):312–8 [discussion: 318].
15. Springer MV, Schmidt JM, Wartenberg KE, et al. Predictors of global cognitive impairment 1 year after subarachnoid hemorrhage. Neurosurgery 2009;65(6):1043–50 [discussion: 1050–1].
16. Broessner G, Lackner P, Hoefer C, et al. Influence of red blood cell transfusion on mortality and long-term functional outcome in 292 patients with spontaneous subarachnoid hemorrhage. Crit Care Med 2009;37(6):1886–92.
17. Naidech AM, Shaibani A, Garg RK, et al. Prospective, randomized trial of higher goal hemoglobin after subarachnoid hemorrhage. Neurocrit Care 2010;13(3):313–20.
18. Diringer MN, Bleck TP, Claude Hemphill J 3rd, et al. Critical care management of patients following aneurysmal subarachnoid hemorrhage: recommendations from the Neurocritical Care Society's Multidisciplinary Consensus Conference. Neurocrit Care 2011;15(2):211–40.
19. Stevens RD, Naval NS, Mirski MA, et al. Intensive care of aneurysmal subarachnoid hemorrhage: an international survey. Intensive Care Med 2009;35(9):1556–66.
20. Broderick J, Connolly S, Feldmann E, et al. Guidelines for the management of spontaneous intracerebral hemorrhage in adults: 2007 update: a guideline from the American Heart Association/American Stroke Association Stroke Council, High Blood Pressure Research Council, and the Quality of Care and Outcomes in Research Interdisciplinary Working Group. Stroke 2007;38(6):2001–23.
21. Kumar MA, Rost NS, Snider RW, et al. Anemia and hematoma volume in acute intracerebral hemorrhage. Crit Care Med 2009;37(4):1442–7.
22. Hemphill JC 3rd, Bonovich DC, Besmertis L, et al. The ICH score: a simple, reliable grading scale for intracerebral hemorrhage. Stroke 2001;32(4):891–7.
23. Diedler J, Sykora M, Hahn P, et al. Low hemoglobin is associated with poor functional outcome after non-traumatic, supratentorial intracerebral hemorrhage. Crit Care 2010;14(2):R63.
24. Sheth KN, Gilson AJ, Chang Y, et al. Packed red blood cell transfusion and decreased mortality in intracerebral hemorrhage. Neurosurgery 2011;68(5):1286–92.

25. Leal-Noval SR, Rincon-Ferrari MD, Marin-Niebla A, et al. Transfusion of erythrocyte concentrates produces a variable increment on cerebral oxygenation in patients with severe traumatic brain injury: a preliminary study. Intensive Care Med 2006;32(11):1733–40.

26. Zygun DA, Nortje J, Hutchinson PJ, et al. The effect of red blood cell transfusion on cerebral oxygenation and metabolism after severe traumatic brain injury. Crit Care Med 2009;37(3):1074–8.

27. George ME, Skarda DE, Watts CR, et al. Aggressive red blood cell transfusion: no association with improved outcomes for victims of isolated traumatic brain injury. Neurocrit Care 2008;8(3):337–43.

28. Duane TM, Mayglothling J, Grandhi R, et al. The effect of anemia and blood transfusions on mortality in closed head injury patients. J Surg Res 2008;147(2):163–7.

29. McIntyre LA, Fergusson DA, Hutchison JS, et al. Effect of a liberal versus restrictive transfusion strategy on mortality in patients with moderate to severe head injury. Neurocrit Care 2006;5(1):4–9.

30. Sena MJ, Rivers RM, Muizelaar JP, et al. Transfusion practices for acute traumatic brain injury: a survey of physicians at US trauma centers. Intensive Care Med 2009;35(3):480–8.

31. Morgenstern LB, Hemphill JC 3rd, Anderson C, et al. Guidelines for the management of spontaneous intracerebral hemorrhage: a guideline for healthcare professionals from the American Heart Association/American Stroke Association. Stroke 2010;41(9):2108–29.

32. Ziai WC, Torbey MT, Kickler TS, et al. Platelet count and function in spontaneous intracerebral hemorrhage. J Stroke Cerebrovasc Dis 2003;12(4):201–6.

33. Akins PT, Guppy KH, Sahrakar K, et al. Slippery platelet syndromes in subdural hematoma. Neurocrit Care 2010;12(3):375–81.

34. Naidech AM, Jovanovic B, Liebling S, et al. Reduced platelet activity is associated with early clot growth and worse 3-month outcome after intracerebral hemorrhage. Stroke 2009;40(7):2398–401.

35. Naidech AM, Bernstein RA, Levasseur K, et al. Platelet activity and outcome after intracerebral hemorrhage. Ann Neurol 2009;65(3):352–6.

36. Naidech AM, Bendok BR, Garg RK, et al. Reduced platelet activity is associated with more intraventricular hemorrhage. Neurosurgery 2009;65(4):684–8 [discussion: 688].

37. Campbell PG, Sen A, Yadla S, et al. Emergency reversal of antiplatelet agents in patients presenting with an intracranial hemorrhage: a clinical review. World Neurosurg 2010;74(2–3):279–85.

38. Naidech AM, Liebling SM, Rosenberg NF, et al. Early platelet transfusion improves platelet activity and may improve outcomes after intracerebral hemorrhage. Neurocrit Care 2012;16(1):82–7.

39. Naidech AM, Bassin SL, Bernstein RA, et al. Reduced platelet activity is more common than reported anti-platelet medication use in patients with intracerebral hemorrhage. Neurocrit Care 2009;11(3):307–10.

40. Mannucci PM, Remuzzi G, Pusineri F, et al. Deamino-8-D-arginine vasopressin shortens the bleeding time in uremia. N Engl J Med 1983;308(1):8–12.

41. Masotti L, Di Napoli M, Godoy DA, et al. The practical management of intracerebral hemorrhage associated with oral anticoagulant therapy. Int J Stroke 2011;6(3):228–40.

42. Flaherty ML, Kissela B, Woo D, et al. The increasing incidence of anticoagulant-associated intracerebral hemorrhage. Neurology 2007;68(2):116–21.

43. Watson HG, Baglin T, Laidlaw SL, et al. A comparison of the efficacy and rate of response to oral and intravenous Vitamin K in reversal of over-anticoagulation with warfarin. Br J Haematol 2001;115(1):145–9.

44. Goldstein JN, Thomas SH, Frontiero V, et al. Timing of fresh frozen plasma administration and rapid correction of coagulopathy in warfarin-related intracerebral hemorrhage. Stroke 2006;37(1):151–5.

45. Pabinger I, Brenner B, Kalina U, et al. Prothrombin complex concentrate (Beriplex P/N) for emergency anticoagulation reversal: a prospective multinational clinical trial. J Thromb Haemost 2008;6(4):622–31.

46. Kuwashiro T, Yasaka M, Itabashi R, et al. Effect of prothrombin complex concentrate on hematoma enlargement and clinical outcome in patients with anticoagulant-associated intracerebral hemorrhage. Cerebrovasc Dis 2011;31(2):170–6.

47. Steiner T, Freiberger A, Griebe M, et al. International normalised ratio normalisation in patients with coumarin-related intracranial haemorrhages—the INCH trial: a randomised controlled multicentre trial to compare safety and preliminary efficacy of fresh frozen plasma and prothrombin complex—study design and protocol. Int J Stroke 2011;6(3):271–7.

48. Guest JF, Watson HG, Limaye S. Modeling the cost-effectiveness of prothrombin complex concentrate compared with fresh frozen plasma in emergency warfarin reversal in the United kingdom. Clin Ther 2010;32(14):2478–93.

49. Mayer SA, Brun NC, Begtrup K, et al. Recombinant activated factor VII for acute intracerebral hemorrhage. N Engl J Med 2005;352(8):777–85.

50. Mayer SA, Brun NC, Begtrup K, et al. Efficacy and safety of recombinant activated factor VII for acute intracerebral hemorrhage. N Engl J Med 2008; 358(20):2127–37.

51. Freeman WD, Brott TG, Barrett KM, et al. Recombinant factor VIIa for rapid reversal of warfarin anticoagulation in acute intracranial hemorrhage. Mayo Clin Proc 2004;79(12):1495–500.

52. Lin J, Hanigan WC, Tarantino M, et al. The use of recombinant activated factor VII to reverse warfarin-induced anticoagulation in patients with hemorrhages in the central nervous system: preliminary findings. J Neurosurg 2003;98(4):737–40.

53. Sarode R, Matevosyan K, Bhagat R, et al. Rapid warfarin reversal: a 3-factor prothrombin complex concentrate and recombinant factor VIIa cocktail for intracerebral hemorrhage. J Neurosurg 2012;116(3):491–7.

54. van Ryn J, Stangier J, Haertter S, et al. Dabigatran etexilate—a novel, reversible, oral direct thrombin inhibitor: interpretation of coagulation assays and reversal of anticoagulant activity. Thromb Haemost 2010;103(6):1116–27.

55. Zhou W, Schwarting S, Illanes S, et al. Hemostatic therapy in experimental intracerebral hemorrhage associated with the direct thrombin inhibitor dabigatran. Stroke 2011;42(12):3594–9.

56. Lin CL, Dumont AS, Lieu AS, et al. Characterization of perioperative seizures and epilepsy following aneurysmal subarachnoid hemorrhage. J Neurosurg 2003; 99(6):978–85.

57. Hart Y, Sneade M, Birks J, et al. Epilepsy after subarachnoid hemorrhage: the frequency of seizures after clip occlusion or coil embolization of a ruptured cerebral aneurysm: results from the International Subarachnoid Aneurysm Trial. J Neurosurg 2011;115(6):1159–68.

58. Butzkueven H, Evans AH, Pitman A, et al. Onset seizures independently predict poor outcome after subarachnoid hemorrhage. Neurology 2000;55(9):1315–20.

59. Naidech AM, Kreiter KT, Janjua N, et al. Phenytoin exposure is associated with functional and cognitive disability after subarachnoid hemorrhage. Stroke 2005; 36(3):583–7.

60. Rosengart AJ, Huo JD, Tolentino J, et al. Outcome in patients with subarachnoid hemorrhage treated with antiepileptic drugs. J Neurosurg 2007;107(2):253–60.

61. Bederson JB, Connolly ES Jr, Batjer HH, et al. Guidelines for the management of aneurysmal subarachnoid hemorrhage: a statement for healthcare professionals from a special writing group of the Stroke Council, American Heart Association. Stroke 2009;40(3):994–1025.

62. Murphy-Human T, Welch E, Zipfel G, et al. Comparison of short-duration levetiracetam with extended-course phenytoin for seizure prophylaxis after subarachnoid hemorrhage. World Neurosurg 2011;75(2):269–74.

63. Bladin CF, Alexandrov AV, Bellavance A, et al. Seizures after stroke: a prospective multicenter study. Arch Neurol 2000;57(11):1617–22.

64. Passero S, Rocchi R, Rossi S, et al. Seizures after spontaneous supratentorial intracerebral hemorrhage. Epilepsia 2002;43(10):1175–80.

65. Messe SR, Sansing LH, Cucchiara BL, et al. Prophylactic antiepileptic drug use is associated with poor outcome following ICH. Neurocrit Care 2009;11(1): 38–44.

66. Ferguson PL, Smith GM, Wannamaker BB, et al. A population-based study of risk of epilepsy after hospitalization for traumatic brain injury. Epilepsia 2010;51(5): 891–8.

67. Brain Trauma F, American Association of Neurological S, Congress of Neurological S, et al. Guidelines for the management of severe traumatic brain injury. XIII. Antiseizure prophylaxis. J Neurotrauma 2007;24(Suppl 1):S83–6.

68. Temkin NR, Dikmen SS, Wilensky AJ, et al. A randomized, double-blind study of phenytoin for the prevention of post-traumatic seizures. N Engl J Med 1990; 323(8):497–502.

69. Haltiner AM, Newell DW, Temkin NR, et al. Side effects and mortality associated with use of phenytoin for early posttraumatic seizure prophylaxis. J Neurosurg 1999;91(4):588–92.

70. Temkin NR, Dikmen SS, Anderson GD, et al. Valproate therapy for prevention of posttraumatic seizures: a randomized trial. J Neurosurg 1999;91(4):593–600.

71. Ma CY, Xue YJ, Li M, et al. Sodium valproate for prevention of early posttraumatic seizures. Chin J Traumatol 2010;13(5):293–6.

72. Manaka S. Cooperative prospective study on posttraumatic epilepsy: risk factors and the effect of prophylactic anticonvulsant. Jpn J Psychiatry Neurol 1992;46(2): 311–5.

73. Naidech AM, Garg RK, Liebling S, et al. Anticonvulsant use and outcomes after intracerebral hemorrhage. Stroke 2009;40(12):3810–5.

74. Shah D, Husain AM. Utility of levetiracetam in patients with subarachnoid hemorrhage. Seizure 2009;18(10):676–9.

75. Szaflarski JP, Sangha KS, Lindsell CJ, et al. Prospective, randomized, single-blinded comparative trial of intravenous levetiracetam versus phenytoin for seizure prophylaxis. Neurocrit Care 2010;12(2):165–72.

76. Jones KE, Puccio AM, Harshman KJ, et al. Levetiracetam versus phenytoin for seizure prophylaxis in severe traumatic brain injury. Neurosurg Focus 2008; 25(4):E3.

77. Cotton BA, Kao LS, Kozar R, et al. Cost-utility analysis of levetiracetam and phenytoin for posttraumatic seizure prophylaxis. J Trauma 2011;71(2):375–9.

78. Pieracci FM, Moore EE, Beauchamp K, et al. A cost-minimization analysis of phenytoin versus levetiracetam for early seizure pharmacoprophylaxis after traumatic brain injury. J Trauma Acute Care Surg 2012;72(1):276–81.

79. Ward MJ, Shutter LA, Branas CC, et al. Geographic Access to US Neurocritical Care Units Registered with the Neurocritical Care Society. Neurocrit Care 2012; 16(2):232–40.

80. Suarez JI, Zaidat OO, Suri MF, et al. Length of stay and mortality in neurocritically ill patients: impact of a specialized neurocritical care team. Crit Care Med 2004; 32(11):2311–7.

81. Varelas PN, Eastwood D, Yun HJ, et al. Impact of a neurointensivist on outcomes in patients with head trauma treated in a neurosciences intensive care unit. J Neurosurg 2006;104(5):713–9.

82. Varelas PN, Schultz L, Conti M, et al. The impact of a neuro-intensivist on patients with stroke admitted to a neurosciences intensive care unit. Neurocrit Care 2008; 9(3):293–9.

83. Lerch C, Yonekawa Y, Muroi C, et al. Specialized neurocritical care, severity grade, and outcome of patients with aneurysmal subarachnoid hemorrhage. Neurocrit Care 2006;5(2):85–92.

84. Samuels O, Webb A, Culler S, et al. Impact of a dedicated neurocritical care team in treating patients with aneurysmal subarachnoid hemorrhage. Neurocrit Care 2011;14(3):334–40.

85. Kurtz P, Fitts V, Sumer Z, et al. How does care differ for neurological patients admitted to a neurocritical care unit versus a general ICU? Neurocrit Care 2011;15(3):477–80.

86. Solomon RA, Mayer SA, Tarmey JJ. Relationship between the volume of craniotomies for cerebral aneurysm performed at New York state hospitals and in-hospital mortality. Stroke 1996;27(1):13–7.

87. Bardach NS, Zhao S, Gress DR, et al. Association between subarachnoid hemorrhage outcomes and number of cases treated at California hospitals. Stroke 2002;33(7):1851–6.

88. Berman MF, Solomon RA, Mayer SA, et al. Impact of hospital-related factors on outcome after treatment of cerebral aneurysms. Stroke 2003;34(9):2200–7.

89. Crowley RW, Yeoh HK, Stukenborg GJ, et al. Influence of weekend versus weekday hospital admission on mortality following subarachnoid hemorrhage. Clinical article. J Neurosurg 2009;111(1):60–6.

90. Bardach NS, Olson SJ, Elkins JS, et al. Regionalization of treatment for subarachnoid hemorrhage: a cost-utility analysis. Circulation 2004;109(18):2207–12.

Interfaces of Sleep and Anesthesia

George A. Mashour, MD, PhD[a,b,c,d], Dinesh Pal, PhD[e],*

KEYWORDS

- Sleep • Anesthesia • REM sleep • Slow wave sleep

KEY POINTS

- Sleep and anesthesia are similar but distinct states.
- Sleep and anesthesia may have a common neurochemical substrate in subcortical nuclei.
- Most anesthetics suppress arousal pathways and excite sleep-related pathways.
- Sleep deprivation affects anesthetic potency and anesthesia affects sleep homeostasis.
- The effect of anesthesia on sleep homeostasis is state-specific and agent-specific.

AN INTRODUCTION TO SLEEP AND ANESTHESIA: METAPHORS AND PHENOTYPES

Sleep is a common metaphor for general anesthesia in the perioperative period, and anesthesiologists can frequently be heard telling their patients that they will soon be "going to sleep." Sleep is useful as a metaphor for anesthesia because it is a reversible state of unconsciousness that every patient has experienced and furthermore carries the positive connotations of restoration. This metaphor is supported by the many phenotypic traits shared by sleep and anesthesia, including unconsciousness, amnesia and immobility.

However, there is no trivial identity relationship between sleep and anesthesia. Critical phenotypes of sleep that are not shared by anesthesia include spontaneous generation and termination, ready reversibility by noxious stimuli, and homeostatic regulation. As opposed to anesthesia, sleep is a highly structured and dynamic state. Electrophysiological recordings, primarily, electroencephalogram (EEG), electrooculogram (EOG), and electromyogram (EMG), allow us to categorize sleep into rapid-eye movement (REM) sleep and non-rapid eye movement (NREM) sleep (**Fig. 1**). REM sleep

Funding sources: Departmental sources only.
Conflict of Interest: None.
[a] Department of Anesthesiology, University of Michigan Medical School, 1H247 University Hospital, SPC-5048, Ann Arbor, MI, USA; [b] Department of Neurosurgery, University of Michigan Medical School, Ann Arbor, MI 48109, USA; [c] Neuroscience Graduate Program, University of Michigan, Ann Arbor, MI 48109, USA; [d] Center for Sleep Science, University of Michigan, Ann Arbor, MI 48109, USA; [e] Department of Anesthesiology, University of Michigan Medical School, 1150 West Medical Center Drive, 7422 Medical Science Building 1, Ann Arbor, MI, USA
* Corresponding author.
E-mail address: dineshp@med.umich.edu

Anesthesiology Clin 30 (2012) 385–398
doi:10.1016/j.anclin.2012.05.003   anesthesiology.theclinics.com

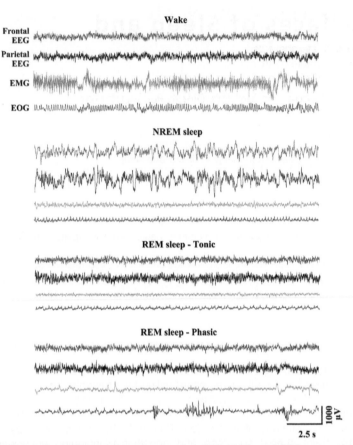

Fig. 1. Representative polygraphic traces showing EEG, EMG, and EOG across sleep-wake states in freely moving rat. The EEG was recorded using a bipolar differential set-up, band-pass filtered between 0.1–100 Hz, and sampled at 250 Hz.

is characterized by low-voltage high-frequency EEG, bursts of rapid eye movements, muscle twitches in extremities, periodic activation of middle ear muscles, and atonia in almost all the skeletal muscles, with the respiratory muscles being a major exception.[1] Low-voltage high-frequency EEG and muscle atonia are tonic features of REM sleep, whereas eye movements, muscle twitches, and middle ear muscle activity are phasic events. The absence or presence of the phasic events differentiates REM sleep into tonic and phasic sub-stages, respectively (see **Fig. 1**). Most dreams have been reported during REM sleep, and thus this phase of sleep is also known as dream sleep.[1]

NREM sleep is characterized by high-voltage low-frequency EEG, low muscle tone, and occasional slow rolling eye movements (see **Fig. 1**). NREM sleep in humans has been subdivided into stage 1 through 4, with a progressive increase in the depth of sleep.[1] The onset of NREM sleep is marked by the shifting of EEG spectrum to lower frequencies (stage 1). Sleep spindles appear during NREM sleep stage 2 whereas stage 3 and 4 are characterized by the presence of slow wave oscillations or delta EEG.[1] Following the recent revision of the human sleep scoring manual by American Academy of Sleep Medicine, the NREM sleep stages 1 and 2 have been reclassified as stages N1 and N2, whereas stages 3 and 4 have been merged into a single stage N3,[2] which in non-human subjects are classified as slow wave sleep.

Despite the apparent behavioral similarity, NREM and REM sleep states are characterized by profound differences at the cellular and physiological levels. NREM sleep is a quiescent state characterized by slow EEG, decrease in body temperature, lowered metabolism, stable heart rate and respiration, and increased parasympathetic tone.[1] In contrast, REM sleep represents a highly aroused state as indicated by activated EEG, increased cerebral blood flow and brain metabolism, almost complete suspension of thermoregulation leading to an increase in core body temperature, irregular heart rate, increased and irregular respiration, and a further decrease in parasympathetic tone as compared with NREM sleep. Further, as might be deduced by the changes in physiological variables like heart rate, respiration and blood pressure, interspersed increases in sympathetic tone occur during phasic REM sleep.[1] Thus, although a convenient and reassuring shorthand for general anesthesia, sleep is unquestionably a distinct state.

SLEEP AND ANESTHETIC MECHANISMS: SUBCORTICAL INTERFACES

In the mid-1990s it was suggested that general anesthetics may act through the subcortical centers involved in the control of sleep-wake states.[3] There is now considerable evidence to support this hypothesis.[4,5] In this section, we will consider a few key hypothalamic and brainstem regions that are critical to sleep regulation and that may mediate anesthetic-induced unconsciousness (**Fig. 2**).

Hypothalamic Sites Involved in Sleep-Wake and Anesthetic Mechanisms

Ventrolateral preoptic and median preoptic nucleus: *γ*-aminobutyric acid–mediated mechanisms
Almost a century ago it was postulated that the anterior hypothalamus/preoptic region is involved in sleep-wake regulation.[6] The experimental evidence gathered since has consolidated the role of preoptic area in sleep promotion.[7] In vivo and in vitro studies have identified γ-aminobutyric acid (GABA) positive neurons in ventrolateral preoptic (VLPO) and median preoptic (MnPO) nuclei that show maximal activity during NREM and REM sleep.[8–12] Although VLPO and MnPO contain sleep-active neurons, the activity profile of VLPO GABAergic neurons correlates with sleep amount, whereas the activity profile of GABAergic neurons in MnPO correlates with sleep pressure or sleep

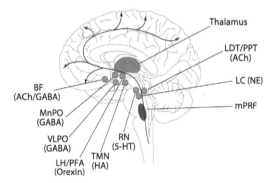

Fig. 2. Important cortical and subcortical nuclei and the associated neurotransmitters underlying sleep-wake and anesthetic mechanisms. Abbreviations: ACh, acetylcholine; BF, basal forebrain; GABA, γ aminobutyric acid; HA, histamine; LC, locus coeruleus; LDT/PPT, laterodorsal tegmentum/pedunculopontine tegmentum; LH/PFA, lateral hypothalamus/perifornical area; MnPO, median preoptic nucleus; mPRF, medial pontine reticular formation; NE, norepinephrine; RN, raphe nuclei; TMN, tuberomammillary nucleus; VLPO, ventrolateral preoptic nucleus; 5-HT, serotonin.

propensity.[7,9–12] Therefore, it has been suggested that VLPO is involved in the maintenance of sleep state, whereas MnPO plays an important role in sleep homeostasis.[7]

The "sleep-ON" neurons in VLPO were attractive candidates as mediators of general anesthetic action. Nelson and colleagues[13] demonstrated that the systemic administration of anesthetic drugs such as propofol and pentothal result in VLPO activation as indicated by c-fos expression, which is a marker for neuronal activity. Activation of VLPO seems to be specific to anesthetics targeting the type A GABA receptors (GABA$_A$) because ketamine does not increase c-fos expression in VLPO.[14] VLPO activation may be mediated by the increased glutamatergic (ie, excitatory) input that is enhanced by general anesthetics.[15] Recently, Eikermann and colleagues[16] lesioned VLPO nucleus in rats and assessed the anesthetic requirements. Contrary to the current paradigm, they found that VLPO lesions *sensitized* the animals to the effects of isoflurane, that is, VLPO was not required for anesthetic-mediated unconsciousness. However, VLPO lesions resulted in chronic sleep deprivation, suggesting that the increased homeostatic pressure for sleep may have overwhelmed the effects of VLPO lesion on anesthetic action. Further work with acutely VLPO-lesioned animals (i.e., those that have not yet encountered severe sleep deprivation) is required to clarify the direct role of VLPO in anesthetic mechanism. Loss-of-function studies associated with MnPO may also provide crucial insights into sleep-anesthesia interfaces.

Tuberomammillary nucleus: histaminergic mechanisms

Tuberomammillary nucleus (TMN) is a histaminergic group of neurons in the posterior hypothalamus and is the only source of histamine in the central nervous system.[17,18] The histaminergic neurons show a behavioral state–dependent profile; the neuronal activity as well as the release of histamine is highest during wake state and lowest during sleep.[17–21] The histaminergic neurons in TMN project to widespread areas in the brain including those involved in sleep-wake regulation. In particular, there is a direct functional relationship between TMN and VLPO.[17,18] The available evidence suggests that histaminergic neurons and VLPO GABAergic neurons share a mutual inhibitory relationship.[7,17,18,22] There is enough evidence to conclude that histamine promotes wakefulness and a reduction in histaminergic neurotransmission decreases wakefulness and increases sleep.[17,18]

In addition to facilitating the activity of sleep-promoting sites, as has been reported with VLPO and MnPO, general anesthetics can also act by inhibiting the wake-promoting areas. Histamine release in the anterior hypothalamus has been reported to decrease during halothane anesthesia and sleep.[23,24] Central administration of histamine decreased pentobarbital-related hypnosis and hypothermia.[25] Nelson and colleagues[13] reported that systemic administration of GABAergic agents-muscimol, propofol, and pentothal-caused a decrease in c-fos expression in TMN whereas the c-fos expression increased in VLPO. Further, central administration or local injection of GABA antagonist into TMN countered the effect of these GABAergic agents.[13] Mutations of the GABA$_A$ attenuate the response of TMN neurons to propofol, suggesting a GABAergic mechanism underlying the reduced TMN activity during general anesthesia.[26] The reduction of TMN activity likely contributes to anesthetic-induced unconsciousness by reducing excitatory histaminergic input to the basal forebrain, which in turn reduces cortical arousal.[27] This may also be the mechanism of the commonly observed sedation that occurs after anti-histaminergic drugs such as diphenhydramine.

Lateral hypothalamus perifornical area: orexinergic mechanisms

Orexins (A and B), also know as hypocretins (1 and 2), are excitatory neuropeptides derived from the same precursor peptide produced by neurons in the perifornical region of the hypothalamus.[17,28] There is widespread orexinergic innervation in the central nervous system, including the monoaminergic and cholinergic arousal centers in forebrain and brainstem.[17,28] Orexinergic neurons show the highest discharge rate during active wake and are silent during sleep, with occasional bursts of activity during phasic REM sleep.[29–31] The activity profile of these neurons shows strong correlation with the muscle activity and the presence of gamma waves as observed during electroencephalographic activation.[29–31] Central and local orexinergic stimulation promote electroencephalographic as well as behavioral arousal, possibly through basal forebrain modulation.[17,28] Loss of orexinergic signaling has been confirmed as a cause of narcolepsy across species, which emphasizes the importance of orexinergic signaling in arousal state.[17,28]

Intracerebroventricular administration of orexin results in EEG activation in rats under isoflurane anesthesia[32] and reduces barbiturate as well as ketamine anesthesia time.[33,34] Local infusion of orexin into basal forebrain caused electroencephalographic arousal in isoflurane- and sevoflurane-anesthetized rats[35,36] and decreased the emergence time from anesthesia.[36] Microinjection of propofol into the perifornical area decreased cortical acetylcholine (ACh) release,[37] which normally mediates behavioral and electroencephalographic arousal. Intracerebroventricular administration of orexin antagonizes the effects of propofol anesthesia as assessed by the time to loss of righting reflex.[26] Recent studies have shown that isoflurane and sevoflurane,[38] but not halothane,[39] decrease c-fos expression in orexinergic neurons. Orexins seem to play a role that is specific to the emergence from sevoflurane and isoflurane anesthesia because the induction of anesthesia does not seem to be affected by the disruption of orexinergic signaling.[38] This suggests a distinct neurobiology underlying the onset and offset of general anesthesia,[40] which may be mediated, in part, by sleep pathways.

Brainstem Sites Involved in Sleep-Wake and Anesthetic Mechanisms

Locus coeruleus: noradrenergic mechanisms

Located in the pons, the locus coeruleus (LC) is a major source of noradrenaline in the central nervous system and has widespread projections throughout the cortex.[41] The activity of the noradrenergic LC neurons is highest during the wake state, decrease during NREM sleep, and decreases yet further during REM sleep.[41–43] A generalized increase in noradrenergic tone is correlated with arousal and cortical activation.[41] Noradrenergic antagonists increase barbiturate anesthesia time whereas agonists decrease barbiturate anesthesia time.[44,45] A direct hyperpolarizing effect of halothane on LC neurons has been shown.[46] Microinjection of dexmedetomidine, α-2 agonist, into LC produced hypnosis that could be prevented through coadministration of α-2 antagonist atipamezole.[47] Further, dexmedetomidine induces c-fos changes comparable to NREM sleep (increases in VLPO and decreases in TMN), including decreased activity in LC.[48] Of note, ketamine increases c-fos expression in the LC,[14] whereas the depletion of LC neurons caused a decrease in ketamine anesthesia time.[49] In contrast, depletion of noradrenergic neurons in LC potentiates thiopental anesthesia.[49] Therefore, arousal-promoting neurons in the LC are a target for the action of some general anesthetics.

Laterodorsal/pedunculopontine tegmentum: cholinergic mechanisms

Laterodorsal/pedunculopontine tegmentum (LDT/PPT) are the major cholinergic neuronal groups in the brainstem.[41] Electrophysiological recordings have confirmed the activation of cholinergic neurons in association with electroencephalographic arousal as observed during wake and REM sleep.[4] There are direct cholinergic projections from LDT/PPT to the thalamus,[41] which has a well-documented role in the generation of spindles and slow wave oscillations.[50] Halothane produces EEG spindles that are similar to the spindles observed during NREM sleep.[51] Microinjection of nicotine, a cholinergic agonist, into centromedial thalamus restored mobility and righting in sevoflurane-anesthetized rats.[52] In addition to thalamus, LDT/PPT also send direct cholinergic projections to medial pontine reticular formation (mPRF), which is important for wake and REM sleep states.[4,41] Microdialysis measurement of ACh in mPRF demonstrated an increase in ACh levels during wake state as well as during REM sleep, which is characterized by electroencephalographic arousal.[4] Inhibition of behavioral and electroencephalographic arousal during halothane and ketamine anesthesia decreases ACh release in mPRF.[51,53,54] GABA in mPRF modulates the local ACh release during wake and REM sleep.[55] A recent report from the same laboratory showed that GABA levels increase during isoflurane anesthesia, which implies that isoflurane decreases ACh levels in mPRF as has been reported earlier for halothane and ketamine.[51,53,54,56] Further, it is becoming increasingly evident that multiple neurotransmitter systems interact in mPRF with the cholinergic projections from LDT/PPT for the regulation of arousal state as well as anesthesia.[4,56,57]

SLEEP AND ANESTHETIC MECHANISMS: THALAMOCORTICAL/CORTICOCORTICAL INTERFACES

The mechanistic interfaces of sleep and anesthesia at the subcortical level are also manifest by similarities in thalamocortical and corticocortical neurophysiology that may mediate the shared trait of unconsciousness. **Fig. 3** shows the electroencephalographic similarity between the slow waves and spindles across sleep, propofol and sevoflurane anesthesia.

Spindles

Stage 2 of NREM sleep is characterized by spindles, which are waxing and waning bursts of activity on the EEG at a frequency of 7–11 Hz. Spindles signal a thalamic hyperpolarization that is thought to block the transfer of sensory information from the periphery to the cortex. In support of the sleep-anesthesia connection, spindles have been observed to occur during exposure to volatile anesthetics,[53,58] propofol,[59] and dexmedetomidine.[60] Spindle activity has been suggested to be of potential utility in assessing anesthetic depth[61] because it signals a breakdown of thalamocortical signaling.

Slow Waves

A recent high-density electroencephalographic study modeled slow waves during NREM sleep and propofol anesthesia in humans.[62] Slow wave activity in the two states shared several features, including the presence in virtually all unconscious epochs, distribution over a high number of channels, consistency of frequency and distribution across subjects, and comparable scalp voltage topography. Both propofol- and sleep-related slow waves seemed to originate in the insular and cingulate cortices, propagating posteriorly along the anterior cingulate, cingulate, and posterior cingulate gyri. Propofol slow waves also demonstrated differences, such as the occasional occipital origin, less demarcated spatial distribution, and lack of the distinctive asymmetries found in sleep.

Cortical Effective Connectivity

Functional connectivity refers to the statistical covariation of neural activity in two brain regions, whereas effective connectivity refers to a causal interaction.[63] Effective

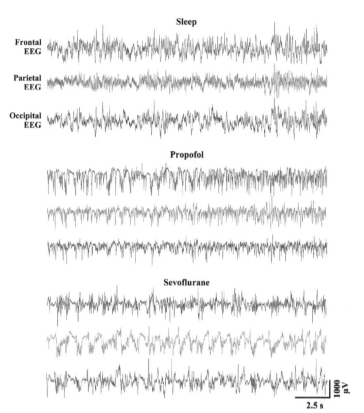

Fig. 3. Monopolar EEG traces showing the presence of slow waves and spindles across sleep (NREM), propofol (800 µg/kg body wt) and sevoflurane (2.0–2.2%) anesthesia in rat. The EEG was bandpass filtered between 0.1–300 Hz, and sampled at 1000 Hz.

connectivity has been regarded as a surrogate for the integration of meaningful information across different brain regions.[64] Using electroencephalography and transcranial magnetic stimulation, Massimini and colleagues[65] demonstrated a breakdown of cortical effective connectivity during NREM sleep. A follow-up study using the same techniques revealed a similar breakdown of cortical effective connectivity during midazolam anesthesia.[66] Thus, both sleep- and anesthesia-induced unconsciousness share similar patterns of communication breakdown in the brain.

FUNCTIONAL INTERFACES OF SLEEP AND ANESTHESIA

The macroscopic phenotypes, mechanistic interfaces, and neurophysiologic similarities of sleep and anesthesia are scientifically and intellectually compelling, but what significance do they have from the functional perspective? We can approach this question by considering the effects of sleep profiles on anesthetic action as well as the effects of anesthesia on sleep profiles.

Effects of Sleep on Anesthesia

Tung and colleagues[67] demonstrated for the first time that alterations of sleep can influence the function of general anesthetics. In one study, rats underwent total sleep deprivation for 24 hours and then were anesthetized with either propofol or isoflurane.

Time to induction was significantly reduced in the sleep-deprived rats compared with non-deprived controls; the sleep-deprived rats also took longer to emerge from each anesthetic. In support of these findings, Pal and colleagues[68] found that 12 hours of total sleep deprivation resulted in a shorter time to induction with sevoflurane. Tung and colleagues[69] showed that the increased sensitivity to anesthesia after sleep deprivation was mediated, in part, by adenosine. During prolonged wakefulness, adenosine accumulates in the basal forebrain and contributes to the homeostatic pressure for NREM sleep.[70]

It is of interest to consider whether this functional relationship between sleep and anesthesia has a genetic basis. *Drosophila melanogaster* (the fruit fly) with mutations of the voltage-gated potassium "Shaker" gene are known to sleep less than their wild-type counterparts.[71] Weber and colleagues[72] found that these same mutants were resistant to the effects of isoflurane. Thus, in *Drosophila*, a single gene controls the complex phenotypes of both sleep and anesthetic sensitivity.

Effects of Anesthesia on Sleep

Tung and colleagues[73] were also the first to show that a general anesthetic could repay sleep debt after sleep deprivation. After 24 hours of total sleep deprivation, rats were administered either propofol or an intralipid control for 6 hours and thereafter electro-physiological sleep-wake recordings were done. Neither REM nor NREM sleep showed a rebound increase in the period after anesthesia, suggesting that propofol satisfied the need for both components of sleep just as well as the *ad libitum* sleep. However, Mashour and colleagues[74] demonstrated that inhaled anesthetics have a distinct profile regarding sleep homeostasis because the REM sleep debt is maintained during the anesthetized state. This finding suggested that functional interfaces of sleep and anesthesia were drug-specific (intravenous vs inhaled) and state-specific (NREM sleep vs REM sleep). Nelson and colleagues[75] found that isoflurane and desflurane satisfied the debt of slow wave sleep, which was confirmed by Pal and colleagues[68] for sevoflurane. The study by Pal and colleagues[68] furthermore showed that sevoflurane had a profound effect on NREM sleep homeostasis, repaying NREM sleep debt twice as fast as ad libitum sleep. Again, REM sleep debt was maintained during the 6-hour sevoflurane exposure and was repaid (rebound increase) after the termination of anesthetic exposure. These state-specific effects of inhaled anesthetics were also reported by Pick and colleagues,[76] who found that mice exposed to halogenated ethers exhibited subsequent REM sleep rebound (ie, a need for REM sleep that was not satisfied during general anesthesia), but no NREM sleep rebound. This finding is in contrast to an earlier study by Tung and colleagues,[77] who found that a 12-hour exposure to propofol did not result in either REM or NREM sleep rebound. The findings from our laboratory and other recent studies have been summarized in **Fig. 4**.

It is important to put these studies in the context of clinical care. All of the experiments described above involved rats subjected to general anesthesia alone. Healthy human volunteers exposed to isoflurane demonstrate suppression of slow wave sleep and reciprocal increases in stage 2 NREM sleep.[78] Surgical stress, pain, and opioid use, among many other perioperative factors, can influence sleep architecture. Knill and colleagues[79] demonstrated that patients undergoing abdominal surgery with the more routine anesthetic management of isoflurane, nitrous oxide, and opioids experience a marked REM sleep rebound at days 2 to 4. REM sleep is associated with cardiovascular instability[80] and, in patients with obstructive sleep apnea, the increased probability of airway obstruction.[81] The drug- and state-specific differences of anesthetic effects on sleep homeostasis forces us to consider which anesthetics are better for patients with sleep deprivation or sleep apnea.

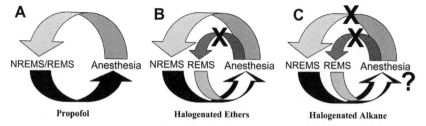

Fig. 4. Schematic to summarize the current state of knowledge about sleep-anesthesia inter-faces. (*A*) Propofol allows the dissipation of sleep debt and thereby allows full recovery from the effects of sleep deprivation.[73] Sleep deprivation potentiates the effects of propofol.[67] (*B*) Halogenated ethers, as a class of inhaled anesthetics, allow the recovery of NREM sleep after sleep deprivation but REM sleep debt is maintained (or can accumulate in the non-deprived animal) during anesthetic exposure ("X" indicating no recovery). The recovery of REM sleep occurs during the period after anesthesia.[68,74,75] Sleep deprivation enhances anesthetic potency as demonstrated by a decrease in the time to loss of righting reflex.[67,68] (*C*) Haloge-nated alkane (halothane) is different compared with propofol and halogenated ethers. Halo-genated alkane causes a suspension of homeostatic mechanisms for both NREM and REM sleep, because of which sleep debt accumulates during anesthesia. Recovery occurs during the period after anesthesia as shown by a rebound increase in NREM and REM sleep.[76]

SUMMARY AND RELEVANCE FOR NEUROANESTHESIOLOGY

Sleep and anesthesia are distinct states with overlapping traits. Although it is patently obvious that there is no identity relationship between the two states, key questions that remain include (1) the contribution of sleep-wake pathways to the mechanism of general anesthesia, (2) the functional and cognitive significance of anesthetic effects on sleep homeostasis, and (3) the optimal anesthetic regimen for patients who present for surgery in a state of sleep deprivation or with disorders such as sleep apnea.

There are also considerations of sleep-wake neurobiology that are particularly rele-vant to neuroanesthesiology although this relationship has received little attention. A central goal that distinguishes neuroanesthetic practice is a rapid and crisp emer-gence from general anesthesia that can facilitate the evaluation of neurologic function after surgical intervention. As discussed previously, there are several nuclei that are critical for cortical arousal, including the TMN (histamine), periformical hypothalamus (orexinergic), locus coeruleus (noradrenergic), and other areas not discussed, such as the basal forebrain (cholinergic), ventral tegmental area/midbrain (dopaminergic), and dorsal raphe (serotonergic) (see **Fig. 2**). Using these pathways to induce emer-gence is starting to be explored and could ultimately be useful for rapid recovery after neurosurgery. For example, methylphenidate, a dopamine agonist that may potentiate the activity of the ventral tegmental area, reverses anesthetic effects in rats.[82] Physo-stigmine, an acetylcholinesterase inhibitor that potentiates cholinergic tone also reverses the effects of anesthesia in humans.[83,84] Instead of passively waiting, neuro-anesthesiologists may one day control the emergence process through pharmaco-logic manipulation of pathways that regulate sleep and wakefulness.

REFERENCES

1. Rechtschaffen A, Siegel JM. Sleep and dreaming. In: Kandell E, Schwartz JH, Jessell TM, editors. Principles of neural science. 4th edition. New York: McGraw-Hill; 2000. p. 936–47.

2. Iber C, Ancoli-Israel S, Chesson A, et al, editors. The AASM manual for the scoring of sleep and associated events: rules, terminology, and technical specification. 1st edition. Westchester (IL): American Academy of Sleep Medicine; 2007.

3. Lydic R, Biebuyck JF. Sleep neurobiology: relevance for mechanistic studies of anaesthesia. Br J Anaesth 1994;72:506–8.

4. Lydic R, Baghdoyan HA. Sleep, anesthesiology, and the neurobiology of arousal state control. Anesthesiology 2005;103:1268–95.

5. Franks NP. General anaesthesia: from molecular targets to neuronal pathways of sleep and arousal. Nat Rev Neurosci 2008;9:370–86.

6. von Economo C. Sleep as a problem of localization. J Nerv Ment Dis 1930;71: 249–59.

7. Szymusiak R, McGinty D. Hypothalamic regulation of sleep and arousal. Ann N Y Acad Sci 2008;1129:275–86.

8. Sherin JE, Shiromani PJ, McCarley RW, et al. Activation of ventrolateral preoptic neurons during sleep. Science 1996;271:216–9.

9. Szymusiak R, Alam N, Steininger TL, et al. Sleep-waking discharge patterns of ventrolateral preoptic/anterior hypothalamic neurons in rats. Brain Res 1998; 803:178–88.

10. Gong H, Szymusiak R, King J, et al. Sleep-related c-Fos protein expression in the preoptic hypothalamus: effects of ambient warming. Am J Physiol Regul Integr Comp Physiol 2000;279:R2079–88.

11. Gong H, McGinty D, Guzman-Marin R, et al. Activation of c-fos in GABAergic neurons in the preoptic area during sleep and in response to sleep deprivation. J Physiol 2004;556:935–46.

12. Suntsova N, Szymusiak R, Alam MN, et al. Sleep-waking discharge patterns of median preoptic nucleus neurons in rats. J Physiol 2002;543:665–77.

13. Nelson LE, Guo TZ, Lu J, et al. The sedative component of anesthesia is mediated by GABA(A) receptors in an endogenous sleep pathway. Nat Neurosci 2002;5:979–84.

14. Lu J, Nelson LE, Franks N, et al. Role of endogenous sleep-wake and analgesic systems in anesthesia. J Comp Neurol 2008;508:648–62.

15. Li KY, Guan YZ, Krnjević K, et al. Propofol facilitates glutamatergic transmission to neurons of the ventrolateral preoptic nucleus. Anesthesiology 2009;111: 1271–8.

16. Eikermann M, Vetrivelan R, Grosse-Sundrup M, et al. The ventrolateral preoptic nucleus is not required for isoflurane general anesthesia. Brain Res 2011;1426: 30–7.

17. Lin JS, Anaclet C, Sergeeva OA, et al. The waking brain: an update. Cell Mol Life Sci 2011;68:2499–512.

18. Thakkar MM. Histamine in the regulation of wakefulness. Sleep Med Rev 2011;15: 65–74.

19. Takahashi K, Lin JS, Sakai K. Neuronal activity of histaminergic tuberomammillary neurons during wake–sleep states in the mouse. J Neurosci 2006;26: 10292–8.

20. Vanni-Mercier G, Gigout S, Debilly G, et al. Waking selective neurons in the posterior hypothalamus and their response to histamine H3-receptor ligands: an electrophysiological study in freely moving cats. Behav Brain Res 2003;144: 227–41.

21. Chu M, Huang ZL, Qu WM, et al. Extracellular histamine level in the frontal cortex is positively correlated with the amount of wakefulness in rats. Neurosci Res 2004; 49:417–20.

22. Liu YW, Li J, Ye JH. Histamine regulates activities of neurons in the ventrolateral preoptic nucleus. J Physiol 2010;588:4103–16.
23. Mammoto T, Yamamoto Y, Kagawa K, et al. Interactions between neuronal histamine and halothane anesthesia in rats. J Neurochem 1997;69:406–11.
24. Strecker RE, Nalwalk J, Dauphin LJ, et al. Extracellular histamine levels in the feline preoptic/anterior hypothalamic area during natural sleep-wakefulness and prolonged wakefulness: an in vivo microdialysis study. Neuroscience 2002; 113:663–70.
25. Kalivas PW. Histamine-induced arousal in the conscious and pentobarbital-pretreated rat. J Pharmacol Exp Ther 1982;222:37–42.
26. Zecharia AY, Nelson LE, Gent TC, et al. The involvement of hypothalamic sleep pathways in general anesthesia: testing the hypothesis using the GABAA receptor beta3N265M knock-in mouse. J Neurosci 2009;29:2177–87.
27. Luo T, Leung LS. Basal forebrain histaminergic transmission modulates electroencephalographic activity and emergence from isoflurane anesthesia. Anesthesiology 2009;111:725–33.
28. Arrigoni E, Mochizuki T, Scammell TE. Activation of the basal forebrain by the orexin/hypocretin neurons. Acta Physiol (Oxf) 2010;198:223–35.
29. Mileykovskiy BY, Kiyashchenko LI, Siegel JM. Behavioral correlates of activity in identified hypocretin/orexin neurons. Neuron 2005;46:787–98.
30. Lee MG, Hassani OK, Jones BE. Discharge of identified orexin/hypocretin neurons across the sleep-waking cycle. J Neurosci 2005;25:6716–20.
31. Takahashi K, Lin JS, Sakai K. Neuronal activity of orexin and non-orexin waking-active neurons during wake-sleep states in the mouse. Neuroscience 2008;153: 860–70.
32. Yasuda Y, Takeda A, Fukuda S, et al. Orexin a elicits arousal electroencephalography without sympathetic cardiovascular activation in isoflurane-anesthetized rats. Anesth Analg 2003;97:1663–6.
33. Kushikata T, Hirota K, Yoshida H, et al. Orexinergic neurons and barbiturate anesthesia. Neuroscience 2003;121:855–63.
34. Tose R, Kushikata T, Yoshida H. Orexin A decreases ketamine-induced anesthesia time in the rat: the relevance to brain noradrenergic neuronal activity. Anesth Analg 2009;108:491–5.
35. Dong HL, Fukuda S, Murata E. Orexins increase cortical acetylcholine release and electroencephalographic activation through orexin-1 receptor in the rat basal forebrain during isoflurane anesthesia. Anesthesiology 2006;104:1023–32.
36. Dong H, Niu J, Su B, et al. Activation of orexin signal in basal forebrain facilitates the emergence from sevoflurane anesthesia in rat. Neuropeptides 2009;43: 179–85.
37. Gamou S, Fukuda S, Ogura M, et al. Microinjection of propofol into the perifornical area induces sedation with decreasing cortical acetylcholine release in rats. Anesth Analg 2010;111:395–402.
38. Kelz MB, Sun Y, Chen J, et al. An essential role for orexins in emergence from general anesthesia. Proc Natl Acad Sci U S A 2008;105:1309–14.
39. Gompf H, Chen J, Sun Y, et al. Halothane-induced hypnosis is not accompanied by inactivation of orexinergic output in rodents. Anesthesiology 2009;111:1001–9.
40. Friedman EB, Sun Y, Moore JT, et al. A conserved behavioral state barrier impedes transitions between anesthetic-induced unconsciousness and wakefulness: evidence for neural inertia. PLoS One 2010;5:e11903.
41. Jones BE. Neurobiology of waking and sleeping. Handb Clin Neurol 2011;98: 131–49.

42. Aston-Jones G, Bloom FE. Activity of norepinephrine containing locus coeruleus neurons in behaving rats anticipates fluctuations in the sleep-waking cycle. J Neurosci 1981;1:876–86.
43. Takahashi K, Kayama Y, Lin JS, et al. Locus coeruleus neuronal activity during the sleep-waking cycle in mice. Neuroscience 2010;169:1115–26.
44. Mason ST, Angel A. Anaesthesia: the role of adrenergic mechanisms. Eur J Pharmacol 1983;91:29–39.
45. Matsumoto K, Kohno SI, Ojima K, et al. Flumazenil but not FG7142 reverses the decrease in pentobarbital sleep caused by activation of central noradrenergic systems in mice. Brain Res 1997;754:325–8.
46. Sirois JE, Lei Q, Talley EM, et al. The TASK-1 two-pore domain K+ channel is a molecular substrate for neuronal effects of inhalation anesthetics. J Neurosci 2000;20:6347–54.
47. Correa-Sales C, Rabin BC, Maze M. A hypnotic response to dexmedetomidine, an alpha 2 agonist, is mediated in the locus coeruleus in rats. Anesthesiology 1992;76:948–52.
48. Nelson LE, Lu J, Guo T, et al. The alpha2-adrenoceptor agonist dexmedetomidine converges on an endogenous sleep-promoting pathway to exert its sedative effects. Anesthesiology 2003;98:428–36.
49. Kushikata T, Yoshida H, Kudo M, et al. Role of coerulean noradrenergic neurones in general anaesthesia in rats. Br J Anaesth 2011;107:924–9.
50. Steriade M. The corticothalamic system in sleep. Front Biosci 2003;8:d878–99.
51. Keifer JC, Baghdoyan HA, Becker L, et al. Halothane decreases pontine acetylcholine release and increases EEG spindles. Neuroreport 1994;5:577–80.
52. Alkire MT, McReynolds JR, Hahn EL, et al. Thalamic microinjection of nicotine reverses sevoflurane-induced loss of righting reflex in the rat. Anesthesiology 2007;107:264–72.
53. Keifer JC, Baghdoyan HA, Lydic R. Pontine cholinergic mechanisms modulate the cortical electroencephalographic spindles of halothane anesthesia. Anesthesiology 1996;84:945–54.
54. Lydic R, Baghdoyan HA. Ketamine and MK-801 decrease acetylcholine release in the pontine reticular formation, slow breathing, and disrupt sleep. Sleep 2002;25:617–22.
55. Vazquez J, Baghdoyan HA. GABAA receptors inhibit acetylcholine release in cat pontine reticular formation: implications for REM sleep regulation. J Neurophysiol 2004;92:2198–206.
56. Vanini G, Watson CJ, Lydic R, et al. Gamma-aminobutyric acid-mediated neurotransmission in the pontine reticular formation modulates hypnosis, immobility, and breathing during isoflurane anesthesia. Anesthesiology 2008;109:978–88.
57. Xi M, Chase MH. The injection of hypocretin-1 into the nucleus pontis oralis induces either active sleep or wakefulness depending on the behavioral state when it is administered. Sleep 2010;33:1236–43.
58. MacKay EC, Sleigh JW, Voss LJ, et al. Episodic waveforms in the electroencephalogram during general anaesthesia: a study of patterns of response to noxious stimuli. Anaesth Intensive Care 2010;38:102–12.
59. Ferenets R, Lipping T, Suominen P, et al. Comparison of the properties of EEG spindles in sleep and propofol anesthesia. Conf Proc IEEE Eng Med Biol Soc 2006;1:6356–9.
60. Huupponen E, Maksimow A, Lapinlampi P, et al. Electroencephalogram spindle activity during dexmedetomidine sedation and physiological sleep. Acta Anaesthesiol Scand 2008;52:289–94.

61. Law CJ, Sleight JW, Barnard JP, et al. The association between intraoperative electroencephalogram-based measures and pain severity in the post-anaesthesia care unit. Anaesth Intensive Care 2011;39:875–80.
62. Murphy M, Bruno MA, Riedner BA, et al. Propofol anesthesia and sleep: a high-density EEG study. Sleep 2011;34:283A–91A.
63. Friston KJ. Functional and effective connectivity: a review. Brain Connect 2011;1: 13–36.
64. Tononi G. Information integration: its relevance to brain function and consciousness. Arch Ital Biol 2010;148:299–322.
65. Massimini M, Ferrarelli F, Huber R, et al. Breakdown of cortical effective connectivity during sleep. Science 2005;309:2228–32.
66. Ferrarelli F, Massimini M, Sarasso S, et al. Breakdown in cortical effective connectivity during midazolam-induced loss of consciousness. Proc Natl Acad Sci U S A 2010;107:2681–6.
67. Tung A, Szafran MJ, Bluhm B, et al. Sleep deprivation potentiates the onset and duration of loss of righting reflex induced by propofol and isoflurane. Anesthesiology 2002;97:906–11.
68. Pal D, Lipinski WJ, Walker AJ, et al. State-specific effects of sevoflurane anesthesia on sleep homeostasis: selective recovery of slow wave but not rapid eye movement sleep. Anesthesiology 2011;114:302–10.
69. Tung A, Herrera S, Szafran MJ, et al. Effect of sleep deprivation on righting reflex in the rat is partially reversed by administration of adenosine A1 and A2 receptor antagonists. Anesthesiology 2005;102:1158–64.
70. Landolt HP. Sleep homeostasis: a role for adenosine in humans? Biochem Pharmacol 2008;75:2070–9.
71. Cirelli C, Bushey D, Hill S, et al. Reduced sleep in Drosophila Shaker mutants. Nature 2005;434:1087–92.
72. Weber B, Schaper C, Bushey D, et al. Increased volatile anesthetic requirement in short-sleeping Drosophila mutants. Anesthesiology 2009;110:313–6.
73. Tung A, Bergmann BM, Herrera S, et al. Recovery from sleep deprivation occurs during propofol anesthesia. Anesthesiology 2004;100:1419–26.
74. Mashour GA, Lipinski W, Matlen L, et al. Isoflurane anesthesia does not satisfy the homeostatic need for rapid eye movement sleep. Anesth Analg 2010;110: 1283–9.
75. Nelson AB, Faraguna U, Tononi G, et al. Effects of anesthesia on the response to sleep deprivation. Sleep 2010;33:1659–67.
76. Pick J, Chen Y, Moore JT, et al. Rapid eye movement sleep debt accrues in mice exposed to volatile anesthetics. Anesthesiology 2011;115:702–12.
77. Tung A, Lynch JP, Mendelson WB. Prolonged sedation with propofol in the rat does not result in sleep deprivation. Anesth Analg 2001;92:1232–6.
78. Moote CA, Knill RL. Isoflurane anesthesia causes a transient alteration in nocturnal sleep. Anesthesiology 1988;69:327–31.
79. Knill RL, Moote CA, Skinner MI, et al. Anesthesia with abdominal surgery leads to intense REM sleep during the first postoperative week. Anesthesiology 1990;73: 52–61.
80. Hanak V, Somers VK. Cardiovascular and cerebrovascular physiology in sleep. Handb Clin Neurol 2011;98:315–25.
81. Mokhlesi B, Punjabi NM. "REM-related" obstructive sleep apnea: an epiphenomenon or a clinically important entity? Sleep 2012;35:5–7.
82. Solt K, Cotten JF, Cimenser A, et al. Methylphenidate actively induces emergence from general anesthesia. Anesthesiology 2011;115:791–803.

83. Meuret P, Backman SB, Bonhomme V, et al. Physostigmine reverses propofol-induced unconsciousness and attenuation of the auditory steady state response and bispectral index in human volunteers. Anesthesiology 2000;93:708–17.
84. Plourde G, Chartrand D, Fiset P, et al. Antagonism of sevoflurane anaesthesia by physostigmine: effects on the auditory steady-state response and bispectral index. Br J Anaesth 2003;91:583–6.

Outcomes After Neuroanesthesia and Neurosurgery
What Makes a Difference

Michael M. Todd, MD

KEYWORDS

- Neuroanesthesia • Neurosurgery • Outcomes • Nitrous oxide

KEY POINTS

- Volatile agents (and nitrous oxide) may be associated with slightly (a few millimeters of mercury) greater intracranial pressures, somewhat greater degrees of cerebral engorgement, lower blood pressures (and hence cerebral perfusion pressures), and brief (but clinically inconsequential) lags in wake-up times.
- Seizures are a known cause of herniation and death in patients with mass lesions, both in the preoperative and postoperative periods. For this reason, anesthesiologists need to be aware of whether their patients have received (or need to receive) anticonvulsants in the perioperative period.
- There is, as yet, no convincing evidence that nitrous oxide is detrimental in any neurosurgical setting.

INTRODUCTION

For almost a century, scientists have explored the cerebrovascular and metabolic physiology of the brain, primarily in animals but also in humans. Some of this work, particularly that done in the late 1940s and in the 1950s, evaluates the impact of both anesthetics as well as other changes of relevance to anesthesia (eg, the cerebral blood flow [CBF] effects of changing carbon dioxide). But until the late 1950s, little of this work was seen to be directly important to clinical practice. Then, in 1957, Furness[1,2] (with later support from Slocum in 1961) demonstrated the value of mechanical ventilation (and hence carbon dioxide control) in neurosurgery. Next were the human studies by Jennett and colleagues[3] in 1969 showing that halothane and other volatile agents (specifically methoxyflurane and trichloroethylene) could increase intracranial pressure (ICP) in patients with central nervous system mass lesions. Adding 1%

Department of Anesthesia, University of Iowa Carver College of Medicine, 6619 JCP 200 Hawkins Drive, Iowa City, IA 52242, USA
E-mail address: michael-todd@uiowa.edu

Anesthesiology Clin 30 (2012) 399–408
http://dx.doi.org/10.1016/j.anclin.2012.06.001
1932-2275/12/$ – see front matter © 2012 Elsevier Inc. All rights reserved.

halothane to a baseline anesthetic of 70% nitrous oxide (N_2O), tubocurarine paralysis increased the ICP by 20 $\pm$ 12 mm Hg in patients who were normocarbic. Since that time, a huge body of literature has been created of frequently excellent studies in humans and animals examining anesthetic-induced changes a wide range of physiologic variables -CBF, ICP, cerebral metabolic rate (CMR), electroencephalography, evoked potentials, arterio-venous oxygen content difference, jugular venous oxygen saturation, autoregulation, and so forth. Extensive discussions of this literature can be found in many comprehensive anesthetic textbooks.[4]

Unfortunately, many of the aforementioned articles draw conclusions based on what are really surrogate variables about the clinical value of different drugs. Too often, we (the author included) have uncritically assumed that drug-related differences in these surrogates are good or bad. This thought process is epitomized by a 1969 anonymous editorial in the British Journal of Anesthesia,[5] suggesting that, based on the work of Jennett and colleagues,[3] halothane was a dangerous agent for use in neurosurgery in spite of more than 5 years of its successful clinical use and its obvious advantages over older drugs, like ether.

The illogic of this approach was beautifully reviewed by Michenfelder[6] in his 1989 Rovenstine lecture at the American Society of Anesthesiologists' annual meeting, who commented, "...I fear that...our achievements (in terms of contributions to the care of neurosurgical patients) have been distorted, abused and misinterpreted by some of our colleagues, including anesthesiologists, neurosurgeons and neurologists...."[6] This author prefers to think that the problem has been one of misinterpretation rather than abuse. But too many times, we have taken a piece of well-done scientific work and carelessly extrapolated it to the clinical arena. We conclude that because intraoperative ICP with drug A is 8 mm Hg but it is 11 mm Hg with drug B, that drug A is better for use in neurosurgical patients. Because a reduction in the metabolic demand of the heart (produced by beta-blockers or anesthetics or preload/afterload reduction) reduces the likelihood of ischemia, we think that any drug-induced reduction in brain metabolism will also protect against an ischemic insult and that if agent A reduces cerebral metabolic rate more than agent B, it is a better protective agent.

What has largely been missing from this discussion is a critical assessment of the clinical impact of our interventions on our patients and a failure to recognize our limited ability to extrapolate measured physiologic changes (even in humans) to the operating room and intensive care unit. Does a drug-induced increase in CBF or cerebral blood volume (CBV) or ICP really matter? If it does matter, in what specific patient groups and when?

This article focuses almost exclusively on human studies of patients undergoing a variety of largely elective neurosurgical procedures; the care of patients with head trauma will not be covered. The author's goal is to demonstrate that much of the cerebrovascular physiology and pharmacology found in our major texts is of limited applicability to the clinical care of neurosurgical patients. The author also tries to point out those aspects of our care that are truly important and that represent our best contributions to our patients' well-being.

TUMOR SURGERY: THINGS THAT DO NOT MATTER
Anesthetic Selection

We have long known that elevations in ICP associated with such disorders as closed head injuries or increasing brain tumor size are strongly associated with poor outcomes. And, as noted, we have long known that certain anesthetic interventions, like the use of volatile anesthetics and N_2O, can produce an increase in ICP. Does it, however, follow that a pharmacologically induced (as opposed to disease-induced) increase in ICP is also likely to be associated with a poor outcome?

In 1990, Crosby and Todd[7] reviewed the literature on the impact of induced changes in ICP. In that article, the investigators pointed out the well-known but well-tolerated ICP increases associated with normal rapid eye movement sleep (even in those with brain tumors); the benignity of artificially increasing ICP in normal subjects, even to values approaching 100 mm Hg; and the comment by Jennett and colleagues in their classic article (noted earlier) that "There was no evidence that the brief periods of raised pressures (exceeding 40 mm Hg in some patients) had any harmful effects, either at the time or subsequently."

There are now several human studies examining the relationship between intraoperative ICP, anesthetic agent choice, and at least short-term outcomes in patients with brain tumors. The first of these, by Ravussin and colleagues,[8] compared intraoperative lumbar cerebrospinal fluid (CSF) pressures, cerebral perfusion pressures (CPP), and wake-up characteristics between neurosurgical patients anesthetized with isoflurane/N_2O and propofol/N_2O. Measured ICPs were slightly greater in the isoflurane/N_2O group (15 vs 12 mm Hg, although not different from preinduction), and patients given propofol woke up (as measured by the Glasgow Coma Scale and orientation to person-place-time) a bit faster but with no meaningful differences by 60 minutes. Fortunately, the investigators limited their conclusions to a statement that propofol seemed to be a suitable alternative to isoflurane, not better.

This study was followed by Todd and colleagues,[9] who compared ICP, intraoperative brain swelling (as assessed by the surgeon), and patient wake up. Three anesthetic regimens were chosen: isoflurane/N_2O (the combination associated with the greatest reported increases in CBF), fentanyl/N_2O, and a pure intravenous anesthetic (propofol/fentanyl). A target $Paco_2$ of approximately 30 mm Hg was maintained in all patients. Surprisingly, the ICPs between the 3 groups were comparable (although there were more patients in the isoflurane/N_2O group with ICPs >20 mm Hg) as were the brain-swelling assessments. Wake-up times (measured as time to eyes open, extubation, following commands, and an Aldrete score of 9) were comparable between the groups. Only the time to orientation was slightly longer in the isoflurane/N_2O group; but when wake-up times were plotted against measured ICPs (which ranged from 0–55 mm Hg), no relationship could be found.

Other studies followed. Talke and colleagues[10] compared the operative and postoperative conditions in patients with tumors receiving propofol/fentanyl, isoflurane, or a combination of isoflurane and propofol. Again, no differences in the rate or quality of postoperative wake up were noted. In 2 related studies, the same investigators observed a measurable increase in intraoperative ICP (measured as lumbar CSF pressure) with isoflurane, sevoflurane, and desflurane. Combining these studies, it can only be concluded that differences in ICP probably do not translate into postoperative differences.

Petersen and colleagues[11] also compared 3 anesthetics in patients with brain tumors: propofol/fentanyl, isoflurane/fentanyl, and sevoflurane/fentanyl. Like Ravussin and colleagues,[8] intraoperative ICPs were slightly higher (and cerebral perfusion pressures lower) in the two groups receiving volatile agents; and the surgical assessment of brain swelling suggested some greater swelling in the volatile-agent groups. However, no mention is made of any differences in the postoperative patient condition. Similarly, Santra and Das[12] compared a propofol/fentanyl anesthetic with isoflurane/N_2O and again found slightly higher ICPs in the isoflurane/N_2O group (10 vs 7 mm Hg) and somewhat greater brain swelling but again make no mention of any differences in wake up or postoperative condition.

In 2 separate studies in patients with tumors, Bilotta and colleagues[13,14] measured postoperative conditions (using the Short Orientation Memory Concentration Test) in patients anesthetized with remifentanil/propofol, sufentanil/propofol (one study), and sevoflurane and desflurane (second study). Although there seemed to be some short-term differences in the return to baseline, all patient groups had comparable baseline scores within 45 minutes after extubation. Lauta and colleagues[15] compared sevoflurane/remifentanil versus propofol/remifentanil in patients with tumors and again found no differences in emergence characteristics based on the time to an Aldrete score of 9.

These observations (albeit inconsistently) suggest that there are differences in the physiologic impact of different agents. Volatile agents (and N_2O) may be associated with slightly greater (a few millimeters of mercury) ICPs; somewhat greater degrees of cerebral engorgement; lower blood pressures and, hence, CPP; and brief, but clinically inconsequential, lags in wake-up times. But no available study suggests any meaningful difference in patient outcomes beyond the early postanesthesia care unit (PACU) period and none have linked even these short-term wake-up differences to the differences in intraoperative conditions. It is far more likely that differences in wake up between agents are simply a reflection of the differing pharmacokinetics and dynamics of the agents and would probably be seen in non-neurosurgical patients, although a direct comparison between neurosurgical and non-neurosurgical patients would be of great value.

Additional Musings

As noted earlier, elevated ICP caused by brain disease is associated with worsened outcomes, although this probably reflects the underlying severity of the disease. However, assuming that a drug-induced (usually small) increase in CBF and ICP is equally detrimental is illogical. Why do volatile agents increase ICP? In most cases, they do so by increasing CBF and CBV (the one exception may be increases in CSF production produced by drugs like desflurane and sevoflurane). Why is an increase in ICP bad? It is bad because it reduces CPP and, hence, may induce tissue ischemia. But then how do we argue that an INCREASE in tissue perfusion induced by a volatile agent can induce ischemia, even when CPP decreases? How can an increase in CBF produce a critical reduction in CBF? We cannot, except in one condition. That condition is when an increase in CBF and CBV in one region of the brain results in a shift in the intracranial contents, producing tissue herniation and critical tissue compression in another region. But brain herniation in the operating room is a rare event and is almost impossible to induce in the course of a well-conducted anesthetic in patients who do not have critically elevated ICPs to begin with. In addition, it is usually quickly reversible (if discovered quickly) with interventions such as hyperventilation and osmotic diuretics. Only a tiny fraction of our patients (eg, those with severe mass effect preoperatively) are at risk for such an event, and it is our task as knowledgeable physicians to recognize when we are dealing with such at-risk patients and when we are not. These patients are usually identifiable by the presence of somnolence, stupor, or a recent alteration in level of consciousness as determined by someone with longitudinal knowledge of their condition. In these rare patients (eg, those who arrive in the operating room somnolent or unresponsive), it may indeed be prudent to avoid the use of vasodilating agents, such as volatile anesthetics or N_2O. But to conclude that we should NEVER use such drugs in neurosurgical patients is neither rational nor logical.

TUMOR SURGERY: THINGS THAT MATTER
Carbon Dioxide

The influence of $Paco_2$ on CBF has long been known.[16] The recognition that controlling $Paco_2$ could be advantageous has already been mentioned. As a result, intraoperative hyperventilation quickly became a mainstay of neuro-anesthetic practice.[a]

However, despite a 40-year history, it was not until 2008 that a formal study of the role of $Paco_2$ on the intraoperative brain was actually completed. In that study, Gelb and colleagues[17] examined, in a large number of patients with tumors, the effects of changing $Paco_2$ (25 vs 37 mm Hg) on ICP and surgeon-assessed brain bulk. Hyperventilation was associated with clearly reduced ICPs (12 vs 16 mm Hg) and a 45% reduction in surgeon-assessed brain bulk. Although quantitative comparisons are difficult (or impossible), the magnitude of these differences seems to match or exceed any ICP or brain-bulk changes associated with anesthetic agents. In the same study, the investigators showed that there were no meaningful differences in ICP or brain bulk between isoflurane and sevoflurane anesthetics.

Tumor Mass Effects and Blood Pressure

Tumor size (and mass effect) seems to be an important factor in postoperative emergence. Schubert and colleagues[18] showed that patients with large lesions were much slower to emerge from anesthesia, by several measures, than those with small lesions. The same investigators demonstrated that postoperative intracranial hemorrhage was associated with an increased likelihood of sustained postoperative systemic hypertension,[19] a finding that confirmed earlier observations from the same institution.[20] Bhagat and colleagues[21] also showed that postoperative hypertension was more common in patients with large intracranial lesions.

Seizure Prevention

Generalized seizures produce some of the largest increases in CBF, CMR, and ICP that can occur; in animals, measured CBF can double or even triple during seizures.[22] These extreme physiologic changes, unlike those produced by anesthetics, may have profoundly detrimental effects, as evidenced by deaths produced by electroconvulsive therapy in patients harboring unknown brain tumors.[23] This is one of the reasons that neurosurgeons use prophylactic anticonvulsants in patients with brain tumors. Also, although the literature is anecdotal (case reports), seizures are a known cause of herniation and death in patients with mass lesions, both in the preoperative and postoperative periods. For this reason, anesthesiologists need to be aware of whether their patients have received (or need to receive) anticonvulsants in the perioperative period. Although such medications are not typically considered as part of the anesthetic, a gentle reminder to the neurosurgeons about their value can be life saving, as can an immediate response to changes in neurologic status that may be caused by seizure activity.

N₂O and Pneumocephalus

The argument regarding the use of N_2O in neurosurgery has persisted for many decades without resolution. There is, as yet, no convincing evidence that N_2O is detrimental in

---

[a] The differences in carbon dioxide control have probably played a role in the differing ICP changes seen by different studies. For example, as noted, the work by Jennett and colleagues,[3] which demonstrated perhaps the largest volatile-agent increase in ICP yet reported, was performed in patients who are normocarbic, whereas almost all subsequent comparative studies were done in patients with hypocarbia.

most neurosurgical settings. The only well-done large randomized trial of N_2O use did include 295 neurosurgical patients but did not provide specific information on these patients.[24] There is also evidence in patients undergoing aneurysm clipping that N_2O is benign.[25,26] There is, however, one situation when N_2O use is detrimental, at least based on anecdote and on our understanding of the physical chemical behavior of N_2O. Even in the best of neurosurgical hands, a fraction of craniotomy patients must be returned to the operating room within hours, days, or weeks of an initial operation to evacuate a clot, to remove an infected bone flap, and so forth. One hundred percent of patients who have undergone an open craniotomy have residual air present in the cranium (pneumocephalus), and the volume of air is quite large for as long as a week.[27] Given the known effects of N_2O-induced bubble expansion,[28] the use of N_2O during a take-back craniotomy should be considered contraindicated unless an immediate preoperative scan demonstrates little or no intracranial air.

THE PRACTICAL ANESTHETIC MANAGEMENT OF PATIENTS WITH INTRACRANIAL MASS LESIONS

The appropriate anesthetic care of patients with a mass lesion begins with a clinical examination and inspection of any imaging studies. Are the patients alert and oriented or are they somnolent or stuporous? Alert patients are unlikely to have severely elevated ICP. Do patients have a focal deficit? How large is the tumor? Is there evidence of major mass effect: midline shift (and how much), ventricular effacement, and hydrocephalus. How much edema surrounds the tumor? Fortunately, in the modern era of readily available brain imaging, far fewer patients arrive in the operating room with critical intracranial hypertension; patients admitted to the hospital with clinically elevated ICPs are frequently subjected to a period of preoperative steroid therapy to reduce edema.

Standard monitors are generally sufficient, with the addition of arterial pressure monitoring. Central venous catheters are rarely indicated. The choice of induction agents should be tailored to the patients' cardiovascular condition. The key goal is the avoidance of severe swings in blood pressure, either high or low, either during endotracheal intubation or during the placement of pin-fixation devices. Similarly, the choice of agent for maintenance should be based on the anesthesiologist's experience and the ability to achieve a rapid emergence postoperatively. The specific selection of agent is unlikely to be important; as noted, there is no meaningful evidence suggesting that one agent is better than any other in most of our patients. In some patients who are deemed at risk for a poor wake up (eg, the elderly, those with large frontal lobe or intraventricular tumors, those in whom extensive frontal lobe retraction is expected), the choice of drugs, like remifentanil and shorter-acting inhaled agents (N_2O and/or desflurane), may offer some advantages simply by eliminating the confusion that may result from residual anesthetic in the early recovery phase. Intraoperative $Paco_2$ control is critical, although there is no evidence that extreme hyperventilation offers any advantage over more moderate hypocapnia. The use of osmotic diuretics, either prophylactically (before opening the dura) or as needed, is common practice, although there is little evidence to support the use of specific agent (ie, mannitol vs hypertonic saline). The use of furosemide seems to be more a matter of personal preference than evidence based. Due attention to appropriate patient positioning is also needed; the head should (if possible) be elevated and the neck kept in as near-neutral a position as possible (if the surgical site is more lateral, turn the patients' trunk using shoulder roles or bolsters). Finally, meticulous attention to blood pressure during emergence and after extubation is critical. The author's practice is to intervene when systolic blood pressure reaches approximately 150 mm Hg, in an effort to avoid pressure exceeding 160 mm Hg. Almost all patients can benefit from at least 24 hours of close postoperative observation in a monitored facility, not because they are critically ill but to permit the immediate detection and evaluation of an intracerebral hemorrhage.

CEREBRAL METABOLISM, ISCHEMIC INJURY, AND BRAIN PROTECTION

Like the issues concerning drug selection and CBF/ICP, there have been a great many misleading conclusions regarding the broad subject of brain protection (ie, the use of anesthetic agents and other drugs to prevent the occurrence of ischemia-induced postoperative neurologic deficit). In some ways, the pursuit of protective interventions (other than just maintaining perfusion) has been a kind of holy grail of our specialty, dating back to the 1950s. Most of this has focused on the concept of metabolic suppression, analogous to the similar approach to myocardial ischemia.

There is no question that essentially all anesthetic agents (with the possible exceptions of N_2O and ketamine), in anesthetic concentrations, reduce the cerebral metabolic rate.[4] There is also a huge body of animal-based literature demonstrating that anesthetics (both intravenous and inhaled) can reduce the amount of tissue damaged by controlled ischemic events (eg, circulatory arrest, focal cerebrovascular occlusion). Unfortunately, as in the broader world of stroke prevention and treatment, efforts to translate such laboratory findings into the clinical arena have failed or have never been subjected to formal trial. In spite of the common belief that drugs producing a greater degree of metabolic suppression are more protective than other agents, there is no human evidence in support of this contention or to support the belief that the use of any drug or combination of drugs or other interventions can protect our patients in the operating room.

A large contributor to this problem is really the woeful lack of human data. To date, there have been only 2 large-scale (and hence adequately powered) randomized clinical trials examining the impact of some anesthesia-related operative interventions in neurosurgery and both of these were resoundingly negative.

The first of these was the Intraoperative Hypothermia for Aneurysm Surgery Trial, which, again based on extensive laboratory data, examined the influence of intraoperative hypothermia (33°C) on the long-term neurologic outcome in patients undergoing aneurysm clipping following subarachnoid hemorrhage.[29] A total of 1001 patients were randomized at 30 centers around the world and followed for 3 months postoperatively. A wide range of outcome measures was assessed, including neuropsychology. However, regardless of the outcome measure, no differences were seen in the hypothermic group relative to a normothermic control group. Subsequent post hoc subgroup studies also failed to demonstrate any adverse effects related to the use of N_2O[25,26] and no benefit to the use of protective drugs (primarily thiopental) during temporary vessel occlusion.[30]

The other study was the large General Anaesthesia versus Local Anaesthesia (GALA) for Carotid Surgery trial, examining the use of general versus local/regional anesthesia for carotid endarterectomy.[31] This study randomly assigned more than 3500 patients to one of the two groups and found no differences in the incidence of stroke or other major complications.

Why did these trials, both of which examined interventions that were strongly supported by the animal ischemic-injury literature, fail to demonstrate a benefit? Both trials were exceptionally well performed and, hence, the lack of protection cannot be attributed to poor quality science. The answer is speculative but may relate to the lack of relevance of the various animal models to clinical medicine. Some evidence for this is found in the success of hypothermia in ameliorating neurologic sequelae following cardiac arrest caused by ventricular fibrillation, a situation that can be almost perfectly modeled in the laboratory and whereby hypothermia was indeed shown to be both protective and therapeutic.[32,33] By contrast, there are no good laboratory models that reflect the pathophysiology of either aneurysmal subarachnoid hemorrhage and surgery or carotid endarterectomy. The problem is not with the physiology of our interventions but with our inadequate understanding of WHY patients with hemorrhagic aneurysmal disease or severe carotid (and systemic) atherosclerosis develop a deficit following operative interventions.

SUMMARY

What we do as neurosurgical anesthesiologists matters a great deal to the well-being of our patients. But the impact is NOT related to the choice of vasoconstricting (eg, propofol, opioids) versus vasodilating (volatile agents, N_2O) drugs or the modest increases in ICP or brain swelling that may accompany those choices, at least in all but the rarest of patients. It is not influenced by our attempts to protect the brain via the use of metabolic depressant anesthetics. In other words, outcomes are not determined by our attempted application of what I have fondly called esoteric brain stuff. Far more important is our understanding of the basics: the role of Pa_{CO_2} and positioning-related differences in venous drainage; the dangers of uncontrolled hypertension; our ability to recognize when we are dealing with patients at greater risk (eg, because of larger tumors, more mass effect, more edema, midline shift, baseline severe ICP increases); and, it can be argued, our understanding of basic neuroanatomy and function and our knowledge of what our neurosurgical colleagues are doing when they operate. As noted, there may be a small group of patients (those with severe preexisting intracranial hypertension as evidenced by a reduced preoperative level of consciousness) in whom the avoidance of vasodilating agents may be reasonable. However, gathering sufficient data in such rare patients (rarer in an era of early tumor diagnosis) to prove this conjecture is nearly impossible. There also may be as-yet unidentified patients in whom as-yet unidentified protective interventions might be beneficial. But it is time that we abandon our belief in the clinically relevant role of metabolic depression by anesthetics as a protective intervention, not because metabolic depression has no protective effects (and protective effects are well known in animals) but because the postoperative deficits we encounter in clinical practice are NOT caused by simple supply-and-demand imbalances but by changes in biology that we do not understand and that are radically dissimilar to what we study in the laboratory.

REFERENCES

1. Furness DN. Controlled respiration in neurosurgery. Br J Anaesth 1957;29:415–8.
2. Slocum HC, Hayes GW, Laezman BC. Ventilator techniques of anesthesia for neurosurgery. Anesthesiology 1961;22:143–5.
3. Jennett WB, Barker J, Fitch W, et al. Effect of anesthesia on intracranial pressure in patients with space-occupying lesions. Lancet 1969;1:61–4.
4. Patel PM, Drummond JD. Cerebral physiology and the effect of anesthetic drugs, Miller's anesthesia. 7th edition. Philadelphia: ChurchillLivingston/Elsevier; 2010. p. 305–39.
5. Anonymous Halothane and neurosurgery. Br J Anaesth 1969;41:277–8.

6. Michenfelder JD. The 27th Rovenstine lecture: neuroanesthesia and the achievement of professional respect. Anesthesiology 1989;70:695–701.
7. Crosby G, Todd MM. On neuroanesthesia, intracranial pressure, and a dead horse. J Neurosurg Anesthesiol 1990;2:143–5.
8. Ravussin P, Tempelhoff R, Modica PA, et al. Propofol vs. thiopental-isoflurane for neurosurgical anesthesia: comparison of hemodynamics, CSF pressure, and recovery. J Neurosurg Anesthesiol 1991;3:85–95.
9. Todd MM, Warner DS, Sokoll MD, et al. A prospective, comparative trial of three anesthetics for elective supratentorial craniotomy. Anesthesiology 1993;78:1005–20.
10. Talke P, Caldwell JE, Brown R, et al. A comparison of three anesthetic techniques in patients undergoing craniotomy for supratentorial intracranial surgery. Anesth Analg 2002;95:430–5.
11. Petersen KD, Landsfeldt U, Cold GE, et al. Intracranial pressure and cerebral hemodynamic in patients with intracranial tumors. Anesthesiology 2003;98:329–36.
12. Santra S, Das B. Subdural pressure and brain condition during propofol vs isoflurane - nitrous oxide anaesthesia in patients undergoing elective supratentorial tumour surgery. Indian J Anaesth 2009;53:44–51.
13. Bilotta F, Caramia R, Paoloni FP, et al. Early postoperative cognitive recovery after remifentanil-propofol or sufentanil-propofol anaesthesia for supratentorial craniotomy: a randomized trial. Eur J Anesthesiol 2007;24:122–7.
14. Bilotta F, Doronzio A, Cuzzone V, et al, PINOCCHIO Study Group. Early postoperative cognitive recovery and gas exchange patterns after balanced anesthesia with sevoflurane or desflurane in overweight and obese patients undergoing craniotomy. J Neurosurg Anesthesiol 2009;21:207–13.
15. Lauta E, Abbinante C, Del Gaudio A, et al. Emergence times are similar with sevoflurane and total intravenous anesthesia: results of a multicenter RCT of patients scheduled for elective supratentorial craniotomy. J Neurosurg Anesthesiol 2010;22:110–8.
16. Gibbs FA, Gibbs EL, Lennox WG. Changes in human cerebral blood flow consequent on alterations in blood gases. Am J Physiol 1935;111:557–63.
17. Gelb AW, Craen RA, Rao GS, et al. Does hyperventilation improve operating condition during supratentorial craniotomy? A multicenter randomized crossover trial. Anesth Analg 2008;106:585–94.
18. Schubert A, Mascha EJ, Bloomfield EL, et al. Effect of cranial surgery and brain tumor size on emergence from anesthesia. Anesthesiology 1996;85:513–21.
19. Basali A, Mascha EJ, Kalfas I, et al. Relation between perioperative hypertension and intracranial hemorrhage after craniotomy. Anesthesiology 2000;93:48–54.
20. Kalfas IH, Little JR. Postoperative hemorrhage: a survey of 4992 intracranial procedures. Neurosurgery 1988;23:343–7.
21. Bhagat H, Dash HH, Bithal PK, et al. Planning for early emergence in neurosurgical patients: a randomized prospective trial of low-dose anesthetics. Anesth Analg 2008;107:1348–55.
22. Plum F, Posner JB, Troy B. Cerebral metabolic and circulatory responses to induced convulsion in animals. Arch Neurol 1968;18:1–13.
23. Maltbie AA, Cavenar JO, Wingfield MS, et al. Electroconvulsive therapy in the presence of brain tumor: case reports and an evaluation of risk. J Nerv Ment Dis 1980;168:400–5.
24. Myles PS, Leslie K, Chan MT, et al, ENIGMA Trial Group. Avoidance of nitrous oxide for patients undergoing major surgery: a randomized controlled trial. Anesthesiology 2007;107:221–31.

25. McGregor DG, Lanier WL, Pasternak JJ, et al, Intraoperative Hypothermia for Aneurysm Surgery Trial Investigators. Effect of nitrous oxide on neurologic and neuropsychological function after intracranial aneurysm surgery. Anesthesiology 2008;108:568–79.

26. Pasternak JJ, McGregor DG, Lanier WL, et al, IHAST Investigators. Effect of nitrous oxide use on long-term neurologic and neuropsychological outcome in patients who received temporary proximal artery occlusion during cerebral aneurysm clipping surgery. Anesthesiology 2009;110:563–73.

27. Reasoner DK, Todd MM, Scamman FL, et al. The incidence of pneumocephalus after supratentorial craniotomy observations on the disappearance of intracranial air. Anesthesiology 1994;80:1008–12.

28. Saidman LJ, Eger EI. Changes in cerebral spinal fluid pressure during pneumoencephalography under nitrous oxide anesthesia. Anesthesiology 1965;26: 67–72.

29. Todd MM, Hindman BJ, Clarke WR, et al, Intraoperative Hypothermia for Aneurysms Surgery Trial Investigators. Mild intraoperative hypothermia during surgery for intracranial aneurysm. N Engl J Med 2005;353:135–45.

30. Hindman BJ, Bayman EO, Pfisterer WK, et al, IHAST Investigators. No association between intraoperative hypothermia or supplemental protective drug and neurologic outcome in patients undergoing temporary clipping during cerebral aneurysm surgery. Anesthesiology 2010;112:86–101.

31. GALA Trial Collaborative Group. General Anaesthesia versus Local Anaesthesia for Carotid Surgery (GALA): a multicentre, randomized controlled trial. Lancet 2008;372:2132–42.

32. Bernard SA, Gray TW, Buist MD, et al. Treatment of comatose survivors of out-of-hospital cardiac arrest with induced hypothermia. N Engl J Med 2002;346: 557–63.

33. The Hypothermia after Cardiac Arrest Study Group. Mild therapeutic hypothermia to improve the neurologic outcome after cardiac arrest. N Engl J Med 2002;346: 549–56.

Index

Note: Page numbers of article titles are in **boldface** type.

A

Ablation, of intracranial aneurysms, anesthesia for, 135–136

Acetaminophen, for postoperative pain, 353, 357
    after craniotomy, 353
    after spine surgery, 357

Acute stroke. *See* Stroke.

Aging brain, anesthetic neurotoxicity in, 215–221

Airway management, in adult traumatic brain injury, 336–337
  in neuroanesthesiology, **229–240**
    after cervical spine surgery, 233–236
      extubation, 233, 236
    for functional neurosurgery, 230–231
    for pituitary surgery, 230
    with the unstable cervical spine, 231–233
      avoiding complications, 231
      clinical precautions and manual in-line stabilization, 232
      implications for airway interventions, 232–233
      rheumatoid arthritis, 231
      traumatic injury evaluation, 231

Alpha-2 adrenergic agonists, for postoperative pain after craniotomy, 354

Analgesia. *See* Pain management.

Anatomy, functional neuroanatomy, 157–161
    cerebellum, brainstem, and posterior fossa, 158
    cranial, 157–158
    spinal, 158–161

Anemia, packed red blood cell transfusions in critically ill neurosurgical patients, 370–372

Anesthesia, interfaces of sleep and, **385–398**
    functional interfaces, 391–393
      effects of anesthesia on sleep, 392–393
      effects of sleep on anesthesia, 391–392
    metaphors and phenotypes, 385–387
    relevance for neuroanesthesiology, 393
    subcortical interfaces, 387–390
      brainstem sites, 389–390
      hypothalamic sites, 387–389
    thalamocortical-corticocortical interfaces, 390–391
      cortical effective connectivity, 390–391
      slow waves, 390
      spindles, 390
  neurosurgical. *See* Neurosurgical anesthesia.

Anesthetic neuroprotection. *See* Neuroprotection.

Anesthesiology Clin 30 (2012) 409–426
http://dx.doi.org/10.1016/S1932-2275(12)00072-9
1932-2275/12/$ – see front matter © 2012 Elsevier Inc. All rights reserved.

anesthesiology.theclinics.com

Moving?

Make sure your subscription moves with you!

To notify us of your new address, find your **Clinics Account Number** (located on your mailing label above your name), and contact customer service at:

Email: journalscustomerservice-usa@elsevier.com

800-654-2452 (subscribers in the U.S. & Canada)
314-447-8871 (subscribers outside of the U.S. & Canada)

Fax number: 314-447-8029

Elsevier Health Sciences Division
Subscription Customer Service
3251 Riverport Lane
Maryland Heights, MO 63043

ELSEVIER

Printed and bound by CPI Group (UK) Ltd, Croydon, CR0 4YY

03/10/2024

01040444-0004